HOMELESSNESS

HOMELESSNESS

A Prevention-oriented Approach

EDITED BY

René I. Jahiel, M.D., Ph.D.

ADJUNCT PROFESSOR OF HEALTH SERVICES RESEARCH AND POLICY
HEALTH SERVICES MANAGEMENT AND POLICY PROGRAM
GRADUATE SCHOOL OF MANAGEMENT AND POLICY
NEW SCHOOL FOR SOCIAL RESEARCH
NEW YORK, NEW YORK

THE
JOHNS HOPKINS
UNIVERSITY PRESS
Baltimore and London

© 1992 The Johns Hopkins University Press

All rights reserved

Printed in the United States of America

The Johns Hopkins University Press
701 West 40th Street
Baltimore, Maryland 21211-2190
The Johns Hopkins Press Ltd., London

The paper used in this book meets the minimum requirements of the American National Standard for Information Sciences—Permanence of Paper for Printed Library Materials, ANSI Z39.48-1984.

Library of Congress Cataloging-in-Publication Data

Homelessness : a prevention-oriented approach / edited by René I. Jahiel.
p.   cm.
Includes bibliographical references and index.
ISBN 0-8018-4313-8 (alk. paper)
1. Homelessness—United States—Prevention.
2. Social service—United States.   I. Jahiel, René I.
HV4505.H6554   1992
363.5′7′0973—dc20   91-40611

CONTENTS

CONTENTS

III. The Social Context of Homelessness

IV. Interventions Directed at the Social Environment

V. Methodology

CONTRIBUTORS

PASQUALE ACCARDO, M.D., professor, Department of Pediatrics, and director of ambulatory pediatrics, Saint Louis University School of Medicine; and medical director, Knights of Columbus Development Center, Cardinal Glennon's Childrens Hospital, Saint Louis, Missouri.

SUSAN MAKIESKY BARROW, PH.D., research scientist, Epidemiology of Mental Disorders Research Department, New York State Psychiatric Institute, New York, New York.

GARY L. BLASI, M.A., attorney, Legal Aid Foundation of Los Angeles, Los Angeles, California.

MARTHA R. BURT, PH.D., director, Social Service Research Program, Urban Institute, Washington, D.C.

PAMELA J. FISCHER, PH.D., assistant professor, Department of Psychiatry and Behavioral Sciences, Johns Hopkins University School of Medicine, Baltimore, Maryland.

JILL HAMBERG, PH.D. cand., urban planning consultant, New York, New York.

KIM HOPPER, PH.D., research scientist, Nathan Kline Institute, Orangeburg, New York.

WILLIAM J. HUTCHISON, PH.D., professor and dean, School of Social Service, Saint Louis University, Saint Louis, Missouri.

RENÉ I. JAHIEL, M.D., PH.D., adjunct professor of health services research and policy, Health Services Management and Policy Program, Graduate School of Management and Policy, New School for Social Research, New York, New York.

JAMES R. KNICKMAN, PH.D., professor of health policy and management and director, Health Research Program, Wagner Graduate School of Public Service, New York University, New York, New York.

PAUL KOEGEL, PH.D., associate behavioral scientist, Department of Social Policy, Rand Corporation, Santa Monica, California.

LARRY W. KREUGER, PH.D., M.S.W., professor, School of Social Work, College of Human Environmental Science, University of Missouri–Columbia, Columbia, Missouri.

ELAINE LOMAS, L.C.S.W., district chief, Child and Youth Services Bureau, Los Angeles County Department of Mental Health, Los Angeles, California.

ANNE M. LOVELL, M.S.W., M.PHIL., PH.D. cand., research scientist, Department of Psychiatry, New York State Office of Mental Hygiene, New York, New York.

KAY YOUNG MCCHESNEY, PH.D., assistant professor, Department of Sociology, University of Missouri, Saint Louis, Missouri.

BEVERLY OVREBO, DR.P.H., associate professor, Department of Health Education, and coordinator, Bay Area Homelessness Program, San Francisco State University, San Francisco, California.

MARJORIE J. ROBERTSON, PH.D., senior scientist, Alcohol Research Group, Medical Research Institute of San Francisco in Berkeley, Berkeley, California.

PRISCILLA SMITH, PH.D., assistant professor, Department of Sociology and Social Work, Southern Illinois University at Edwardsville, Edwardsville, Illinois.

JANE M. SPRANKEL, M.S.W., medical social worker, Saint John's Mercy Medical Center, Saint Louis, Missouri.

LOUISA R. STARK, PH.D., executive director, Community Housing Partnership, Phoenix, Arizona; adjunct professor of anthropology, Arizona State University, Tempe, Arizona; founding president, National Coalition for the Homeless, Washington, D.C.

JOHN J. STRETCH, PH.D., M.B.A., professor, School of Social Service, Saint Louis University, Saint Louis, Missouri.

ELMER L. STRUENING, PH.D., associate professor of epidemiology, School of Public Health, Columbia University; and director, Epidemiology of Mental Disorders Research Department, New York State Psychiatric Institute, New York, New York.

EZRA SUSSER, M.D., PH.D., assistant professor of clinical psychiatry, Columbia University and New York State Psychiatric Institute, New York, New York.

BETH C. WEITZMAN, PH.D., assistant professor of public and health administration, Wagner Graduate School of Public Service, New York University, New York, New York.

CONTRIBUTORS

BARBARA Y. WHITMAN, PH.D., associate professor, School of Social Service, and associate professor, Department of Pediatrics and Adolescent Medicine, School of Medicine, Saint Louis University, Saint Louis, Missouri.

ROBERTA YOUMANS, B.A., Government Programs Advocate, National Housing Law Project, Washington, D.C.

PREFACE

The contemporary increase in poverty and homelessness in the United States is a national tragedy that our society has failed to confront. Policies have been ineffective in reversing or even slowing it. Despite the procurement of much information on this problem in the past decade, inaccurate explanations of homelessness and unrepresentative stereotypes of homeless people continue to abound. There is still a wide gap between what we know of the problem and what we are doing to solve it, that is, to prevent people from becoming homeless or, until that can be done, to alleviate the damage done to them. The intent of this book is twofold: to present a thorough, critical, scholarly review of current knowledge on the subject, and to use this knowledge to construct preventive approaches to homelessness.

Scholarly interest in homelessness has evolved over the years, from investigations of the characteristics of homeless people to a much broader field of inquiry. Homelessness—life without one's own home—is now viewed as a modality of life in poverty. This modality occurs as a single episode in an individual's life; or as a series of recurrent episodes, with shuttling back and forth among poor settings; or as a prolonged, perhaps permanent condition. Diverse groups of people have been plunged into this life in large numbers. They have brought with them their past experiences and their human assets and deficiencies, they have reacted and adapted in various ways to the situation of homelessness, and they have been categorized and labeled by professionals and the public. Thus, a large number of factors relevant to the individuals and their microenvironment have to be examined in scholarly studies to understand the dynamics of homelessness and the adaptations of standard interventions which are necessary to help homeless people It is also necessary to examine broader factors in the areas of poverty and housing which determine the size and nature of the homeless population.

The prevention-oriented approach of this book is borrowed from the field of public health. The prevention of homelessness and of its ill effects can be primary (preventing homelessness from occurring or recurring), secondary (returning homeless people to a stable existence in homes of their own as soon as possible), or tertiary (preventing or minimizing the damage done by homelessness to the individual). To implement primary, secondary, or tertiary prevention of any condition, one must have knowledge of the affected individual or the individual at risk and of the physical and social environments so as to understand the relative contributions of personal and environmental factors to the condition, and the expected impact of interventions directed at the individual and at the environment.

Accordingly, the material in this book is organized into five parts. The first two parts focus on homeless people and the next two parts on the social environment. Parts One and Three review our knowledge of homeless people and of the environmental factors relevant to homelessness, respectively. Parts Two and Four deal with interventions directed at the individual and at the environment, respectively. Part Five discusses some critical methodological problems.

Chapters 1 and 2 introduce the two main subjects of the book—homelessness and prevention—and place them within the complex set of social interactions that govern their impact.

Part One, "Homeless People in Their Environment," presents our knowledge of homeless people. Chapter 3 gives a historical survey of the homeless population in the United States. Chapter 4 reviews the knowledge acquired in quantitative surveys of homeless populations. Three chapters focus on salient issues concerning homeless people: their mental status (chapter 5), their criminal and victimization experiences (chapter 6), and the development of homeless children (chapter 7). Ethnographic methods are brought in to understand the way in which the environment, past experience, and "an insider's perspective" explain homeless people's behavior (chapter 8) and reveal their needs (chapter 9) and the barriers they are subject to (chapter 10).

Part Two, "Interventions Directed at Homeless People," draws on the knowledge of the homeless population gained in Part One to assess services in relation to needs. Chapter 11 surveys the various services available for the three types of prevention and assesses them quantitatively by comparison with the volume of services actually needed. Chapters 12 through 14 take a more qualitative approach to assessing the adaptations of services which are needed in the homeless situation and with specific groups of homeless people.

Part Three, "The Social Context of Homelessness," examines the social factors associated with the rise of homelessness. After an introductory perspective on the demographic and social factors that preceded the contemporary rise of homelessness (chapter 15), the role of increasing poverty and decreasing affordable housing is examined in detail in chapters 16 and 17. For a fuller understanding of these factors and of the potential resistance to measures to prevent homelessness, chapter 18 presents an overview of how the societal factors that are the direct causes of homelessness actually benefit various people or groups.

Part Four is entitled "Interventions Directed at the Social Environment." Advocacy and legal intervention in the courts may aim at tertiary prevention, to improve homeless people's microenvironment; at secondary prevention, to provide housing and job opportunities so that people can climb out of homelessness; or at primary prevention, to prevent loss of benefits, evictions, other forms of displacement, or neighborhood gentrification (chapter 19). When they create precedents or are conducted as class actions, such interventions may affect more than the individual concerned. However, more fundamental social changes are needed to protect all people at risk. Chapter 20 shows that a broad approach, as opposed to an individual approach, is needed to achieve that end, since only an increase in the total amount of low-income housing and/or the number of households with incomes that enable them to afford such housing can reduce the size of the homeless population. The quantitative features of such changes (the size of the target population, the resources and funding needed) are assessed in the first part of chapter 21; the remainder discusses social and political strategies for short-term and long-term prevention of homelessness.

The lack of appropriate methods with which to study homelessness remains an impediment to the development of policies on prevention. Part Five, "Methodology," assesses some critical methodological problems of studies of homelessness (chapters 22–24).

HOMELESSNESS

CHAPTER 1

The Definition and Significance
of Homelessness in the United States

René I. Jahiel, M.D., Ph.D.

Homelessness and hunger exist in the face of abundance. Therein
lies the outrage.
Graffito on the sidewalk of East 10th Street
New York City, October 1990

Homeless people are people who have no home. In general, they are extremely poor. The simplicity of these statements stands in contrast to the
lack of general agreement on a definition of homelessness or of homeless
people in the numerous monographs on the subject published in the 1980s in the
United States (1–18) and in Great Britain (19) and other European countries
(20). Perhaps this inability to reach a consensus reflects the difficulty of differentiating homeless people from other people who live in extreme poverty.
Perhaps it also reflects our society's difficulty in coming to grips with homelessness in its midst.

The various definitions of homelessness which have been advanced will not
be compiled here, since this has been done elsewhere (19). Suffice it to say that
they fall into two groups: some of them try to incorporate a concept of the social
meaning or causes of homelessness, thus associating the definition with theories of homelessness; others, discussed in this chapter, propose criteria of place
to to be used in designating people as homeless. After presenting place-based
definitions, I will discuss the significance of homelessness for the individual
and society.

Place-based Definitions of Homelessness

Place-based definitions of homelessness focus on an individual's place of residence on a given night or nights. Because these definitions are objective and
provide specific criteria, they are useful in empirical studies of homeless people
and in the formulation and administration of policies. One such definition, that

of the McKinney Act, has considerable impact because it sets homeless people's eligibility for programs supported by the act.

The Stuart B. McKinney Homeless Assistance Act (PL 100-77) was passed in 1987 as an emergency measure, but it remains the main federal support program for homeless people (chapter 11). It defines homelessness as follows:

For purposes of this Act, the term . . . homeless individual includes:

1. an individual who lacks a fixed, regular and adequate nighttime residence, and,
2. an individual who has a primary nighttime residence that is:
   A—a supervised publicly or privately operated shelter designed to provide temporary living accommodations (including welfare hotels, congregate shelters, and transitional housing for the mentally ill); or,
   B—an institution that provides a temporary residence for individuals intended to be institutionalized; or
   C—a public or private place not designed for, or ordinarily used as a regular sleeping accommodation for human beings. (21:Title I)

The McKinney Act definition includes those people described by Rossi et al. as "literal homeless" (22)[1] but excludes others who may be called homeless, such as those who "double up" with other households. Furthermore, it lacks a unifying concept. Finally, along with other place-based definitions, it creates a sharp distinction between homeless people and other very poor people. Alternative formulations have been proposed which meet some of these criticisms.

People who double up with other households because they have nowhere else to go constitute a larger group than all of the McKinney Act categories taken together (chapter 22). Roth et al. included them among homeless "resource people" (23).[2] HomeBase, an advocacy organization located in San Francisco, added to the McKinney Act categories a fourth group, namely, people who have "D—an accommodation with friends or others that is understood by both parties to be a last resort and temporary solution, the alternative to which is the street or refuge in one of the facilities listed above" (24).

The definitions given above specify categories of homeless people. They do not provide a concept of homelessness which would link these categories and which might help in defining boundaries. A few years ago, I proposed a definition of homelessness as "life without a home of one's own" (25:99). Elaborating on that definition, I would now say, "Homelessness is life without one's own home, exclusive of the instances when a home is shared with others because of custom or free choice." Further specifications are needed to remove ambiguities:

• The term *one's own home* refers to a residence that is legally sanctioned, as when a person owns a house or rents an apartment. Thus, squatters do not have their own homes.

- In our culture, the basic household unit is the family. All family members in the household have their own home, even if only one is the legal owner or tenant. However, when spouses or children flee because of abuse or are thrown out, they become homeless until they secure another home.
- Sharing a residence with another family or individual who is its legal occupant may come about by free choice (as in communal living) or may be forced by circumstances (e.g., lack of money to pay one's rent). The term *doubling up* will be used in this book only to refer to the latter instance, and doubled-up individuals or families are considered homeless.
- The concept of one's own home implies a certain degree of stability. Thus, people who have no homes and are able to pay for hotel rooms for only a few days or weeks—like some of those included by Roth et al. (23) in the category of resource people—are considered homeless.
- Residents of shelters are homeless even if they pay token fees. Families who live in hotel rooms paid for entirely by public or private agencies are homeless, regardless of the length of the stay. However, individuals who live in single-room occupancy hotels and pay on their own, even if much or all of their income comes from public support programs, are not homeless.
- Individuals who are in hospitals, jails, or other institutions and who have no homes to go to upon discharge are homeless.

These specifications are needed because the transition between homelessness and marginal home situations is not sharp. However, the boundaries were not drawn arbitrarily. The guide was the intuitive concept of a home as a residence to which one is entitled; for which one has responsibility; over which one exerts control, including the right to decide whom to admit; and which has a certain degree of permanency. This guide may be used to develop decision rules in ambiguous situations (for instance, when an adult returns to his or her parents' home because no other residence is available but those listed in the McKinney Act definition).

To define a homeless person as one who is without a home at a given point in time is like taking a snapshot of an individual. It shows where that individual is at a certain point in his or her life, but it leaves out the groups of which the individual is part, as well as his or her past life.

There are dangers in this approach. One is that the definition may turn into a label, a "master status" that sets homeless people apart from other people and disregards their personalities. There is abundant evidence (chapters 3 and 4) that homeless people have diverse characteristics and become homeless for different reasons, along differing trajectories, although a common characteristic is severe poverty. To define an individual by homelessness alone not only eliminates a considerable amount of information but also dehumanizes the person and invites prejudice.

Another danger exists when the definition is intended specifically to separate people who are homeless from other people. The benefits provided by the McKinney Act are directed mainly at people who are homeless. Not only is there no actual sharp separation between homeless people and other very poor people, but in many instances the inadequate or dangerous housing and community environment of poor people and their lack of resources lower their quality of life to a level near or even below that of some homeless people. Studies or policies targeted exclusively to homeless people do not deal with the underlying problem of severe poverty in our society.

Finally, a definition of homelessness focused on homeless people alone tends to promote an approach that seeks causes for homelessness predominantly in the personal characteristics of those who become homeless. While many homeless people have characteristics that increase their vulnerability to losing a home (chapter 4), that is only part of the process. The homeless-making processes (i.e., processes that create homelessness) involve parties, individuals as well as institutions, who tend to profit from the events that make other people homeless and who are often the prime movers of these events (chapter 18). Research or policies that aim to be effective in preventing homelessness have to address all parties involved in its creation.

The preceding discussion shows that the general concept of homelessness is simple, involving poverty and the loss of a home, but the social interactions and constructions related to this concept are complex. I will now discuss these matters with regard to the role of the home in our society, the place of homelessness in the life of an individual, and the significance of large-scale homelessness in our society.

The Significance of Homelessness

A home is a place that fulfills several functions and establishes relationships between its residents and their social environment. Table 1.1 shows the functions of a home and the impact on the person when these functions are lost. These functions give the home a great biological, psychological, legal, economic, and social utility. Because of this utility, the home has become, in our competitive society, a contested commodity.

Aware of the utility of the home to households (and of buildings and land to business), banks, landlords, developers, and others invest in this commodity and try to achieve high financial returns, thus creating a supply-side pressure to increase the cost of housing (chapter 18). Affluent people are often willing to commit a large part of their resources to have a home in a desirable location or to maximize the functions of their home, thus creating a demand-side pressure to increase the cost of housing. Business and not-for-profit corporations exert similar demand-side pressures with regard to their offices and other buildings (chapter 18). As a result of these pressures, there is a shortage of inexpensive

TABLE 1.1 THE FUNCTIONS OF A HOME

Function	Hazard(s) When the Function Is Lost
1. Protection from the elements	1. Dehydration, heat stroke, hypothermia, exposure, discomfort
2. Protection from crime	2. Increased risk of robbery, beating, rape, or murder
3. A place to rest, sleep, recuperate from stress, wash, toilet, clean one's clothes	3. Stress, fatigue, lack of sleep, poor judgment, irritability, slow reactions, poor hygiene, dirty clothing, so-called "homeless appearance," dependent edema, peripheral vascular disease
4. A place to keep one's possessions	4. Need to carry one's remaining possessions
5. A place to be alone; one's "personal space"	5. Stress and tension, demoralization, exposure to respiratory infections, etc.
6. Control of entry; a place to be with friends	6. Intrusion of people who may be disruptive, exploitative, or abusive; lack of social life in the ordinary sense
7. One's own place; a place that reflects one's personality, taste, and creativity; a place to prepare one's meals	7. Anonymity, demoralization, increased exposure to alcohol and drugs
8. A place where one lives with and raises one's family; which provides role models for children; where children do homework	8. Interference with family life; emotional stress and demoralization; poor role models and bad influences for children; poor progress of children in school; sometimes, separation of parents from children
9. An address; a place where one can be reached by mail or phone; a place near work or recreation	9. Interference with searching for a job or receiving benefits
10. A symbol of one's belonging to a community; facilitation of political action	10. Decreased ability to participate in mainstream politics; in some states, inability to vote
11. A place that confers social status	11. Low social status and consequent risk of lowered self-esteem or self-image
12. Economic value of the home; home as investment; home as a place to engage in gainful work	12. Low economic status; decreased ability to improve one's economic status

housing. Because the functions of a home listed in Table 1.1 are so significant and the damage done is so great when they are missing, tens of millions of households strive to keep their homes by spending an excessive part of their income on rent, mortgage, and utilities, thus contributing further to the demand-side pressure to increase the cost of housing, even though they endure considerable deprivation to do so (chapter 18).

People who lose their homes attempt to retain as many of the functions of a home as they can. Table 1.1 reveals what may be lost in the various alternatives to one's own home. Often, the first reaction to the loss of a home is to double up with friends or relatives; this generally maintains the first four functions, but it interferes at least to some extent with functions 5–7 and 10–12. Squatting in a house behind closed doors maintains in part the first six functions, but it interferes severely with the last four. Being placed in a hotel usually means that a family has to live in one room, often in squalid conditions and with a hazardous environment (chapter 11). This often interferes severely with the functions related to family life, respite, and safety.

When these "solutions" fail, shelters and the street are the alternatives. Environments rife with violence and unhygienic conditions have to be contended with (chapter 11). As very few functions of the home are left, the decision between street and shelter often revolves upon a single major factor, such as the fear of violence in a shelter or on the street, the need for privacy, the ability to remain together with one's spouse or children, the need for warmth and the comfort of a bed, or the need for or aversion to a structured environment. Often, there is little or no choice. When there is nobody to double up with and shelters and welfare hotels cannot meet the demand, "the street," in its various aspects (such as building entrances, sidewalks, alleyways, parks, beaches, underpasses, train or bus stations, subway platforms, underground tunnels or rooms, roofs, hospital emergency rooms, other public buildings, parking lots, parked vehicles, moving subway or freight trains, fields, forests, caves or barns) is the only recourse.

Homelessness may be benign or malignant (25:100–106). In benign homelessness, the state of homelessness is short, the subsequent domiciled state is stable, and homeless individuals incur relatively little hardship. In malignant homelessness, the state of homelessness is long or it recurs with periods of marginal housing in the interval, and homeless persons incur considerable hardship and damage to the person. There is a self-perpetuating element in malignant homelessness, because the hardship, demoralization, demands on one's time for survival needs, lack of address, change in appearance, stigma, and low-paying casual jobs associated with homelessness mitigate against gaining the stable and sufficient income needed to maintain a home. A striking feature of the recent epidemic of homelessness in the United States is that it has involved a marked increase in the number of people experiencing malignant homelessness (25:100).

Malignant homelessness seldom develops suddenly. Rather, it happens to poor people, and it is usually the culmination of a long process of marginal living and precarious housing (chapter 4). A survey of homeless people revealed a high prevalence of adverse life events in the year preceding homelessness (26). By the time they become homeless, people (whether runaway or thrown-away youths, unemployed workers, mentally ill people, women with children, or others) have already endured considerable pain or stress, they are left with few if any resources, and the type of social support needed to get up the social ladder is gone if it ever was present.

On top of that, they are faced with, to paraphrase Beverly Ovrebo, an environment for which nothing in their previous lives has prepared them (chapter 9). The homeless environment is generally brutal, demoralizing, and stigmatizing (27). There is increased risk of death, disease, and physical disability for all (chapter 4), and of impaired development for children (chapter 7). People adapt, attend to the functions needed for survival even though this may leave little time for anything else (chapter 10), and develop their own social and communication networks on the street or in shelters (28,29) with homeless or other very poor people, who may be good resources for survival in the homeless state but not for reintegration into society's mainstream. Many homeless people are very resilient, and such resilience, along with favorable environmental conditions, allows a few to make spectacular recoveries. For instance, John Major, the British prime minister, was once homeless. However, for the majority, recovery from homelessness means climbing up to marginal housing (chapter 9) and remaining very poor in a fragile economic situation with a high risk of recurring homelessness (30). A significant number of homeless people need some form of support in addition to a home, because one or more overwhelming conditions such as mental disorder, substance abuse, illiteracy or lack of word skills, and frail old age provide handicaps to earning a living and in a few instances to managing a home. Thus, homelessness is usually not an isolated event in the life of an individual but part of a stressful and damaging process associated with poverty and vulnerability—before and after the homeless episode.

The societal changes of the 1970s and 1980s associated with the growth of homelessness are reviewed in chapter 15. Here I highlight one factor that has been rather neglected in the literature on homelessness, though not in the literature on poverty: the changing power relationships and growing conflicts of interest between the more affluent members of society and poor people which have occurred since the mid-1970s. In broad lines, the developments were as follows. The rise in the nation's productivity came to a virtual stop in the 1970s (31), setting the conditions for a "zero-sum society" (32), that is, the economic gains of some occur at the expense of losses by others. Edsall described how the business community became organized for effective political action, and how the Democratic party moved politically rightwards and ceased to provide an effective barrier to the demands of the affluent part of the population (33). The shift of political power to the Right was apparent in 1978 when poverty and consumer protection programs of the preceding decades were rolled back and the attack on property taxes began at the state level. Under Reagan, that shift continued and intensified, with attacks on poor people's interests, on welfare

(34, 35), and on housing for poor people (chapter 17). Legislation on taxes and on regulation favored business and affluent people and helped them to increase their wealth and power, while low-income workers and poor people lost both (36). Thus a vast transfer of power and money, which is still in progress, is disempowering and impoverishing the lower-income segment of society. Homelessness is only the most extreme of many aspects of the increased severity of poverty.

There is not much difference between the Right and the Left concerning this sequence of events. Where the two differ is over the justification of what is happening. The Right, which now has political ascendancy, believes that the provision of capital for business will bring a prosperity that, as it increases, diffuses down the socioeconomic scale. The responsibility for homeless people's fate is attributed to their own ways of life, which in turn are seen as due to cultural changes (e.g., the drug culture, the culture of the 1960s, the underclass) rather than to economics. The Left believes that the prosperity of a large part of the nation has been accompanied by errors of great magnitude, such as the collapse of the savings and loan associations and the growing national debt, which are weakening the economy and creating mounting problems for the future. Homeless people are seen as defenseless victims of these economic forces.

This argument has been going on for 10 years, and there is no sign of prosperity trickling down the income scale. Much to the contrary, there has been a widening of the distance between rich and poor, and a steady growth of poverty and homelessness. The capital growth that was supposed to bring back high productivity has not done so; instead, capital has often been squandered on real estate speculation or poor financial decisions while programs for poor people were being cut. This is a clear instance of the "outrage of homelessness in the face of abundance."

The destitution and suffering of homeless people has not evoked a public reaction to prevent homelessness. The majority of the public is indifferent or downright hostile to homeless people (37). The minimal emergency step represented by the McKinney Act has not been followed by significant additional steps (chapter 11), as if society has accepted homelessness in its midst. This is not the first time that a societal phenomenon that will be looked at later with abhorrence is accepted by the contemporary population. Slavery or the gross abuse of retarded persons in institutions or of elderly persons in nursing homes was tolerated for decades or centuries until people eventually decided to come to grips with the social institutions responsible for these social ills. This has not yet happened in the instance of homelessness.

Notes

1. Rossi et al. (22) coined the term *the literal homeless* to refer to homeless people who spend the night in the streets or in shelters. However, in the remainder of this book, the term *literally homeless people* will be used instead.

2. Roth et al. (23) used the term *resource people* to refer to homeless people who have lodging resources that make it possible for them to spend the night in places other than shelters or the streets, such as the homes of relatives or friends (doubling up) or hotel rooms for which they can pay for a limited number of days.

References

1. Lamb HR (ed.). *The Homeless Mentally Ill.* Washington, D.C.: American Psychiatric Association, 1984.

2. Brickner PW, et al. (eds.). *Health Care of Homeless People.* New York: Springer, 1985.

3. General Accounting Office. *Homelessness: A Complex Problem and the Federal Response.* Washington, D.C.: Government Printing Office, 1985.

4. Erikson J, Wilhelm C (eds.). *Housing the Homeless.* New Brunswick, N.J.: Center for Urban Policy Research, Rutgers University, 1986.

5. Hope M, Young J. *The Faces of Homelessness.* Lexington, Mass.: Lexington Books, 1986.

6. Redburn FS, Buss TF. *Responding to America's Homeless: Public Policy Alternatives.* New York: Praeger, 1986.

7. Morse GA. *A Contemporary Assessment of Urban Homelessness: Implications for Social Change.* St. Louis: Center for Metropolitan Studies, University of Missouri at St. Louis, 1986.

8. Bingham RD, Green RE, White SB (eds.). *The Homeless in Contemporary Society.* Newbury Park, Calif.: Sage Publications, 1987.

9. Wright J, Weber E. *Homelessness and Health.* Washington, D.C.: McGraw-Hill Health Care Information Center, 1987.

10. Institute of Medicine. *Homelessness, Health, and Human Needs.* Washington, D.C.: National Academy Press, 1988.

11. Ropers RH. *The Invisible Homeless: A New Urban Ecology.* New York: Human Sciences Press, 1988.

12. Burt MR, Cohen BE. *America's Homeless: Numbers, Characteristics, and Programs That Serve Them.* Washington, D.C.: Urban Institute, 1989.

13. Wright JD. *Address Unknown: The Homeless in America.* New York: Aldine de Gruyter, 1989.

14. Rossi P. *Without Shelter: Homelessness in the 1980s.* New York: Priority Press Publications, 1989.

15. Lang MH. *Homelessness amid Affluence: Structure and Paradox in the American Political Economy.* New York: Praeger, 1989.

16. Momeni J (ed.). *Homelessness in the United States: State Surveys.* New York: Praeger, 1989.

17. Momeni J (ed.). *Homelessness in the United States: Data and Issues.* New York: Praeger, 1990.

18. Brickner PW, et al. (eds.). *Under the Safety Net: The Health and Social Welfare of the Homeless in the United States.* New York: W. W. Norton, 1990.

19. Watson S, Austerberry H. *Housing and Homelessness: A Feminist Perspective*. London: Routledge and Kegan Paul, 1986.

20. Friedrichs J. *Affordable Housing and the Homeless*. Berlin: Walter de Gruyter, 1988.

21. *Stuart B. McKinney Homeless Assistance Act*. 42 USC 11301, July 22, 1987.

22. Rossi PH, et al. The urban homeless: Estimation of composition and size. *Science* 235:1336–1341, 1987.

23. Roth D, et al. *Homelessness in Ohio: A Study of People in Need*. Columbus: Ohio State Department of Mental Health, 1985.

24. HomeBase. *A Place for Everyone: Community-Based Planning for the Provision of Housing and Human Services to Homeless People*. San Francisco: HomeBase, 1990.

25. Jahiel RI. The situation of homelessness. In Bingham, Green, White (eds.), *The Homeless in Contemporary Society*, pp. 99–118. See ref. 8.

26. Morse G, et al. *Homeless People in St. Louis: A Mental Health Program Evaluation, Field Study, and Follow-up Investigation*. Jefferson City: State of Missouri Department of Mental Health, 1985.

27. Joe Homeless. My own story. *Newsday Magazine*, October 28, 1990.

28. Boner W. Life on Lower Broad. *Nashville Magazine*, August 1984.

29. Hevesi D. Running away. *New York Times Magazine*, October 2, 1988.

30. Farr RK, Koegel P, Burnam A. *A Study of Homelessness in the Skid Row Area of Los Angeles*. Los Angeles: County Department of Mental Health, 1986.

31. Krugman P. *The Age of Diminished Expectations*. Cambridge, Mass.: MIT Press, 1990.

32. Thurow LC. *The Zero-Sum Society*. New York: Basic Books, 1980.

33. Edsall TB. *The New Politics of Inequality*. New York: W. W. Norton, 1984.

34. Katz MB. *The Undeserving Poor*. New York: Pantheon Books, 1989.

35. Piven FF, Cloward RA. *The New Class War*, 2d ed. New York: Pantheon Books, 1984.

36. Phillips K. *The Politics of Rich and Poor*. New York: Random House, 1990.

37. Waxman LD, Reyes LM. *A Status Report on Hunger and Homelessness in America's Cities, 1990*. Washington, D.C.: United States Conference of Mayors, December 1990.

CHAPTER 2

Preventive Approaches
to Homelessness

René I. Jahiel, M.D., Ph.D.

The prevention-oriented approach of this book is an adaptation of the methods of preventive medicine, but instead of disease, the condition dealt with is a social ill, homelessness. The nature, feasibility, and effectiveness of the various prevention methods are determined by technical and political factors. This chapter has three objectives. The first objective is to describe the prevention paradigm as it applies to homelessness. The second objective is to sketch three types of technical factors influencing prevention efforts related to homelessness: empirical data regarding homeless people and homelessness; theories of homelessness; and the tools with which different types of prevention may be implemented. The third objective is to review briefly the political factors and policy priorities that have influenced preventive approaches to homelessness in the 1980s.

The Prevention Paradigm Applied
to Homelessness

The objectives of prevention are to minimize harm to the individual and the community and to maintain economic productivity. These objectives may be achieved in three ways: by preventing the harmful condition from occurring (primary prevention), by detecting the condition soon after it occurs and taking steps to eliminate it (secondary prevention), or by minimizing the harmful effects of an existing condition (tertiary prevention).

The definition of the condition that is targeted for preventive measures determines the scope and nature of the measures. For instance, if the definition of homelessness is "being without a roof over one's head," the solution is shelter; if it is "being without one's own home," the solution is a home; if it is "being without resources to make a living," the solution is income or empowerment.

The timing of preventive intervention is also significant. One may intervene during an extended period of homelessness (tertiary prevention or late secondary prevention), shortly after the onset of homelessness (secondary prevention), when homeless is imminent (late primary prevention), or long before homelessness would occur (primary prevention). Another important dimension is the target of the intervention, that is, whether the intervention is directed at the affected individual (i.e., a homeless person or a person at risk of homelessness) or at the environment (e.g., people or agencies that cause homelessness [chapter 18] or serve homeless people). Decisions about preventive approaches depend upon technical factors (e.g., knowledge of the population; causal factors; and state-of-the-art intervention methodology) and political factors (e.g., cost, motivation, and power relationships).

Technical Factors

EMPIRICAL DATA

There is general agreement that the number of homeless people has increased markedly and steadily since 1980, as the demand for shelter has risen by an average of 20 percent per year for the period, but there is disagreement about the actual size of the population. Estimates of the number of literally homeless people given in the literature in 1987–88 range from 600,000 to 1 million. However, the analysis presented in chapter 22 suggests that the number on any given day of 1990 was higher, possibly 1.5 million. The number of doubled-up homeless people is estimated at 7.5 million on the basis of very soft data (chapter 22).

Numerous surveys show that the literally homeless population is very heterogeneous. About 25 percent of literally homeless people are children, and more than one-third are in family groups. The median age has decreased since the 1970s, as the representation of homeless youths and young adults has increased, but there are still elderly homeless people. The population is heterogeneous with respect to the duration of homelessness, marital history, ethnicity, education, previous occupation, socioeconomic status, welfare experience, geographic mobility, current means of subsistence, health status, alcohol or drug use (chapter 4), mental disorder (chapter 5), and history of criminal actions or victimization (chapter 6). About the only common feature is extreme poverty.

The paths to homelessness are varied, usually involving a conjunction of several factors, and recurrent homelessness is frequent. A relatively large number of homeless adults have a history of foster care as children or of never having had a home (chapter 4). Homelessness is damaging to children's development (chapter 7). For adults, the homeless situation is an experience that outsiders are ill-prepared to understand. Ethnographic studies, which combine ecological, processual, and insiders' perspectives (chapter 8), help to understand the actions of homeless (chapter 8), and near-homeless (chapter 9) people and the barriers to services in the homeless situation (chapter 10).

Demographic and economic changes during the 1970s and 1980s (chapter 15), especially changes in income statistics, unemployment statistics, and welfare subsidies (chapter 16), and low-income housing programs (chapter 17), are associated with the increased severity of poverty of a large part of the population and an increased risk of homelessness. Pressures toward homelessness and processes that cause people to lose their homes have been identified, along with the role of individuals who profit from the very events that make other people homeless (chapter 18).

THEORIES OF HOMELESSNESS

Four main theories explain the causation and growth of homelessness and provide rationales for preventive measures.

HOMELESSNESS BY CHOICE, BY NATURE, OR BY PERSONALITY.   The theory that people become homeless by choice or by "constitution" goes back to the nineteenth century (chapter 24). In the 1980s, little evidence was found for that theory as originally stated (chapter 4). Yet this explanation is still widely believed (1).

More recent interpretations of the "homeless by nature" hypothesis have examined the personality of homeless people. Levinson gives the following description of a homeless person: "We thus find a man who values his leisure, his partial retirement from life and his independence of any institutional control. This man does not look for security, for a place to remain and to stay for a long time. He prefers his freedom, even if it is only freedom to starve and to beg" (2:597). Levinson posits that these features are not inborn characteristics of homeless men but rather, that they developed out of the experiences that these men had in their dealings with society, as he states, "The homeless man has lost out in the battle for acceptance" (2:596) and "These are the byproducts of our society. They have gone through aversive learning experiences which we have provided for them" (2:597). One finds some support for this theory in studies showing that homelessness is preceded in many instances by a long period of marginal subsistence, losses, and failures (chapter 4). Ethnographic studies of the paths to homelessness are needed to assess and develop this theory.

A related hypothesis presents homelessness from the perspective of the underclass. Referring to homeless people, Schiff stated,

Almost all lack the sense of personal "structuring" necessary to maintain steady employment. . . . Why do such people become homeless? Can it even be a rational decision? To understand why, it requires viewing them from the perspective of the underclass, not the middle class. To someone with at least a decent high-school education, possessing at least some of the middle class values, and capable of steady work paying say $25,000, homelessness is not an option. On the other hand, to slum-dwellers with different values, poorly or not educated, not capable of high earnings (except in illegal enterprise), not capable of affording more than substandard housing, often in drug-infested areas—to such people, living in the streets, subways, bus terminals or shelters is a viable alternative. And while middle class people consider the streets and shelters to be extremely dangerous, they are *that* dangerous only in comparison with wealthier areas, not with the areas from which most of the homeless come. . . . In reality, many (though not all) of the shelters are much safer than most ghetto neighborhoods. . . . Shelter may in fact be the ultimate form of "affordable housing." . . . In plain English, the welfare state is in essence providing, for a large percentage of the homeless a life-style that would cost roughly $10,000 to $12,000 were it to be purchased on the open market. (3:35)

This explanation assumes that most homeless people belong to an underclass with a culture of its own—a new version of the "culture of poverty." According to this concept, the rise in homelessness in the 1980s was due in part to the welfare policies of the 1960s and to neglect of education in the inner city, by which a whole generation came to adulthood without the skills or desire to earn a living independently. The evidence that the homeless population is very heterogeneous and comes from different socioeducational groups (chapter 4) mitigates against this theory; however, it does not rule out its applicability to part of the homeless population.

Hopper, Susser, and Conover (4) suggest that episodic homelessness is part of a repertoire of adaptations to a state of severe poverty. People become homeless when other ways of subsisting are rejected for specific reasons or are impossible. Becoming homeless requires some action on the part of individuals, but this action is forced upon them by the social forces that create their extreme poverty. This interpretation shifts the focus from homelessness to poverty, since the former is considered a modality of poverty.

SOCIAL DISAFFILIATION.   Recognizing the heterogeneity of homeless populations, Bahr and Caplow suggested nearly 20 years ago that social disaffiliation, a faulty relationship between homeless people and society, might be the one explanatory factor of homelessness common to all homeless people. Social disaffiliation can be the result of external changes, such as an economic depression, when society "withdraws" from the individual; the adoption by the individual of a deviant role, such as chronic alcoholism, which leads to rejection by society; or "unsocialization," with lifelong isolation, as in chronic mental illness (5). This theory, which was based in part on empirical studies in Philadelphia's Skid Row and New York's Bowery during the 1960s (chapter 3), would attribute the growth of homelessness in the 1980s to several processes that increased the number of socially disaffiliated individuals in the community. Among such processes are deinstitutionalization of mentally ill people without appropriate community services, the economic recession of 1981–82, the rise in immigration, and the growth of an underclass with decreased ties to social institutions. There is evidence that some homeless people have deficient social networks (chapter 4). However, comparative studies of homeless and other poor populations, cohort studies of populations before and after they become homeless, and sophisticated social network analysis are needed to critically test this theory. Empirical studies with such methods are in progress (chapter 4).

HOUSING AND POVERTY.   In this theory, homelessness is the end result when people lack the money to pay for housing. Characteristics found with increased frequency among homeless people (e.g., mental disorder, substance abuse, unemployment, and racial or ethnic minority status) are merely vulnerability factors, that is, conditions that make the individual unable to earn enough money. Further, people with these features are often discriminated against in the competition for the limited number of jobs and affordable housing units. According to this theory, the rise in the size of the homeless population during the 1980s was due to the increased severity of poverty and the decreased amount of low-income housing, which caused a "housing affordability gap" (6–9). The strong evidence in favor of this theory includes the nearly universal poverty of homeless people and certain developments in welfare and employment (chapter 16) and in low-income housing (chapter 17) in the 1980s. The main argument that can be directed against this theory is the ecological fallacy critique. Therefore, macroeconomic approaches (chapter 16) must be combined with ethnographic approaches (chapter 8) to test this theory.

SOCIETAL DISINVESTMENT.   This theory accepts the premises of the housing and poverty theory but carries them one step further, asserting that the people who are vulnerable to homelessness were the object of specific decisions to disinvest societal resources from them. These decisions, often made long before the affected people become homeless, are usually coupled with increased societal investment in other people. They reflect conflicts of interest and differential power among societal groups. The rise of homelessness in the 1980s is explained by the growing power of affluent individuals and corporations and their increasing demands on the government, starting in the mid-1970s, along with the disinvestment of people who had been dependent on the government for support or who had to be sacrificed to allow investment in other people (10). This theory has not yet been specifically tested with empirical studies. However, empirical studies of housing, welfare, and unemployment are compatible with it (chapter 18). Critical empirical testing would involve the identification of the relevant decision networks, and it would require policy research at the macro and micro levels.

These theories are not mutually exclusive; for instance, Ropers presented displacement from a job and housing as "the contemporary path to mass disaffiliation" (11). Also, they may be integrated in various ways into broader political frameworks. (For instance, the last two theories could be elaborated from the viewpoint of Marxism or of interest group politics.) However, they are useful in their present form because of their distinctive implications for prevention.

IMPLICATIONS FOR PREVENTIVE ACTION.   Tertiary prevention is relatively insensitive to the theoretical context. Homeless people are in need, and services should be provided to them for that reason only. However, the "homeless by nature" theory, which presents homeless people as part of an underclass for which many people have relatively little sympathy and/or as people whose actions have made them responsible for their homelessness, provides a rationale for providing only minimal services.

Secondary prevention involves, in all instances, facilitating the recovery of a stable home. The theories emphasize different approaches to this aim. In the "homeless by nature" theory, homeless people are required to change their ways, with little help or with coercion (e.g., in "workfare" requirements for assistance). The social disaffiliation theory suggests a "therapeutic" approach that would reconnect individuals with social organizations by providing remedies to the conditions responsible for the disaffiliation (e.g., help in getting a job or welfare allowance, supported work and housing for individuals with mental disorder or substance abuse, and reestablishment of family ties). The last two theories suggest that secondary prevention requires intervention with the community as well as the homeless individual, for instance, the creation of jobs or low-income housing or the overcoming of community resistance to homeless people.

The differences among the theories are greatest with regard to primary prevention. The "homeless by nature" theory would rely on antidrug policies, education, and training for work skills in low-income neighborhoods. The social disaffiliation theory would require the early detection and treatment of the conditions that cause deviance or lifelong disaffiliation, and the prevention of economic depression or other large-scale social changes that have disaffiliating consequences. The housing and income theory would emphasize action at the societal level to increase poor people's income, the amount of affordable housing, or both. The societal disinvestment theory would use the same approach but would emphasize the empowerment and organization of poor people or people at risk of impoverishment to increase their influence on societal decisions.

The significance of theories with regard to homelessness-prevention policies is threefold. First, they may be incorporated into policy makers' ideologies and knowledge base and thereby influence their policies. Second, theoretical analysis may be used to assess the likelihood that given policies will succeed. Third, theories may be used after the fact to defend or promote existing policies.

The tools of implementation include the instruments, tactics, and strategies used in the three types of prevention.

The instruments for tertiary prevention are services that provide shelter; meals; health, mental health, or substance abuse care; protection; education of children; and so on in order to improve the safety and quality of homeless life (chapter 11). Like services to any other population, they have to be available, accessible, and acceptable. Tactics and strategies to that effect include overcoming the resistance of the community to the services; finding and mobilizing resources (e.g., capital, technology, and trained staff); adapting the services to make them acceptable to homeless people (chapters 12 and 13); and advocating improvements in the availability, accessibility, and quality of services (chapter 19).

The instruments for secondary prevention are services (e.g., rehabilitation, remedial education, job training, and job finding); the initial provision of income and housing; and the provision of protected work or housing when needed (chapter 11). Tactics include fitting the sequence of interventions to the situation and needs of homeless people, and using a networking approach to provide them with appropriate services at the appropriate time (chapter 14). Strategies include administrative or legislative approaches to the initial provision of services, income, and housing (chapter 21) and court actions (chapter 19).

The instruments for primary prevention include providing education and training to people at risk; providing early treatment for mental disorders or substance abuse; preventing disability; preventing housing or job displacement; raising individuals' income (wages or welfare); extending the duration of or eligibility for unemployment benefits; and increasing the supply of low-income housing. The selection of instruments, tactics, and strategies depends upon the policy makers' theoretical orientation (chapter 21). The tactics or strategies of primary prevention usually involve much more extensive policy changes, competition among interest groups, and intervention at the macrosocietal level than do the other forms of prevention (chapters 19, 20, and 21).

Policies on Homelessness

Policies on homelessness are determined in part by pressures of competing policies, by ideology, by political exigencies (i.e., the need to do something about a problem either to satisfy constituents' demands or to use the issue for political purposes), by legal exigencies (i.e., the need to conform with existing laws), and by the information available to policy makers. This information comes from many sources, including personal experience and hearsay, the media, "action research" (i.e., research performed in the course of an action, such as a program or a lawsuit, to obtain the information needed to guide or assess the particular action), and "formal research" (i.e., research performed by scientists according to the norms of the scientific research community). In the 1980s, the main actors were advocates and governments.

ACTIONS BY ADVOCATES

Actions by advocates for homeless people played a critical role in giving visibility to the situation of homeless people and in stimulating court and legislative interventions, as well as certain private programs. In 1979, Robert Hayes advocated for homeless men in *Callahan* v. *Carey,* which compelled New York City to provide appropriate shelter for homeless adults (12). In 1981, ethnological research by Baxter and Hopper brought attention to the plight of homeless people (13), and the following year, Hombs and the late Mitch Snyder, of the Community for Creative Non-Violence (CCNV) in Washington, D.C., reported, following a national telephone survey, that there were more than 2 million homeless people in the United States, bringing attention to the magnitude of the problem (14). In the following years, Hayes, Hopper, and others organized the Coalition for the Homeless (CFH), an advocacy organization with chapters in several states and headquarters in New York and in Washington, D.C. In addition to its local functions, the CFH serves as a clearinghouse of information with its newsletter and is an advocate for legislation at the federal level. In the mid-1980s, a homeless person, Chris Sprowal, began to organize homeless people and other poor people into the Union of the Homeless. Hope and Young have described in detail the development of these movements (15).

A different type of advocacy involved professional action in response to the lack of services for homeless people. Brickner and his team at Saint Vincent's Hospital and Medical Center in New York City developed in the early 1970s an approach to primary health care for homeless people (16) which was then used as a model by the Robert Wood Johnson Foundation and Pew Trust's Health Care for the Homeless projects (JP/HCH), which were active in 19 cities from 1985 to 1989 and in turn became the model for the federal Health Care for the Homeless program under the McKinney Act (McK/HCH), which began operations in 1988 (chapter 11). The JP/HCH program stimulated the formation of local coalitions of providers, administrators, and advocates, and the McK/HCH program's evaluation component, under the National Association for Community Health Centers (NACHC), continued to provide a nucleus for those active in services for homeless people.

POLICIES OF LOCAL AND STATE GOVERNMENTS

The emergence of homelessness as a public problem took place in the states between 1980 and 1984. The sequence of events in New York illustrates some of the issues faced by the nation. Max Stern (17) analyzed it with Blumer's five-step model of the development of a public problem as a process of collective definition: emergence; legitimization; the mobilization of forces; the development of an "official solution"; and the implementation of the plan (18). The emergence phase, as described by Stern, was marked by *Callahan v. Carey* (12); Rousseau's (19) and Baxter and Hopper's (13) monographs on homeless people; newspaper reports; pressures from merchants concerned with the effects of homeless people on their business; and the harsh winter of 1981–82. The rapid legitimization and mobilization phases that followed were at first focused on homeless people who were mentally ill. This would have made the state (which is responsible for mental health services) responsible to provide for them. But resistance by the state, court orders addressed to the city, evidence that chronically mentally ill people are only one group in the homeless population, and the rise in unemployment-driven homelessness during the recession of 1981–82 made this approach untenable and gave New York City the "ownership" of the problem. In the conservative atmosphere of the early 1980s, when taxes were being cut and federal funds for housing were being curtailed, a consensus quickly arose not to attack the fundamental causes of the problem but merely to provide food and shelter to homeless people—that is, tertiary prevention was the main "solution." The problem had become "owned" by the providers of tertiary homelessness services and their public and private funders, and was defined as providing services to the literally homeless, especially those who were single. The New York City Human Resources Administration became the main city agency dealing with it. Massive shelters emerged as the intermediate solution.

Thus, the initial public response was focused on shelter rather than housing. The emergence of housing as a solution to the problem came later, and only in relation to homeless families with children. In the mid-1980s, homeless families were housed in welfare hotels and shelters (chapters 7 and 11). At that time they began to emerge as a separate public problem. A sequence similar to the one described by Stern took place. Advocates described the intolerable environment homeless children were exposed to (20) and went to court with lawsuits against the city (21); newspapers ran articles about homeless families; a book (22) helped to raise public consciousness; and the cost of welfare hotels to the city (over $20,000 per room yearly in the lowest-grade hotel) became generally known. In October 1987, new federal regulations limited AFDC's share of reimbursement to the first 30 days the family stayed in the hotel, leaving the full cost afterwards to the city (23). Responding to these pressures, and in line with its stated intention, after two terms oriented toward business interests, to work on the problems of poverty (24), the Koch administration in August 1988 announced a new policy. Over a two-year period, families with children were to be resettled in tier 2 shelters (shelters where a family had its own bedrooms, bath, and kitchen) or in apartments made available by the rehabilitation of city-held vacant property or by new construction, at a cost of over $85,000 per unit (23:334). A different city agency, the Department of Housing Preservation and Development, took charge of that program. The plan was based on estimates of the number of homeless families. When a larger-than-expected demand for the housing developed, in 1991, hotels were used again. New York is unusual in having planned and begun to develop a major housing program for homeless families. Most cities relied on shelters and have minimal if any housing initiatives.

There were also modest efforts, in New York and other cities, to help prevent evictions through legal advice, mediation, or short-term grants; and to keep single-room occupancy hotels (SROs) open as an alternative to homelessness, by means of moratoria on SRO conversion or programs to open new SROs (25,26). As of 1991, at the time of this writing, these efforts have been too minimal or intermittent to result in significant sustained primary prevention (chapter 21).

POLICIES OF THE FEDERAL GOVERNMENT

The position of the federal government during the first half of the 1980s was that the problem was best handled by the private sector and local government. In 1982–83, an interagency task force was established and funds were appropriated for emergency food and shelter programs run by the Department of Agriculture (USDA) and the Federal Emergency Management Agency (FEMA) (27). They were minor programs with little national impact. The federal government undertook two research projects. The first was conducted by the Department of Housing and Urban Development (HUD). After CCNV had estimated that there were, in 1982, 2–3 million homeless people (14), HUD early in 1984 did a national survey of providers and local administrators which yielded an estimate one-tenth to one-fifth as large (28). Despite severe methodological problems that raised doubts about its validity (29,30), the HUD report was widely circulated and used for secondary data analysis. The second project was a peer-reviewed three-year research grant program sponsored by the National Institute of Mental Health (NIMH), starting late in 1983, to do surveys of the adult homeless population to learn about their characteristics, their needs, and the services available to them (31). Congress early showed an interest in homelessness, evidenced by several hearings (32–35), yet no significant congressional action occurred during the first half of the 1980s.

The private sector made some attempts to respond to the need on a national scale, including the JP/HCH project (chapter 11) and expanded services by private organizations such as Travelers Aid and the Salvation Army. By the mid-1980s it was clear that neither these efforts nor those of local governments were meeting the need. Pressures grew for greater federal involvement. Several advocacy organizations spearheaded by CFH pressed for legislative initiatives and contributed to a bill addressing the long-term needs of homeless people, the Homeless Persons' Survival Act of 1986, which was introduced in Congress by Senator Gore and Representative Leland but did not pass.

With the prospect that homelessness would be an important issue in the 1988 elections, members of Congress, including the then Speaker of the House, Jim Wright, joined in these pressures, and in 1987 another bill, providing emergency rather than long-term measures, the Stuart B. McKinney Homeless Assistance Act (PL 100-77), was passed. It defined the problem in terms of providing comprehensive services (planning, shelter, food, health, mental health and substance abuse, social services, education, job training, and employment assistance) to literally homeless people through grants to states, cities, or private nonprofit agencies (chapter 11). Funding was very limited, underlining the position that city and state governments and private providers still "owned" the problem. It was clear from the 1987 bill that the "solution" was still to be found in tertiary prevention. When the McKinney Act was reauthorized in 1989, a modest attempt was made to include housing—in the form of SRO programs and supported housing for families with children, or for mentally ill persons—in the solution. However, funding was very low (chapter 11). The various federal initiatives are coordinated by the Interagency Council on the Homeless, which publishes a yearly report (36). The "Goals and Objectives of the Federal Plan to Help End the Tragedy of Homelessness," which it adopted late in 1990, identifies preventing nonhomeless families and individuals from becoming homeless as one of its two goals (37:1003). It remains to be seen whether and how this proposal will be implemented.

POLICY PRIORITIES

It is clear from the preceding analysis that the main preventive approach used in the 1980s by government, at all levels, and by private agencies was tertiary prevention—shelter, food, and other subsistence services. The growth of a "homelessness industry" (chapter 11) was associated with this approach. It may be surmised that tertiary prevention was given the highest priority for several reasons: it provided an answer to the most urgent needs; it seemed to be the cheapest of the three prevention approaches, although this inference may not be warranted in general, and especially in the long run; and it helped homeless people while giving funds for the purpose to various categories of providers. Of the three forms of prevention, it is the one that provides the greatest control over the homeless populations, as well as the one that requires the least social change involving other societal groups.

Secondary prevention efforts have been directed mainly at families with children, and these efforts began relatively late. When done on a scale commensurate with the need, as in New York City, they involve a considerable initial expense in housing (at least $85,000 per housing unit, i.e., per household). Such expense may be reduced to some extent by selecting more modest housing objectives or using nonprofit housing, as discussed in detail in chapter 21. Furthermore, the problem of maintaining housing (i.e., ensuring an income sufficient to pay for the rent and basic necessities, and preventing various forms of displacement) has not yet been faced. This approach would involve a significant redistribution of resources or income in favor of homeless people, and as long as the economy appears to be of the zero-sum variety (chapter 1), it means that some other social group(s) would have something to lose. Finally, the stratification of secondary prevention (most for families with children, less for mentally ill people, and little if any for families without children, or single adults or youths) suggests that differing values are attached to different groups of homeless people.

Primary prevention requires that one take a position about which theory of homelessness will provide a rationale for the intervention. Depending on the theory, the intervention may be limited to antidrug programs and education and training programs for the selected population, with a very long latency period before the results, if any, can be seen ("homeless by nature" theory); or it would involve considerable interaction with numerous organizations (social disaffiliation theory); or it would involve sizeable redistribution of economic resources (housing and poverty theory) with, additionally, the redistribution of power over certain societal decisions (societal disinvestment theory). Each of these approaches would require significant structural change in our society and would elicit the opposition of those groups who are favored under the status quo and have the greatest political power.

The Outlook for the Future

The low level of primary and secondary prevention of homelessness in the 1980s may be attributed in part to governmental policies that caused a marked aggravation of poverty (chapters 1, 15–18), forcing the selection of tertiary prevention as the "solution" of the "homelessness problem." Homelessness was treated as a phenomenon distinct from severe poverty. Criticism of the policies is emerging as a main political theme in the 1990s. Increasingly, homelessness is approached in the context of poverty. The information base for the primary and secondary prevention of severe poverty and of homelessness is growing as a result of empirical research within and outside the field of homelessness studies. While it has not yet been translated into effective antipoverty programs, approaches are being formulated and proposals are beginning to emerge (chapter 21).

References

1. Roberts SV. Reagan on homelessness: Many choose to live in the streets. *New York Times,* December 23, 1988, p. A26.
2. Levinson BM. The homeless man: A psychological enigma. *Mental Hygiene 47:* 590–601, 1963.
3. Schiff L. Would they be better off in a home? *National Review 42(4):*33–35, 1990.
4. Hopper K, Susser E, Conover S. Economies of makeshift: Deindustrialization and homelessness in New York City. *Urban Anthropology 14(1–3):*183–236, 1985.
5. Bahr H, Caplow T. *Old Men Drunk and Sober.* New York: New York University Press, 1973.
6. Hartman C (ed.) *America's Housing Crisis: What Is to Be Done?* Boston: Routledge and Kegan Paul, 1983.
7. Hopper K, Hamberg J. The making of America's homeless: From Skid Row to the New Poor. In Bratt RG, Hartman C, Meyerson A (eds.), *Critical Perspectives on Housing.* Philadelphia: Temple University Press, 1986, pp. 12–40.
8. Andrews N. *The Challenge of Affordable Housing: A Perspective for the 1980s.* New York: Ford Foundation, 1986.
9. Wright JD, Lam JA. Homelessness and the low-income housing supply. *Social Policy 17(4):*48–53, 1987.
10. Jahiel RI. Selective disinvestment theory of homelessness. Manuscript, 1989.
11. Ropers RH. *The Invisible Homeless: A New Urban Ecology.* New York: Human Sciences Press, 1988.
12. Hopper K, Cox LS. Litigation in advocacy for the homeless: The case of New York City. *Development: Seeds of Change 2:*57–62, 1982.
13. Baxter E, Hopper K. *Private Lives, Public Spaces: Homeless Adults in the Streets of New York.* New York: Community Service Society, 1981.
14. Hombs ME, Snyder M. *Homelessness in America: A Forced March to Nowhere.* Washington, D.C.: Community for Creative Non-Violence, 1982.
15. Hope M, Young J. *The Faces of Homelessness.* Lexington, Mass.: Lexington Books, 1986.
16. Brickner PW, et al. *Health Care of Homeless People.* New York: Springer, 1985.
17. Stern MJ. The emergence of the homeless as a public problem. *Social Service Review 58:*291–301, 1984.
18. Blumer H. Social problems as collective behaviors. *Social Problems 18:*298–306, 1969.
19. Rousseau AM. *Shopping Bag Ladies: Homeless Women Speak about Their Lives.* New York: Pilgrim Press, 1981.
20. Wackstein N. *Seven Thousand Homeless Children: The Crisis Continues.* New York: Citizens' Committee for Children of New York, 1984.
21. *Yvonne McCain et al. v. Edward I. Koch.* Court of Appeals, State of New York, no. 41023/83, November 14, 1986. Reprinted in Hayes RM (ed.), *The Rights of the Homeless.* New York: Practising Law Institute, 1987, pp. 205–301.
22. Kozol J. *Rachel and Her Children: Homeless Families in America.* New York: Crown Publishers, 1988.

23. Tobier E. The homeless. In Brecher C, Horton RD (eds.), *Setting Municipal Priorities, 1990*. New York: New York University Press, 1989, pp. 307–338.

24. Brecher C, Horton D. Introduction. In Brecher, Horton (eds.), *Setting Municipal Priorities*, pp. 1–23. See n. 23.

25. Nenno MK. *Assistance for Homeless Persons: A NAHRO Resource Book for Housing and Community Development Agencies*. Washington, D.C.: National Association of Housing and Redevelopment Officials, 1988.

26. Schwartz DC, Glascock, JH. *Combating Homelessness: A Resource Book*. New Brunswick, N.J.: Rutgers—State University of New Jersey, American Affordable Housing Institute, 1989.

27. Health and Human Services Working Group on the Homeless. The homeless: background, analysis, and options. Report transmitted to the President by Margaret M. Heckler, Secretary, Department of Health and Human Services, on August 15, 1984.

28. U.S. Department of Housing and Urban Development. *A Report to the Secretary on the Homeless and Emergency Shelters*. Washington, D.C.: HUD, May 1984.

29. House Committee on Banking, Finance, and Urban Affairs, and Committee on Government Operations. *HUD Report on Homelessness*. Joint Hearing before the Subcommittees on Housing and Community Development and on Manpower and Housing, 98th Cong., 2d sess., May 24, 1984. Washington, D.C.: Government Printing Office, 1984.

30. House Committee on Banking, Finance, and Urban Affairs. *HUD Report on Homelessness—II*. Hearing before the Subcommittee on Housing and Community Development, 99th Cong., 1st sess., December 4, 1985. Washington, D.C.: Government Printing Office, 1986.

31. Morrissey JP, Dennis DL. *NIMH Funded Research Concerning Mentally Ill Persons: Implications for Policy and Practice*. Washington, D.C.: U.S. Department of Health and Human Services, 1986.

32. House Committee on Banking, Finance, and Urban Affairs. *Homelessness in America*. Hearings before the Subcommittee on Housing and Community Development, 97th Cong., 2d sess., December 15, 1982. Washington, D.C.: Government Printing Office, 1983.

33. House Committee on Banking, Finance, and Urban Affairs. *Homelessness in America—II*. Hearings before the Subcommittee on Housing and Community Development, 98th Cong., 2d sess., January 25, 1984. Washington, D.C.: Government Printing Office, 1984.

34. House Committee on Government Operations. *The Federal Response to the Homeless Crisis*. Hearings before the Subcommittee on Intergovernmental Relations and Human Resources, 98th Cong., 2d sess., October 1, November 20, and December 18, 1984. Washington, D.C.: Government Printing Office, 1985.

35. Senate Special Committee on Aging. *Living between the Cracks: America's Chronic Homeless*. Hearing held in Philadelphia before the Special Committee on Aging, 98th Cong., 2d sess., December 12, 1984, Serial no. 98-20. Washington, D.C.: Government Printing Office, 1985.

36. Interagency Council on the Homeless. *1990 Annual Report*, Parts I and II and Executive Summary. Washington, D.C.: Interagency Council on the Homeless, 1991.

37. Lindblom EN. Toward a comprehensive homelessness prevention strategy. *Housing Policy Debate 2(3): 957–1025*, 1991.

PART I

Homeless People in
Their Environment

CHAPTER 3

Demographics and Stereotypes of Homeless People

Louisa R. Stark, Ph.D.

At about a quarter to six, the Irishman led me to the spike. . . . It
looked much like a prison. Already a long queue of ragged men had
formed up, waiting for the gates to open. They were of all kinds and
ages, the youngest a fresh-faced boy of sixteen, the oldest a
doubled-up mummy of seventy-five. Some were hardened tramps,
recognizable by their sticks and billies and dust-darkened faces;
some were factory hands out of work, some agricultural laborers,
one a clerk in collar and tie, two certainly imbeciles.

George Orwell
Down and Out in Paris and London (1933)

This chapter examines the demographics of homelessness in the urban United
States from the end of the nineteenth century to the present. In the past, the
popular perception was that all homeless individuals were alcoholics. A decade
or so ago this perception changed, and today the general homeless population is
more often labeled mentally ill. Although it might appear that these perceptions
mirror actual changes in the demographic composition of our homeless population, a historical study of homelessness reveals that all the distinctive categories
of homeless people that are present today have been evident throughout our
nation's history.

The Face of Homelessness:
Continuity and Change

Beginning in the 1870s, run-down city neighborhoods, often called mainstems
or Skid Rows, began to evolve as poor inner-city enclaves with lodging houses,
hotels, restaurants, saloons, and other services dedicated to fulfilling the needs
of single, mostly male, transient workers (1). The mainstems soon began to
inspire studies that attempted to describe the residents of these areas and their
needs. In the early 1890s, J. J. McCook sent batches of questionnaires to the

mayors of 40 cities, to be given to homeless men to fill out. Returns were received from 1,349 participants in 14 cities. On the basis of these self-reports, 9 percent of the homeless men were older than 50 and 8.5 percent were in bad health, while 38.5 percent had been arrested for drunkenness at least once. Furthermore, 57.4 percent of the respondents were people with trades or professional skills (including weavers, 3.6% of the sample, who had lost their jobs because of the mechanization of the textile industry), 41.4 percent were unskilled laborers, and 1.5 percent had no regular calling. After reviewing these statistics, McCook concluded that the most important causes of homelessness were "economic influences" (2).

After the panic of 1907–8, which caused more unemployment and homelessness, a number of studies were undertaken to find out who the homeless people were (3). What was probably the earliest study of New York City's Skid Row was carried out in 1910 by H. S. Cook, social secretary of the Municipal Lodging House. In contrast to the popular opinion of the times—that homeless people were all criminals and should be imprisoned—Cook found that most of the men he interviewed were recently unemployed, with good references from former employers. He concluded that "we are the guilty ones, we are the criminals" for treating homeless people so badly (4:5).

The earliest study of homeless men in Chicago, by Alice Solenberger, was published in 1911. She based her conclusions on interviews with 1,000 homeless men, whom she divided into four categories: "self-supporting," "temporarily dependent," "chronically dependent," and "parasitic." Economically self-supporting individuals amounted to 13 percent. Chronically dependent persons formed the largest group and included 5.2 percent who were defined as "insane," 1.9 percent who were feebleminded, 16.7 percent who were crippled, and 9.8 percent who were "addicted to the excessive use of drink." Thirteen and two-tenths percent were over 65 years old. Solenberger blamed industry for the fact that so many homeless workers were then congregated in the nation's urban areas. She noted that to be continuously employed, a man had to move constantly from one urban area to another and rarely had the opportunity to put down roots (5).

Solenberger compared the results of her study with data collected on 200 homeless men in Minneapolis. Of the people in the Minneapolis sample, 11.5 percent were over age 60. About 40 percent of the sample were in "good mental and physical condition"; the remaining 60 percent, in "defective physical and mental condition," included 7 percent who were insane, 2 percent who were feebleminded, 17.5 percent who were crippled, and 46.5 percent who "drank to excess" (5).

Another early study was a doctoral dissertation published in 1916 by Frank Laubach (6), which was based on interviews with 100 New York City Skid Row men. Of the men interviewed, 48 percent were classified as "bad alcoholics" and 12 percent as "mentally disqualified" to work. Of those with mental problems, there appear to have been equal numbers of people with schizophrenia and those with personality disorders. This is consistent with figures that he cites from the Municipal Lodging House in the same year, where the rate of mental disability was also estimated at 12 percent. Laubach found that 18 percent of the men he interviewed haa physical disabilities (4% "deformed" and 14% "maimed"). His estimate that 16 percent of the men were "past the age of usefulness for laboring men" compares with similar estimates of 12 percent in 1909–10 and 13.2 percent in 1913 at the Municipal Lodging House. Like Solenberger, Laubach criticized the organization of industry during the early twentieth century. He believed that more than anything, economic conditions drove men to "vagrancy." He wrote at length about the exploitation of unskilled laborers, especially by employment agencies, which, he said, in league with employers, "keep their employees for a week and then discharge them on some pretext, in order to get fees for the same jobs from other applicants" (6:79). He concluded, "It is almost impossible for those who live within a wide margin of economic safety to realize how close the ordinary unskilled worker is to that social abyss called 'vagrancy'" (6:80).

In 1918, Stuart Rice, who had worked for many years as superintendent of the New York Municipal Lodging House, published an article entitled "The Homeless." Although he did not present any statistics, Rice echoed Solenberger's classification of homeless people as self-supporting, temporarily dependent, chronically dependent, or parasitic. He noted, "That more men and women of the first two groups do not actually pass into the third and fourth is a sure evidence of fundamental human character. Everything in the lives of homeless men and women drives them in the direction of chronic dependency and parasitism. Many fight against the odds, day after day, to retain their precarious foothold upon the social ladder; others go down in the struggle, their spirits unbroken to the end" (7:142).

Rice also emphasized the role of homeless people in the economy of the time:

Homeless men are demanded to build the bridges and tunnels, the irrigation systems and railroads, to harvest our forests and embank our rivers. They are the pioneers of modern industry. . . . Homeless women are preferred to do the "dirty work" in our public institutions and to scrub and clean at night in our hotels. Generally, only they are willing to accept the work and hours demanded. . . . Homelessness and intermittent labor go hand in hand. This reserve is highly essential. . . . Men or women without money are docile. How otherwise would they be induced to return to jobs affording no chance of normal living? (7:141)

In 1921–22, Nels Anderson wrote about homeless men in Chicago. He described some as suffering "defects of personality," referring to psychotic symptoms as well as "low intelligence." He noted that 212 (30%) of the 707 men he interviewed were alcoholic. However, Anderson's broadest characterization of homeless people was as unemployed individuals who were unable to keep up with the pace demanded by modern large-scale industry, or who were physically handicapped or old. He concluded that the causes of homelessness have "roots in the very core of our American life, in our industrial system, in education, cultural and vocational, in family relations, in the problems of racial and immigrant adjustment, and in the opportunities offered or denied for the expression of the person" (8:86).

The Depression brought many more people to Skid Row. In a study of 119 homeless men who were "sleeping out" in the streets of Chicago in 1933, Max Stern found that 17 percent were over the age of 60. Those with physical or mental problems included 24 percent described as having a "serious physical condition," 13 percent with a "minor physical ailment," and 9 percent who exhibited a "serious mental abnormality or condition." It is of interest that Stern did not mention alcoholism as a problem in the group he interviewed (9).

In a somewhat more ambitious study of 20,000 unemployed men sheltered in Chicago in 1934, Edwin H. Sutherland and Harvey J. Locke found that while the average age of their homeless respondents was 45, 2 percent were over 65. Psychiatric examination of 265 men revealed that 18 percent suffered from "problems of psychosis, neurosis, or psychopathic personality." Physical examination of 665 men showed that 34 percent were "incapacitated for hard work by chronic or frequent illness" or because of physical disability. An additional 12 percent were described as "chronic alcoholics" (10).

In collecting the life histories of 320 of the homeless men, Sutherland and Locke found that 14 percent supported themselves by "casual labor" (odd jobs). Another 14 percent were migrant workers, primarily railroad track laborers, harvest hands, and lumberjacks. The authors described 28 percent of the men as steady unskilled laborers: "During most of their lives, they have worked steadily at common labor and have made relatively few changes in occupation or in the communities in which they resided. A few of them have worked for 20 or 25 years for one company. To be a 'good worker' has been their chief ambition and pride" (10:58).

The authors described some of the 19 percent who were skilled workers as "men averaging about 45 years of age [who] have been replaced as a result of technological change or the depression, and have found it impossible to get work at their trades" (10:59). Finally, the authors described 24 percent of those from whom they collected life histories as white collar workers. Overall, the authors estimated that only 5 percent of the men staying at the shelters could be classified as "bums . . . who will not work except on rare occasions" (10:52).

Another study conducted during the Depression was based on interviews with 136 male residents of a shelter in Palo Alto, California. Its author, Benjamin Culver, noted that 9.6 percent of the men were over the age of 50, and 5.2 percent had permanent physical disabilities. Although 14.5 percent claimed that they were unemployed because of excessive use of alcohol, Culver concluded that "it cannot be claimed that more than 7 or 8% have been rendered unemployed or homeless because of alcoholic intemperance" (11:531).

In 1934, Eric Hoffer spent a month in a federal transient camp in California. Of the 200 residents in the camp, 25 percent were veterans, 25 percent were "aged men," 21 percent were physically disabled, 2 percent were "mildly insane," and 30 percent he termed "confirmed drunkards." Forty percent were unemployed workers. Hoffer, like Rice before him, defined many of these unemployed workers as "pioneers": "I saw them fell lumber, clear firebreaks, build rock walls, put up barracks, build dams and roads, handle steam shovels, bulldozers, tractors, and concrete mixers. I saw them put in a hard day's work after a night of steady drinking. They sweated and growled but they did the work. . . . In short, it was not difficult to visualize the tramps as pioneers" (12:147).

There are very little data on the demographic composition of the nation's homeless population during the 1940s. Studies from that period tend to focus on the relation between homelessness and substance abuse (13,14). Some homeless men enlisted in the armed forces during World War II. However, this did not cause a decline in the numbers of single people living in Skid Rows. On the contrary, the areas grew during the 1940s because of the lack of housing for single people during and after the war. This acute shortage of housing forced many single people who would not normally have lived in the deteriorating central cities to look for housing there (15). Furthermore, many veterans found themselves unable to reintegrate into civilian life despite their government benefits, and they too migrated to Skid Row. There they joined the employable yet unemployed, the physically and mentally handicapped, and the alcoholic, the last-named group estimated at one-third of the total population (16).

By the late 1950s, inner-city homeless people came to be of interest to those involved in urban redevelopment. In 1958, in preparation for a central area redevelopment project, the city of Chicago commissioned a study of homeless men living on its Skid Row. Of the 614 men interviewed, 16.6 percent were alcoholic, 18 percent were mentally ill or had mental or nervous problems, 9.4 percent were physically handicapped, and 8.8 percent were too old to work. The last group were described as "captive residents," people who were forced to live on Skid Row because it was the only place they could afford on their meager Social Security checks. On the other hand, 40 percent of those interviewed had worked during the previous week, and 84 percent had worked at some time during the previous year. Such individuals were described as " 'lost souls' economically, and most of them at the present time can only look forward to a life of economic hardship. They are the men hardest hit by inflation, the losers in the competition for steady jobs" (17:504).

The authors concluded that there were five major reasons for unemployment among the men living on Skid Row: (a) many of the men had occupations in industries where involuntary or seasonal unemployment was a chronic condition; (b) a high percentage of them were physically handicapped; (c) many were over the age of 40 and were discriminated against by employers, who hired younger workers; (d) some drank heavily and were irregular in their work habits; and (e) many lacked the necessary education or employment skills, in addition to having the stigma of a Skid Row address (17).

The director of the Chicago study was Donald J. Bogue, who published his own study of Chicago's Skid Row from data collected during the late 1950s (18). Bogue estimated, on the basis of 613 interviews, that 10.2 percent of the men were too old to work, 9.4 percent were severely physically handicapped, and 20 percent were mentally ill or had mental or nervous problems. Counted with the mentally disabled group were the 4 percent Bogue described as severely psychotic, who, he added, were generally "picked up rather promptly by the police, and the screening process in the courts causes them to be institutionalized" (18:383). He also defined 35 percent of the population as drinking heavily. Bogue discovered that 40 percent of the men had had some steady employment at the time they were interviewed. However, most were exploited by unscrupulous employers who had found loopholes in the nation's minimum wage laws and unemployment compensation programs. Bogue suggested that "one of the ways to shrink Skid Row is to patch some of the leaks in the 'floor' of social legislation that seeks to establish minimum employment conditions" (18:197). Otherwise, he concluded, Skid Row would continue to grow, even during times of economic prosperity (18).

As urban redevelopment continued, so did studies of the residents of the urban areas to be affected. Such a study was begun in 1960 in Philadelphia (19). In surveying the homeless people of the inner city, the authors discovered that "in general, Skid Row men subscribe to a positive work ethic and are little different in this respect from the working class population of which they were a part before moving to Skid Row. That work did not touch the lives of many of the men in the same way as it did those of other workers was a consequence of their alcohol behavior, poor health, and difficulties in overcoming these problems" (19:95).

Specifically, the authors, Leonard Blumberg, Thomas E. Shipley, Jr., and Irving W. Shandler, found that 18 percent of the men they interviewed were over 65 years of age, and 29–30 percent were "spree drinkers" who chronically lost control when drinking. An additional 20 percent had mental problems, including 8 percent with personality disorders, 5 percent with brain disorders, 4 percent with psychoneurosis, 2 percent with psychosis, and 1 percent defined as mentally deficient (19).

A comparable study of men living in New York's Bowery was carried out between 1963 and 1968 by Howard M. Bahr and Theodore Caplow. They found that 21 percent of those interviewed were over the age of 65, 44 percent were in poor health, 51 percent currently had or previously had had some form of physical disability, and 26–36 percent could be classified as drinking heavily (20).

In the 1970s, much of what was written was concerned with the "disappearance" of Skid Rows (21). Some authors asserted that the areas and their populations were vanishing with the onslaught of urban redevelopment, while others proposed that homeless people, having been displaced from traditional Skid Rows, were simply moving into other urban areas. A few writers from this period commented on the demographic changes that were taking place. They noted that the homeless population was becoming younger, included many Vietnam veterans, and was beginning to encompass more members of minority groups. Coincidentally, the number of homeless people who used drugs or were mentally ill was beginning to rise (22,23). However, specific demographic data on homeless people appear to be scarce for the decade.

The first half of the 1980s is noted for the large number of publications with detailed descriptions of the demographics of homelessness. Many of these studies can be classified as "advocacy literature," literature that explains to policy makers and human service providers who the homeless people are and what their needs may be (24). These studies, like those that preceded them, showed that homeless people were a very heterogeneous group, representing all ages and all ethnic groups, as well as employable and currently unemployable people (the last including those who were physically disabled, mentally ill, or substance abusers). A survey of the literature between 1982 and 1984 indicates that the prevalence of alcoholism, alcohol abuse, or problem drinking varied between 16 and 43 percent, and the prevalence of daily or regular alcohol use was between 21 and 35 percent (25). On the other hand, data on mental health from the period indicate that 28–37 percent of the nation's homeless individuals could be characterized as having severe mental disorders (26). Of those homeless people who were employed or employable, a 12-city survey in 1983–84 showed numbers varying from 6 to 43 percent, with the highest percentages reported in New York City and in Phoenix, Arizona (27).

More data were collected on homeless people during the middle to late 1980s, in surveys conducted under the National Institute of Mental Health (28), in the records of the Robert Wood Johnson and Pew Trust Health Care for the Homeless program (29), and in other studies (30,31). These studies (reviewed in chapter 4) show that 1–23 percent of homeless interviewees were holding full-time or part-time jobs; 12–39 percent had worked within the previous month, and only a very small minority had never held a job. The prevalence of alcohol abuse generally was 30–40 percent among men and approximately 15 percent among women. Mental health status varied considerably across studies (chapter 5), in part because of differences in the criteria and instruments used (chapter 5 and 24). The studies reviewed in chapter 5 are compatible with a gross estimate that 30 percent of homeless adults in the streets and shelters (i.e., literally homeless people) might have some mental disorder.

Most significantly, the 1980s saw a dramatic increase in the number of homeless families. Review of the historical literature shows that, with the exception of the Depression years, homelessness has been associated primarily with single males. In 1984, an estimated 21 percent of the homeless population was composed of members of homeless families (27). In 1989, the proportion was about 30 percent (32).

Discussion

From the data examined, we may conclude that during the past century, the U.S. urban homeless population has been a relatively heterogeneous group. Even with the availability of public facilities for chronically mentally ill people and (since the 1930s) a welfare system that is supposed to care for disabled and elderly people, there have always been individuals from these populations who are homeless and live on Skid Row. And there have always been employable people, those who migrated to the inner cities in search of work. Yet until recently, homeless people were most often characterized as alcoholic. As J. P. Wiseman stated, "To the average person, the term Skid Row immediately brings to mind . . . society's cast-offs, poverty-stricken men who have failed to make it in the competitive world and are now eking out an existence in an alcoholic haze amid environmental squalor and human misery" (33:3).

There is also the belief that these individuals do not want to work. As Ronald Vander Kooi pointed out, "Most Americans think of all Skid Rowers as drunken bums who won't work" (34:68). However, this stereotype does not coincide with the heterogeneous makeup of the homeless population.

Since the turn of the century, the proportion of homeless people classified as alcoholic has generally remained at only about 30–33 percent (35). Part of the problem may have to do with the definition of the term *alcoholic*. Street life and the Skid Row subculture encourage the consumption of alcohol. For homeless individuals, drinking is often a way to get through the tensions of a day (36) or to forget failure (33). Unlike domiciled people who drink in the privacy of their homes, homeless people who drink are highly visible. Should they drink too much, their comportment is seen by all. The public perception that all homeless people are alcoholic may result from the visibility of homeless people who have been drinking in the streets. Employable homeless people who do not drink are ignored; they simply blend into the crowd of other poor people.

Until the 1960s, an alcoholic person was generally considered "morally degenerate" rather than sick and in need of treatment. As a result, alcoholism was considered a crime, with the homeless alcoholic individual often thrown in jail when caught drinking in public. (Those who drank in private were, of course, neither considered to be engaging in a criminal activity nor jailed when they drank too much.) The justice system was used to manage publicly inebriated people, with the courts using the jails to remove alcoholic people from the streets and provide a place to dry out (36). What happened, however, was that, stereotyping all homeless individuals as alcoholic, the powers that be often arrested Skid Row people who did not drink, sometimes according to a quota system, and charged them with being drunk when in fact they were sober (20). In other words, homeless people were often arrested because of their perceived status (alcoholic) rather than their overt behavior (16).

Conceivably, homeless people could have stereotyped differently: as unemployed people who needed jobs or job training, as elderly people who needed concern and care, or as individuals who were disabled or had mental problems. Stereotyping them instead as alcoholic and criminal meant that society did not have to deal with the structural problems that were causing homelessness. Throwing homeless people into jail on perceived or actual public drunkenness charges negates the necessity for examining the underlying issues of homelessness in a society where the family as a support unit was all but disappearing and where there were serious structural problems, including unemployment, a lack of affordable housing, a lack of care for elderly people, and a lack of medical attention for disability or mental illness.

In the 1960s, alcoholism was seen as a disease requiring specialized medical treatment rather than as a vice of individuals who could stop drinking if they wanted to. Although this change in the perception of alcoholism was accepted by much of the general public, albeit with some moral ambivalence (16), homeless people continued to be stereotyped as alcoholic. Rather than being arrested and jailed for public inebriation, homeless individuals were referred to publicly funded detoxification programs, where they received some form of treatment. Ideally, these programs would have both medical and social components of detoxification as well as follow-up case management, including job training and/or placement, and help in securing housing. This has rarely been the case. In general, publicly funded programs for treating alcoholism have dealt with the symptoms of the disease but did not or could not go beyond them. To do so, they would have had to tackle some of the structural problems of homelessness.

At the same time that alcoholism was being redefined as a disease, new policies concerning chronic mental illness came about. The Mental Health Act of 1964 paved the way for the deinstitutionalization of hundreds of thousands of mentally ill people. Although community health centers were expected to care for most of them, the money never followed the patients out of the hospital. As a result, funding was never provided to set up enough community health centers to care for former patients. To compound the issue, many of those who were released had little in the way of discharge planning or follow-up case management. This, coupled with a lack of affordable housing for the better-functioning individuals who might be able to live independently, has meant that thousands of former mental patients are currently living in our streets. Additionally, some homeless people have become seriously mentally disturbed as a result of not being able to gain access to appropriate care. Although no accurate estimate exists of the number of chronically mentally ill homeless people (chapter 5), many researchers accept the assessment that mentally ill individuals account for one-third of the homeless population. Yet since the early 1980s, this group has become synonymous with homelessness. One stigmatized illness (alcoholism) has been replaced by another (mental disorder) as a stereotype for homeless people.

Several factors tend to inflate estimates of the number of homeless people with mental disorder: studies based in mental health clinical settings have yielded estimates of 60–90 percent (however, as discussed in chapter 5, homeless people in such settings are not representative of the homeless population at large); alcohol or drug use has often been included as a criterion of mental illness; and assessment methods have been used which tend to increase the number of people scored as mentally ill, because the instruments are not adapted to the situation of homelessness (chapter 24) or because diagnostic interviewers did not consider the effect of a lack of sleep or other crisis-associated factors in people who have just been admitted to a shelter (K. Hopper, personal communication, March 12, 1985). Inflation of the number of homeless mentally ill people is analogous to inflation of the number of homeless individuals classified as alcoholic.

Also, the lifestyle of the mentally ill homeless person, like that of the alcoholic homeless person, is visible to the general public. As a result, the public is willing to create a stereotype of all homeless people based on the distinctive outward appearance and actions of what may be a few individuals. It should be noted that this stereotype has often been supported by community mental health centers, which have used it, often successfully, to leverage funding for programs for chronically mentally ill homeless people. However, these programs, like those set up earlier for alcoholic homeless people, are often long on treatment and short on case management or any attempt to reintegrate the individual into the community—steps that, again, would mean society's having to come to grips with problems such as job training, employment and housing.

Finally, like homeless alcoholic people, chronically mentally ill homeless people have often been relegated to our country's jails. The justice system is now being used to manage chronically mentally ill homeless people, just as in the past it was used to manage publicly inebriated individuals. Today there is also the belief that our correctional systems are not the place for psychiatric treatment, and that what mentally ill homeless people really need is some sort of institutionalization, whether a reentry to a state hospital (37) or placement in a supervisory care facility. Rarely is there any attempt to reintegrate the individual more fully into the socioeconomic system.

Conclusion

By stereotyping homeless people as chronically mentally ill or as substance abusers, we are asserting that the solution to the problem of homelessness lies in some sort of treatment or institutionalization, which in turn makes it easier for us to ignore the structural defects in our society that cause homelessness in the first place. This means that we do not have to come to grips with a socioeconomic system that has denied jobs to those who need them, housing to those without shelter, medical care to those who are sick and disabled, refuge in their later years to elderly persons, and dignity and independence to those with mental illness. Homeless people are a daily reminder of a society that has based its economic and social morality on principles that have failed the majority of its citizens. These people are an affront to such a system, the most visible manifestation of its failure: "They tell us that in the late twentieth century, the American dream—the belief that anyone who tried hard enough in the competitive struggle could prosper—has become an illusion" (38:293).

There are two ways to solve the problem of homelessness. The first is to recognize the problems of the system and confront them head on. We can begin by reforming the inequitable distribution of wealth in our society through revision of the tax structure. And we can continue by constructing affordable housing for poor people, developing a universal system of health care, renewing the drive to unionize people who are not organized, establishing a minimum living wage, and guaranteeing income above the poverty level for those who cannot work. Or we can be embarrassed about the implications of homelessness for our present system of values and try to wish the problem away. How better to do this than to stereotype the poorest of our poor as having stigmatized illnesses and then to hide them away from public view? This has been our answer in the past. As it now appears, it may well be our solution in the future.

References

1. Erickson J, Wilhelm C (eds.). *Housing the Homeless*. New Brunswick, N.J.: Rutgers University, Center for Urban Policy and Research, 1986.
2. McCook JJ. A tramp census and its revelations. *Forum 15*:753–66, 1893.
3. Ringenbach PT. *Tramps and Reformers, 1873–1916: The Discovery of Unemployment in New York*. Westport, Conn.: Greenwood Press, 1973.
4. Cook HS. *Report of the Social Security of the Municipal Lodging House for October 1910*. New York: Papers of the New York Charity Organization Society, 1910.
5. Solenberger AW. *One Thousand Homeless Men*. New York: Russell Sage Foundation, 1911.
6. Laubach FC. Why they are vagrants: A study based upon an examination of one hundred men. Manuscript, 1916.

7. Rice S. The homeless. *Annals of the American Academy of Political and Social Sciences* 77:140–153, 1918.

8. Anderson N. *The Hobo: The Sociology of the Homeless Man.* Chicago: University of Chicago Press, 1923.

9. Stern M. The transfer of single men to relief in Chicago. *Social Science Review 10:* 277–287, 1936.

10. Sutherland EH, Locke HJ. *Twenty Thousand Homeless Men: A Study of Unemployed Men in the Chicago Shelters.* Philadelphia: J. B. Lippincott, 1936.

11. Culver BF. Transient unemployed men. *Sociology and Social Research 17:*519–535, 1933.

12. Hoffer E. *The Ordeal of Change.* New York: Harper and Row, 1964.

13. Straus R. Alcohol and homeless men. *Quarterly Journal of Studies on Alcohol 7:* 360–404, 1946.

14. Stearns AW, Ulman AD. One thousand unsuccessful careers. *American Journal of Psychiatry 105:*801–810, 1949.

15. Rose AM. Living arrangements of unattached persons. *American Sociological Review 12:*429–435, 1947.

16. Rubington E. The chronic drunkenness offender on Skid Row. In Gomberg E, White HR, Carpenter JA (eds.), *Alcohol, Science, and Society Revisited.* Ann Arbor: University of Michigan Press, 1982, pp. 322–335.

17. Chicago Tenants Relocation Bureau. *The Homeless Man on Skid Row.* Chicago: City of Chicago, 1961.

18. Bogue DJ. *Skid Row in American Cities.* Chicago: University of Chicago Press, 1963.

19. Blumberg L, Shipley TE Jr., Shandler IW. *Skid Row and Its Alternatives: Research and Recommendations from Philadelphia.* Philadelphia: Temple University Press, 1973.

20. Bahr HM, Caplow T. *Old Men Drunk and Sober.* New York: New York University Press, 1973.

21. Lee BA. The disappearance of Skid Row. *Urban Affairs Quarterly 16:*81–107, 1980.

22. Cohen CI, Briggs F. A storefront clinic on the Bowery. *Journal of Studies on Alcohol 37:* 1336–1340, 1976.

23. Reich R, Seigal L. The emergence of the Bowery as a psychiatric dumping ground. *Psychiatric Quarterly 50:*191–201, 1978.

24. Blau J. The homeless of New York: A case study in social welfare policy. Diss. proposal, Columbia University School of Social Work, 1985.

25. Mulkern V, Spence R. *Alcohol Abuse/Alcoholism among Homeless Persons: A Review of the Literature.* Rockville, Md.: National Institute on Alcohol Abuse and Alcoholism, 1984.

26. Morrissey JP, Dennis DL. *NIMH Funded Research Concerning Homeless Mentally Ill Persons: Implications for Policy and Practice.* Rockville, Md.: Alcohol, Drug Abuse, and Mental Health Administration, 1986.

27. U.S. Department of Housing and Urban Development. *A Report to the Secretary on the Homeless and Emergency Shelters.* Washington, D.C.: HUD Office of Policy Development and Research, 1984.

28. Tessler RC, Dennis DL. *A Synthesis of NIMH-Funded Research Concerning Persons Who Are Homeless and Mentally Ill.* Rockville, Md.: National Institute of Mental Health, 1989.

29. Wright JD, Weber E. *Homelessness and Health.* New York: McGraw-Hill, 1987.

30. Sosin MR, Colson P, Grossman S. *Homelessness in Chicago: Poverty and Pathology, Social Institutions and Social Change.* Chicago: Chicago Community Trust, 1988.

31. Burt MR, Cohen BE. *America's Homeless: Numbers, Characteristics, and Programs That Serve Them.* Washington, D.C.: Urban Institute, 1989.

32. Reyes LM, Waxman LD. *A Status Report on Hunger and Homelessness in America's Cities, 1989*. Washington, D.C.: United States Conference of Mayors, 1989.

33. Wiseman JP. *Stations of the Lost: The Treatment of Skid Row Alcoholics*. Chicago: University of Chicago Press, 1979.

34. Vander Kooi R. The main stem: Skid Row revisited. *Society 10:*64–71, 1973.

35. Stark L. A century of alcohol and homelessness. *Alcohol, Health, and Research World 11:*8–13, 1987.

36. Morgan R, et al. Alcoholism and the homeless. In Brickner PW, et al. (eds.), *Health Care of Homeless People*. New York: Springer, 1985, pp. 131–150.

37. Lamb HR. Deinstitutionalization and the homeless mentally ill. In Lamb HR (ed.), *The Homeless Mentally Ill*. Washington, D.C.: American Psychiatric Association, 1984, pp. 55–74.

38. Hope M, Young J. *The Faces of the Homeless*. Lexington, Mass.: Lexington Books, 1986.

CHAPTER 4

Empirical Studies
of Homeless Populations
in the 1980s

René I. Jahiel, M.D., Ph.D.

T hree general questions dominated empirical research on homelessness in the 1980s: How many homeless people are there? What are their characteristics? Why are they homeless, and what is the relative importance of individual versus societal factors in causing homelessness?

How Many Homeless People
Are There?

There is no accurate estimate of the number of homeless people (chapter 22). This is due to a lack of general agreement on the definition of homelessness (i.e., who should be included in the count?) and to obstacles to counting homeless people (i.e., difficulties in sampling, locating, and identifying homeless people). Therefore the discussion of the various estimates that have been advanced is deferred till chapter 22, where the matter can be presented in the context of a methodological analysis. Only a brief summary is given here. As noted earlier, homeless people consist of two fairly distinct groups: the "literal homeless" (1), who spend most of their nights in shelters, welfare hotels, or the streets, and the "resource people" (2), who have resources that allow them to spend most nights in other places (e.g., doubling up with other households). Most of the studies have been targeted to the "literal homeless" or to "service-using" homeless people (i.e., those who use shelters or meal services), a category that overlaps markedly with the literally homeless. Current estimates of the number of literally homeless people range from 0.5 million to 3 million. Current estimates of the doubled-up population are based on fewer studies; they range from 2 million to 10 million people (chapter 22).

What Are the Characteristics of Homeless People?

The information available in 1991, at the time of this writing, came from three sources: the homeless persons surveys (HPS) sponsored by the NIMH and other agencies and published between 1983 and 1989 (1–14); the data retrieved in 1984–86 from the Robert Wood Johnson Foundation and Pew Trust's Health Care for the Homeless projects (JP/HCH) (15,16) and the McKinney Act's Health Care for the Homeless projects (McK/HCH) (17); and the yearly surveys of city officials conducted each year by the United States Conference of Mayors, (COM) (18–22). The HPS data are from 10 large cities, three counties, and two statewide studies. JP/HCH has data from 16 projects, all in large cities. McK/HCH has data from 109 projects in large cities and some small cities. COM has data from 25–27 mostly large cities each year.

The HPS studies consist of interviews of homeless adults in shelters, meal service sites, congregating sites, or street sites. They vary greatly in population and sampling design (Table 4.1). As a whole, there is overrepresentation of adults, single individuals, men, and Skid Row or central-city locations; and underrepresentation of children (they are not represented at all), youths, family groups, women, the major residential and peripheral parts of cities, suburban, rural, and small-town areas, and the less visible homeless people (e.g., doubled-up families, squatters, people in very small shelters, and people who do not have the typical "homeless appearance").

The JP/HCH and McK/HCH data are derived from homeless patients who present themselves for health services at ambulatory care centers or outreach sites (e.g., services in shelters and mobile units). The JP/HCH data were retrieved and tabulated for the following categories: all patients; patients seen more than once; and a group of patients seen more than three times whose charts were analyzed in greater detail with the Case Assessment and Review Questionnaire (CARQUEX). The authors estimated that the comprehensiveness and accuracy of diagnosis improved as the number of visits increased (15). The McK/HCH data were given for all patients. On the night before the first McK/HCH contact, the patients' housing status was: shelters, 47 percent; street, 11 percent; doubled up, 11 percent; transitional housing, 11 percent; other sites, 9 percent; and unknown, 10 percent (17). Thus, literally homeless people form a large majority of McK/HCH patients. This also appears to be true of JP/HCH patients. Both HCH populations can be expected to underrepresent homeless people who seldom need health services, have access to other health services, or tend not to use professional health services when they are sick.

In some respects, the COM data (18–22) are the "softest," since they represent estimates given by city personnel (in contrast with interview data, as in the HPS studies, or data retrieval from records, as in the HCH studies). However, they are based on reports by the various types of providers who serve homeless people, and therefore they are likely to deal with a more representative popula-

41

TABLE 4.1 HPS STUDY DESIGNS

Location/Year of Survey[a]	N	Kind(s) of Interview Site[b]			Location(s) of Interview Site	Shelters[c]		Site Sampling Method
		SH, H	MS, CS	S		Included	Excluded	
CA-Rand/87 (13)	315	+	–	+	Countywide	NA	NA	Stratified, random
LA-SR/85 (11)	374	+	+	–	Skid Row	M, D, R, H	W, F, Y	Representative
LA-SR + WS/84 (6)	238	+	+	+	Skid Row and West Side	M, BW, R	F, Y, D, MI	Convenience
Phoenix/83 (4)	195	+	–	+	Downtown	M, W, F	BW, D, MI	Convenience
Texas/88 (14)	2,836	+	–	–	Statewide, 25 cities	M, W, BW	NA	Attempted census
St. Louis/84 (5)	248	+	–	–	Citywide	M, W, F	NA	Stratified, random
Milwaukee/85 (7)	237	+	+	+	Part of downtown	M, W	BW, Y, D, MI	Convenience
Chicago/86 (12)	722	+	–	+	Citywide	NA	BW, Y, D	Stratified, random
Detroit/85 (9)	75	+	–	–	Four shelters	M, W, F	BW, Y, D, MI	Convenience
Ohio/84 (2)	979	+	+	+	Statewide	M, W, F	BW, >45 days	Systematic
Boston/84 (8)	327	+	–	+	Selected areas of the city[d]	M, W, MI	BW, F, Y, D	Convenience
Baltimore/85 (10)	55	+	–	–	Four shelters	M, W	BW, F, Y, D, MI	Convenience

[a]The number in parentheses is a reference citation. Locations: CA-Rand, California, Rand Corporation study; LA-SR, Los Angeles, Skid Row; LA-SR + WS, Los Angeles, Skid Row and West Side (Venice). Year is year of completion of survey.

[b]Interview sites: SH, shelter; H, voucher hotel; MS, meal service; CS, congregating sites; S, street sites; +, included in study; –, excluded from study.

[c]Types of shelter: M, men; W, women; BW, battered women; F, family; Y, youth; H, voucher or welfare hotel; D, detoxification center; MI, shelter for mentally ill clients; R, rehabilitation facility; >45, client not counted as homeless if stay was longer than 45 days; NA, information not available.

[d]Areas of high homeless population density were selected.

tion than do the two other sets of data. The COM data, like the HPS and HCH data, underrepresent homeless people who are doubled up or use few if any services.

DEMOGRAPHY

Family status is best represented in the COM surveys. People who are homeless as families constituted 28 percent of the homeless population in 1985 (18) and 1986 (19), 34 percent in 1988 (20), 36 percent in 1989 (21), and 34 percent in 1990 (22). Slightly under 40 percent of the 1989 COM population (21) and 37 percent of the 1988 McK/HCH population (including children) were female.

All adult age groups are represented in the HPS population. Age distribution varied across studies. This is reflected in the median age, which ranges from 29 to 39. Compared to the local domiciled population, the median age of the homeless study population was older in Baltimore, about the same in Chicago, and younger in Ohio and Los Angeles (Table 4.2). The percentage of those older than 55 was smaller among homeless people than in comparable domiciled populations (2,6,11,12).

All HPS studies show fewer married individuals in the homeless population than in comparable domiciled populations and a marked excess of people who were never married or who were separated, divorced, or widowed (Table 4.2). Selection factors such as the low representation of shelters for battered women and the overrepresentation of downtown areas in the samples may contribute in part to this finding. For example, 37 percent of homeless respondents who had no severe mental disorder (SMD) in suburban Orange County were married, compared to 3 percent of respondents without SMD in Los Angeles's Skid Row (13).

The percentages of blacks and American Indians varied from city to city, reflecting local population differences. When comparisons with local domiciled populations were available, the homeless population was found to have a greater percentage of blacks and a markedly greater percentage of American Indians (Table 4.2).

The number of years of schooling showed considerable dispersion in each HPS study. From 35 percent to 59 percent of homeless respondents had less than 12 years of schooling, versus 30–46 percent in domiciled comparison groups. From 12 percent to 38 percent homeless people had some education beyond high school, compared with 25–40 percent in the domiciled groups (Table 4.2).

WORK AND INCOME

Table 4.3 shows that 87–99 percent of HPS respondents had had a steady job at some time in the past and 37–88 percent had had a job at some time during the

Table 4.2 Demographic Variables of HPS Studies

Location/Year of Survey[a]	% Male	Median Age	Marital Status (%)			Ethnicity (%)			Years of Schooling (%)			
			Never Married	SDW[b]	Married	Black	Indian	White	0–8	9–11	12	>12
Ca-counties/87 (13)	73	31	49	31	21	29	NA	53	NA	NA	NA	NA
LA-SR/85 (11)	95	35	59	38	4	39	5	27	22	27	28	23
(LA census)[c]	(48)	(38)	(35)	(13)	(53)	(11)	(<1)	(58)	(17)	(13)	(30)	(40)
LA-SR + WS/84 (6)	77	35	55	38	7	30	6	51	13	22	26	38
Phoenix/83 (4)	86	37	46	41	13	9	9	64	17	23	26	34
Texas/88 (14)	74	36	NA[d]	NA	NA	28	3	50	NA	NA	NA	NA
St. Louis/84 (5)	(50)	29	52	39	8	64	NA	35	12	31	36	21
Milwaukee/85 (7)	87	35	36	53	11	32	4	60	NA	NA	NA	NA
Chicago/86 (12)	76	39	57	36	7	53	5	31	8	37	32	24
(Chicago census)[c]	(46)	(40)	(35)	(22)	(43)	(36)	(0.1)	(55)	(14)	(30)	(28)	(28)
Detroit/85 (9)	71	33	51	43	6	73	NA	26		57e		43f
Ohio/84 (2)	81	34	45	43	9	30	NA	65	17	37	30	15
(Ohio census)[c]	(47)	(40)	(25)	(16)	(59)	(9)	(NA)	(90)	(14)	(22)	(39)	(25)
Boston/84 (8)	81	36	61	34	5	23	NA	70	49e		29	23
Baltimore/85 (10)	94	38	61	39	0	47	NA	53	20	39	20	20
(Balt. Males >18)[g]	(100)	(34)	(35)	(17)	(48)	(39)	(NA)	(61)	(17)	(29)	(29)	(25)

aLocations: CA-counties, California counties (Alameda, Yolo, Orange); LA-SR, Los Angeles Skid Row; LA-SR + WS, Los Angeles, Skid Row and West Side (Venice). The year given is the year when interviews were completed. The number in parentheses is a reference citation. bSDW, separated, divorced, or widowed. cLA census, Chicago census, Ohio census, data from general (domiciled) population in 1980 census. dNA, information not available. eYears of schooling: 0–11. fYears of schooling: 12 or more. gBalt. Males >18, data from males more than 18 years of age in the Eastern Baltimore Epidemiologic Catchment Area.

previous two years, but only 1–18 percent had a steady job at the time of the interview. This suggests a relatively long process of falling out of the job market before becoming homeless. The homeless people did mainly daywork or other sporadic work (Table 4.3). Only 3 percent (12), 6 percent (2,6), or 11 percent (14) of respondents currently had full-time jobs. The type of work done was documented in two studies. In Phoenix, 55 percent of respondents did farm work or unskilled work, despite the fact that only 40 percent had no high school degree (4). In Chicago, 12 percent of respondents with current earnings were doing skilled work, while 34 percent of these respondents had done skilled work in their last steady job (12).

Table 4.3 shows that 8–24 percent of HPS respondents were receiving Supplemental Security Income (SSI), Social Security Disability Insurance (SSDI), or other federal assistance, and 9–27 percent were on welfare. In Los Angeles (11) and Chicago (12), many ostensibly eligible individuals were not receiving such benefits because they had applied and had been turned down, had been unable to provide all the needed documents, had found the forms too difficult, or had been discouraged from applying. In the JP/HCH study, the results of multiple regression analysis were compatible with the hypothesis that denial of eligibility by state laws or administrative decisions was the greatest contributing factor to failure to receive benefits (15).

The most pervasive finding of all the studies is the extreme poverty of homeless people. Not only did 13–65 percent of them have no income at all (Table 4.3) but the remainder received a very inadequate income. In Chicago, more than half of the respondents had a monthly income below $100; the estimated average monthly income, given according to source, was $131 from welfare, $247 from AFDC, $251 from SSI, $73 from temporary jobs, or $336 from steady jobs (12). Only a small percentage of homeless people received income from more than one source.

In each HPS study, many of the homeless respondents had been born in the study city, and except in Phoenix, a majority had lived there for more than 12 months (Table 4.3). In a study in Ogden, Utah, recent arrivals were in the majority (23). In general, homeless people who had recently arrived in the city had come to get a job, be with family, or obtain services. There were relatively few "drifters" (8).

MEDICAL AND SOCIAL PATHOLOGY

HPS respondents ranked their health as fair or poor more often than did comparable domiciled adults (2,6,11,12). Several acute or chronic diagnoses occurred markedly more often among patients seen at the JP/HCH (15) or McK/HCH (17) programs than among patients included in the National Ambulatory Medical Care Survey (NAMCS) (15,17), a nationally representative sample of ambulatory care visits. Homeless children in the HCH programs had more devel-

TABLE 4.3   PERCENTAGE DISTRIBUTION OF HOMELESS POPULATION BY WORK, INCOME, AND MIGRATION IN HPS STUDIES

Location/Year of Study[a]	Work				Income[b]					Migration	
	Once Had Steady Job	Had Job in Last Two Years	Is Disabled	Is Looking for Work	Has Current Employment		Has SSI[e] or SSDI	Has GA	Has No Income[f]	Was Born in County or City	Has Lived >12 Months in County or City
					Steady[c]	Sporadic[d]					
LA-SR/85 (11)	99	88	16	66	5	11	11	9	NA	13	66
LA-SR + WS/84 (6)	91	53	21	49	11[g]	10	12	11	33	14	75
Phoenix/83 (4)	99	NA	NA	NA	3	6	24[h]		13	5	42
St. Louis/84 (5)	NA	53	NA	91	9	NA	8	23	62	NA	56
Milwaukee/85 (7)	NA	NA	NA	NA	2	NA	11	20	65	29	69
Chicago/86 (12)	NA	37	28	NA	3	32[i]	9	22	17	46[j]	89
Detroit/85 (9)	93	45	NA	NA	1	12	29[h]		47	NA	92
Ohio/84 (2)	87	48	13	33	12[k]	13	13	24	37	NA	64

| Boston/84 (8) | 93 | NA | NA | 64 | 11 | NA | 24 | 27 | 13 | 29 | 76 |
| Baltimore/85 (10) | NA | NA | 14 | NA | 18 | NA | 20 | 18 | NA | NA | NA |

[a] Locations: LA-SR, Los Angeles, Skid Row; LA-SR + WS, Los Angeles, Skid Row and West Side (Venice). The number in parentheses is a reference citation.

[b] Excludes categories such as no answer, multiple sources of income, selling blood, money from family, begging; stealing, etc.

[c] "Steady" includes full-time (FT) or part-time (PT) work described as steady or regular, except in the Baltimore study, where it was described as "salaries."

[d] "Sporadic" includes work described as sporadic, occasional, day labor, for room and bed, for voucher.

[e] SSI, Supplemental Security Income; SSDI, Social Security Disability Insurance; GA, general assistance; NA, information not available.

[f] The restrictiveness of this category varied widely across the different studies, as some—but not all—studies considered individuals to have income if they received even small amounts of money from the excluded sources listed in note b. For instance, in Milwaukee the 65 percent who has no regular income included those who were selling blood, asking for change, recycling things, doing irregular day labor, or having illicit earnings. In contrast, in Phoenix individuals who sold their blood, recycled things, obtained money from their families, or received food stamps were not included in this category.

[g] Six percent FT, 5 percent PT.

[h] Has SSI, SSDI, or GA.

[i] In the Chicago study, all PT work was included in the "sporadic" category.

[j] Was born in Illinois.

[k] Six percent FT, 6 percent PT.

opmental or immunization delays than did children in nationally representative samples (16,17). In other studies, homeless youths had increased frequencies of venereal diseases and serious chronic illnesses (24). A very high frequency of human immunodeficiency virus (HIV) infection was reported in some shelters (25). Infants born of homeless women in New York City had a low-birthweight rate markedly higher than that of a citywide sample and significantly higher than that of a comparison group in low-income housing (26). Thus, there is ample evidence that the liberally homeless population has a much higher morbidity than does the nation's population. The analysis of disease patterns in homeless people shows that much of the excess morbidity is attributable to the combined effect of poverty and homelessness (27).

The prevalence of mental disorders in homeless populations is discussed at length in chapters 5 and 24. Although rates of mental disorder of 15–50 percent have been suggested for nonclinical samples of literally homeless or service-using homeless populations, the validity of diagnostic instruments and the significance of psychiatric diagnoses and hospitalization history have been severely questioned (chapter 5 and 24), so that the prevalence of mental disorder cannot be estimated accurately with the data at hand (chapter 5). There is evidence for a higher prevalence of mental disorder in homeless adult samples than in nationally representative samples (chapter 5), for a lower prevalence of mental disorder among adults who are homeless in family groups than among single homeless adults (chapter 5), and for a high prevalence of developmental delays and emotional problems among homeless children (chapters 5 and 7) and of emotional problems and suicide attempts among homeless youths (chapter 5). Although mental disorder often precedes the onset of homelessness, in some instances it follows it. Furthermore, the conditions of homeless life may contribute to the emergence or aggravation of mental disorder by causing demoralization and stress, interruption of psychotropic drug therapy, or brain damage due to malnutrition, alcohol, or trauma.

A recent review of alcohol abuse among literally homeless men and women yielded a prevalence range of 15–80 percent, with a median of 33 percent, versus 7 percent in the general population (30). The methodological problems in estimating the frequency of alcohol abuse are similar to those encountered in the estimation of mental disorder. There may be a selection of people with increased alcohol use in the HPS studies (due to an overrepresentation of single men and of Skid Row residents) and in the HCH studies (due to an increased prevalence of alcohol abuse among people seen in ambulatory care centers). Alcohol abuse started before the first episode of homelessness in 75 percent of alcohol-abusing respondents, and afterwards in 25 percent (11). Homeless people who began to abuse alcohol after the onset of homelessness were, as a group, young adults (28,29). A literature review through the mid-1980s yielded a 3–31 percent prevalence of other drug abuse (30). Rates are expected to be significantly higher at present because of the crack epidemic.

Crime and victimization occur at very high rates in the homeless population, although many of the arrests are for minor offenses or reasons other than criminal activity (chapter 6). Snow and colleagues suggest that the greater frequency of arrests of homeless people for minor offenses may be accounted for by three processes: the criminalization of street life; the stigmatization of homeless people; and the role of criminal activities as an adaptation for survival (31).

Morse and colleagues found that the mean number of stressful life crises homeless people reported having had in the year preceding their initial homelessness was 3.3 times greater than that seen in the general population and 1.9 times greater than that seen among depressed psychiatric patients (5).

MORTALITY RATES

There is consensus among most professionals who work with homeless people that their mortality rate is considerably higher than that of domiciled people. However, it is difficult to obtain data regarding this assertion. The mortality rate is the ratio of the number of people dying during a given period of time to the total number of people in the population being studied, and is usually expressed as the number of deaths per 10,000 people. A major difficulty is that the denominator—the size of the homeless population—is not known accurately. Another difficulty is that it is not always possible to determine from the death certificate whether the person was homeless at the time of death. In Sweden, where these barriers are partly removed by a registry for homeless men, the mortality of 6,032 men registered with the Bureau of Homeless Men was studied over a three-year period (1969–71). The observed mortality rate for a given age group (age-adjusted mortality rate) was compared with that expected in men from the same age group in the general Swedish population. The observed:expected age-adjusted mortality ratio among homeless men of all ages was 4:1; among those aged 20–39, it was 9:1. The largest differential was for death from accidents—a 12:1 ratio (32). The JP/HCH study has some corroborative evidence. Of 61 clients who died during a two-year study period, the cause of death was murder or accidents in 39.3 percent and drugs and/or alcohol in 16.4 percent, far in excess of the relative frequency of death from these causes in the general population of the same age range (15).

Patterns and Causal Factors of Homelessness

PATHS TO AND DURATION OF HOMELESSNESS

There are numerous paths to homelessness, a better understanding of which would require more ethnographic studies. Homelessness is often preceded by a prolonged period without steady employment or with inadequate social benefits (11,12). Another frequent pattern is a long period of dependency for lodging upon friends or relatives, which is suddenly interrupted by events or conflicts (chapter 20). From 32 percent to 67 percent of HPS respondents had been homeless before the current episode, many of them several times (Table 4.4). Thus, in many if not most instances, homelessness is part of a prolonged pattern of social or economic marginality.

The duration of the current episode of homelessness ranged from less than a month to more than five years (Table 4.4). However, those who have been homeless for one or two months are not necessarily "new homeless," since many of them have been homeless before (11). Those who have been continuously homeless for a long period, for instance, more than two years, are thought by some to constitute a distinct group. However, some of them too have a history of more than one episode of homelessness (11).

Literal homelessness is preceded in many instances by doubling up with another household (33). In interviews with literally homeless people in the HPS studies, the frequency of doubling up during the previous week or month was low—usually less than 10 percent. This suggests that a relatively small minor-

TABLE 4.4   HISTORY OF HOMELESSNESS IN HPS STUDIES

	Percentage Homeless by									
	Duration of Current Homeless Episode							Number of Previous Homeless Episodes		
	(months)					(years)				
Survey Site[a]	<1	<2	<6	<12	<24	≥2	≥5	0	1–4	≥5
LA-SR (11)	NA[b]	NA	55	70	80	20	NA	33	41	26
LA-SR + WS (6)	NA	NA	43	64	NA	NA	8	69	16[c]	16[d]
Phoenix (4)	31	NA	58	72	81	18	10	65	27[e]	8[f]
St. Louis (5)	35	52[g]	NA	NA	NA	16	NA	47	40	13
Milwaukee (7)	NA	32	NA	NA	70[h]	30	NA	NA	NA	NA
Chicago (12)	13	NA	46	61	75	25	NA	NA	NA	NA
Ohio (2)	39	49	NA	73	80	15	NA[i]	NA	NA	NA

[a]LA-SR, Los Angeles, Skid Row; LA-SR + WS, Los Angeles, Skid Row and West Side (Venice). The numbers in parentheses are reference citations.
[b]NA, data not available.
[c]One or two previous episodes.
[d]Three or more previous episodes.
[e]One to three previous episodes.
[f]Four or more previous episodes.
[g]Less than 3 months.
[h]Less than 18 months.
[i]No answer by 5 percent of interviewees.

TABLE 4.5 PERCEIVED CAUSES OF HOMELESSNESS IN HPS, JP/HCH, AND COM STUDIES

Perceived Cause	Percentage of Homeless Respondents by the Principal Cause They Selected in Survey Cities[a]						Percentage of Homeless Patients by Most Important Cause(s) according to Staff of JP/HCH (15)[b]	Percentage of Cities Whose Officials Cited Cause in	
	LA-SR (11)	LA-SR + WS (6)	Phoenix (4)	Milwaukee (7)	Ohio (2)	Boston (8)		1986 (19)	1989 (21)
Economic[c]	69.8	42.0	53.0	31.0	48.0	40.0	30.2	100	100
Personal[d]	11.4	15.7	9.0	32.0	21.3	26.0	20.1	24	26
Disability[e]	3.8	10.4	3.0	24.0	9.8	24.0	52.1	NA	70[f]
Alcohol and/or drugs	3.8	7.3	3.0	—	7.3	14.0	31.6	36	52
Mental health	—	3.1	—	24.0	2.5	3.0	17.4	56	52
Physical disability	—	—	—	—	—	7.0	3.1	—	—
Own choice[g]	—	—	4.0	—	6.0	3.0	—	—	—
Other	15.0	31.8	30.0	11.0	14.9	7.0	7.1	36	NA

[a]The numbers in parentheses are references citations.

[b]Numbers add up to more than 100 because some reviewers gave more than one most important cause per person.

[c]Includes unemployment or loss of job; government benefits stopped; no money; problems paying rent; eviction (unless it is specifically stated that eviction was for behavioral cause).

[d]Includes loss of relationship, being thrown out, running away, physical abuse, sexual abuse.

[e]Sum of causes given as alcohol and/or drugs, mental health problems, and physical disability.

[f]Percentage of cities citing alcohol and/or mental illness as cause.

[g]Includes own choice, "like it better."

ity of homeless people alternate frequently between doubling up and living on the streets or in shelters, and that most remain either doubled up or literally homeless for a long period of time.

CAUSES OF HOMELESSNESS SUGGESTED IN THE SURVEY STUDIES

Rosnow, Shaw, and Concord group the factors that contribute to homelessness into stage setting (housing and job markets), mediating conditions (history of mental illness, substance abuse, or criminal condition), and precipitating factors (loss of job, loss of support by welfare or family, or personal conflicts) (7). Morse classifies the factors as follows: cultural (e.g., discrimination against minorities), institutional (e.g., unemployment, a shortage of low-income housing, deinstitutionalization, and cuts in financial assistance), community (e.g., urban redevelopment), organizational (e.g., inadequate provision, accessibility, and appropriateness of services), group (e.g., lack of social support, and family conflicts), and individual (e.g., impairment or disability, and personal choice) (34).

In Table 4.5, the causes of homelessness perceived by respondents of the three sets of studies are grouped into several categories: economic factors (lack of low-cost housing or depressed job market—at the stage-setting level—or displacement, eviction, or loss of job or benefits—at the precipitating level); personal factors (breakup of relationship, physical or sexual abuse, running away or being thrown out); disability (alcohol or other drug abuse, mental disorder, physical condition); and own choice (likes to move around, does not want a home). The results differ in the three sets of studies. The predominant factor is economic in the HPS studies (at the precipitating level) and in the COM studies (at the stage-setting level), while it is disability in the JP/HCH study; disability is a poor third in the HPS studies. These differences may be related to the respondents' differing perspectives. Thus the areawide administrative perspective of the COM respondents may lead them to highlight stage-setting economic factors; the clinical perspective of the HCH respondents may favor highlighting the mediating disability factors; and the self-involvement of HPS respondents may lead them to emphasize precipitating factors rather than the mediating factors with which they had lived long before becoming homeless. These findings are compatible with multiple interacting factors, yet few studies (15) have attempted to assess the various factors acting on an individual in terms of their relative contributions to homelessness.

Curiously, the factor of social isolation was not mentioned among perceived causes. Yet there was evidence of some isolation in many HPS studies. From 8 percent to 31 percent of respondents had no relatives; 20–40 percent had not seen a blood relative for more than a year; and 25–45 percent stated either that they had no friends or that they had not been in contact with a friend for over a year (6,8,11,12). However, the standard questions asked in these surveys to assess complex phenomena such as social networking or relationships are crude tools. Two approaches might yield more meaningful results. The first would use instruments that focus on functionality, intensity, continuity, and other specific features of interactions within the network (35–37). The second would use ethnographic studies in conjunction with a network instrument (38–41). In a society as marginal, stressed, and different from the norm as that formed by groups of homeless people and their contacts, it becomes necessary to redefine role relationships, the meaning of exchange interactions, and even the use of language, through ethnographic approaches (41). For instance, the terms *associate* (39) and *hanging out* (42) were used instead of *friend* by the homeless people who were interviewed. The early results of such research (35–42) show that most homeless people have diverse social networks involving, in general, poor people or people with limited resources. This might suggest that efforts be directed toward integrating homeless people in networks of people with less limited resources.

DETERMINANTS OF HOMELESSNESS

Comparison and longitudinal studies have much greater analytical power than does survey research. They have come to this field relatively late.

COMPARISON STUDIES. The first major comparison study of a homeless population in the 1980s was done in Chicago by Sosin and colleagues (43). Its fundamental premise is that homeless people must be studied in the context of poverty. The population consisted of three groups of very poor people who used soup kitchens: those who had never been homeless; those who had been homeless in the past but were not at the time of the study, and and those who were currently homeless.

The domiciled-poor sample overrepresented single men and minorities by comparison with the general population. A majority of the respondents rated their family backgrounds as average or slightly below average economically. Most of them had had good working-class jobs at one time but had not had their best jobs in many years, as if "they fell from the blue collar jobs as the economy changed" (43:344). A moderate proportion had few or no social contacts, and there was moderate overrepresentation of alcoholics and people who had been in mental hospitals.

The homeless respondents did not differ from the domiciled poor people in education, symptoms of mental disorder, work experience, or jail history. They had higher rates of mental hospitalization and of military service. They were more likely to have been in out-of-home care as children. They were much more likely to have lower monthly earnings and to have paid higher rent. They were less likely to receive welfare, and more likely to have lived alone.

These results must be interpreted cautiously because the assumption that the two groups were initially part of the same population has not been validated. They may well have been members of two distinct populations who converged for free meal services. Notwithstanding this caveat, the study identifies factors that are associated with homelessness and are distinct from those associated with the broad context of severe poverty. Sosin et al. propose an interactional view of homelessness—individual deficiencies (low human capital related to lack of education, pathology, or social isolation) combine with environmental factors (higher rent payments, poor income, no current work, nonreceipt of welfare, or lack of relatives) to push poor people into homelessness (43).

Several comparison studies are in progress. Knickman and Weitzman worked with women on welfare who had just become homeless, and with other women on the same welfare lists. They identified pregnancy as a precipitating factor of homelessness in that population (44). They review the methodology of comparison studies of the homeless population in chapter 23.

LONGITUDINAL STUDIES. Belcher followed 132 patients for six months after release from a midwestern state hospital to compare those who became homeless and those who did not. Functional level, employment patterns, and psychiatric diagnostic categories were not significant discriminators, but financial support was significantly higher in those who remained domiciled. A history of prior homelessness or of being released homeless, of decreased family involvement, or of poorer compliance with medication was associated with becoming homeless during the study period. Belcher classified his homeless sample into four groups—wanderers, tenuous planners, the socially disadvantaged, and dropouts—according to their patterns of becoming homeless (45). A comprehensive longitudinal study by Piliavin and Robertson of a panel of psychiatric patients is under way.

Some investigators have looked into homeless people's pasts, sometimes as far back as childhood. Piliavin and Sosin reported from Minneapolis that many homeless people had been reared in foster homes and had no families to rely on (46). A similar finding has been reported by other workers (47–49). McChesney in Los Angeles (chapter 20) found that many homeless young women had never had homes of their own.

References

1. Rossi PH, et al. The urban homeless: Estimation of composition and size. *Science* 235:1336–1341, 1987.

2. Roth D, et al. *Homelessness in Ohio: A Study of People in Need.* Columbus: Ohio Department of Mental Health, 1985.

3. Burt MR, Cohen BE. *American's Homeless: Numbers, Characteristics, and Programs That Serve Them.* Washington, D.C.: Urban Institute, 1989.

4. Brown C, et al. *The Homeless of Phoenix: Who Are They? And What Should Be Done?* Phoenix, Ariz.: South Phoenix Community Mental Health Center, 1983.

5. Morse G, et al. *Homeless People in St. Louis: A Mental Health Program Evaluation, Field Study, and Follow-up Investigation.* Jefferson City: Missouri Department of Mental Health, 1985.

6. Robertson MJ, Ropers RH, Boyer MA. *The Homeless of Los Angeles County: An*

Empirical Evaluation. Los Angeles: University of California–Los Angeles, School of Public Health, Psychiatric Epidemiology Program, 1985.

7. Rosnow MJ, Shaw T, Concord CS. *Listening to the Homeless: A Study of Homeless Mentally Ill in Milwaukee.* Madison: Wisconsin Office of Mental Health, 1985.

8. Mulkern V, et al. *Homelessness Needs Assessment Study: Findings and Recommendations from the Massachusetts Department of Mental Health.* Boston: Human Services Research Institute, 1985.

9. Mowbray CT, et al. *Mental Health and Homelessness in Detroit: A Research Study.* Lansing: Michigan Department of Mental Health, 1986.

10. Fischer PJ, et al. Mental health and social characteristics of the homeless: A survey of mission users. *American Journal of Public Health 76:*519–524, 1986.

11. Farr RK, Koegel P, Burnam A. *A Study of Homelessness in the Skid Row Area of Los Angeles.* Los Angeles: Los Angeles County, Department of Mental Health, 1986.

12. Rossi PH, Fisher GA, Willis G. *The Condition of the Homeless in Chicago: A Report of Surveys Conducted in 1985 and 1986.* Amherst: University of Massachusetts, Social and Demographic Research Institute, 1986.

13. Vernez G, et al. *Review of California's Program for the Homeless Mentally Disabled.* Santa Monica, Calif.: Rand Corporation, 1988.

14. Andrade SJ. *Living in the Gray Zone: Health Care Needs of Homeless Persons.* San Antonio, Tex.: Benedictine Health Resource Center, 1988.

15. Wright JD, Weber E. *Homelessness and Health.* New York: McGraw-Hill, 1987.

16. Wright JD. Poverty, homelessness, health, nutrition, and children. In papers of the conference Homeless Children and Youth: Coping with a National Tragedy, held at Johns Hopkins University, Institute for Policy Studies, in Baltimore, Md., April 25–28, 1989.

17. Lewin ICF. *The Health Needs of the Homeless: A Report on Persons Served by the McKinney Act's Health Care for the Homeless Program.* Washington, D.C.: National Association of Community Health Centers, 1989.

18. Waxman LD, Reyes LM. *The Growth of Hunger, Homelessness, and Poverty in American Cities in 1985.* Washington, D.C.: United States Conference of Mayors, 1986.

19. Reyes LM, Waxman LD. *The Continued Growth of Hunger, Homelessness, and Poverty in American Cities, 1986.* Washington, D.C.: United States Conference of Mayors, December 1986.

20. Waxman LD, Reyes LM. *A Status Report on Hunger and Homelessness in America's Cities, 1988.* Washington, D.C.: United States Conference of Mayors, 1989.

21. Reyes LM, Waxman LD. *A Status Report on Hunger and Homelessness in America's Cities, 1989.* Washington, D.C.: United States Conference of Mayors, December 1989.

22. Waxman LD, Reyes LM. *A Status Report on Hunger and Homelessness in America's Cities, 1990.* Washington, D.C.: United States Conference of Mayors, December 1990.

23. Maurin JT, Russell L. Homelessness in Utah. In Momeni J (ed.), *Homelessness in the United States: State Surveys.* New York: Praeger, 1990.

24. Yates GL, et al. A risk profile comparison of runaway and non-runaway youths. *American Journal of Public Health 78:*820–821, 1988.

25. Partnership for the Homeless. *AIDS—The Cutting Edge of Homelessness in New York City: A Survival Plan for People with AIDS Who Are Homeless.* New York: The Partnership, 1989.

26. Chavkin W, et al. Reproductive experience of women living in hotels for the homeless in New York City. *New York State Journal of Medicine 87:*10–13, 1987.

27. Jahiel RI. Health and health care of homeless people. In Greenblatt M, Robertson MJ (eds.), *Homelessness: The National Perspective.* New York: Plenum, in press.

28. Koegel P, Burnam MA. Traditional and non-traditional homeless alcoholics. *Alcohol, Health, and Research World 2:*28–34, 1987.

29. Shandler IW, Shipley TE Jr. New focus for an old problem: Philadelphia's response on

homelessness. *Alcohol, Health, and Research World 2:*54–56, 1987.

30. Fischer PJ. Substance abuse in contemporary homeless populations. In Dennis DL (ed.), *Research Methodology Concerning Homeless Persons with Serious Mental Illness or Substance Abuse.* Rockville, Md.: Alcohol, Drug Abuse, and Mental Health Administration, 1987.

31. Snow DA, Baker SG, Anderson L. Criminality and homeless men: An empirical assessment. *Social Problems 36:*532–549, 1989.

32. Alstrom CH, Lindelius R, Salum I. Mortality among homeless men. *British Journal of Addiction 70:*245–252, 1975.

33. Waxman LD, Reyes LM. *A Status Report on Homeless Families in America's Cities.* Washington, D.C.: United States Conference of Mayors, 1987.

34. Morse GA. *A Contemporary Assessment of Urban Homelessness: Implications for Social Change.* St. Louis, Mo.: University of Missouri at St. Louis, Center for Metropolitan Studies, 1986.

35. Sokolovsky J. Network Methodologies in the study of aging. In Fry C, Keith J (eds.), *New Methods for Old Age Research.* South Hadley, Mass.: Bergin and Garvey, 1986.

36. Solarz A. Social support among the homeless. Paper presented at the 113th annual meeting of the American Public Health Association, Washington, D.C., November 17–21, 1985.

37. Lovell AM. Networks, mental health status, and the context of homelessness in New York City. Paper presented at the 116th annual meeting of the American Public Health Association, Boston, Mass., November 16, 1988.

38. Cohen CI, Sokolovsky J. *Old Men of the Bowery: Strategies for Survival among the Homeless.* New York: Guilford Press, 1989.

39. Martin MA. Strategies of adaptation: Coping patterns of the urban transient female. Ph.D. diss., Columbia University School of Social Work, 1982.

40. Lovell A, Sokolovsky J. Social networks and social supports. In Morrissey JP, Dennis DL (eds.), *Homelessness and Mental Illness: Toward the Next Generation of Research Studies.* Rockville, Md.: National Institute of Mental Health, Office of Programs for the Homeless Mentally Ill, 1990.

41. Lovell AM, Barrow S, Hammer M. *Social Support and Social Network Interview.* New York: New York State Psychiatric Institute, 1984.

42. Robertson MJ. Homeless youth: An overview of recent literature. In papers of the conference Homeless Children and Youth: Coping with a National Tragedy, held at Johns Hopkins University, Institute for Policy Studies, Baltimore, Md., April 25–28, 1989.

43. Sosin MR, Colson P, Grossman S. *Homelessness in Chicago: Poverty and Pathology, Social Institutions and Social Change.* Chicago: Chicago Community Trust, June 1988.

44. Knickman JR, Weitzman BC. *A Study of Homeless Families in New York City: Risk Assessment Models and Strategies for Prevention.* Final Report, vol. 1. Prepared for the New York City Human Resources Administration. New York: New York University, Robert F. Wagner Graduate School of Public Service, Health Research Program, September 1989.

45. Belcher JR. On becoming homeless: A study of chronically mentally ill persons. *Journal of Community Psychology 17:*173–185, 1989.

46. Piliavin I, Sosin M, Westerfeld H. Tracking the homeless. *Focus 10(4):*20–24, 1987–88.

47. Susser E, Struening E, Conover S. Childhood experiences of homeless men. *American Journal of Psychiatry 144:*1599–1601, 1987.

48. Wood D, et al. Homeless and housed families in Los Angeles: A study comparing demographic, economic, and family function characteristics. *American Journal of Public Health 80:*1049–1052, 1990.

49. Barth RP. On their own: The experiences of youth after foster care. *Childhood and Adolescent Social Work Journal 7:*419–440, 1990.

CHAPTER 5

The Prevalence of Mental Disorder among Homeless People

Marjorie J. Robertson, Ph.D.

In recent years, a multitude of reports, articles, books, special projects, and conferences have addressed the issue of mental health status among homeless people in the United States. However, there is little agreement on the extent of mental disorder in this group (1–7). In light of this controversy, we will examine the literature to address three major questions:

• What is the extent of mental disorder among homeless people in the United States?
• Is there evidence that homeless people exhibit higher rates of mental disorder than nonhomeless people?
• How does mental disorder vary across subgroups of the homeless population?

A Critique of National Prevalence Estimates

In 1984, the American Psychiatric Association (APA) Task Force on the Homeless Mentally Ill estimated that "between 25 and 50% [of the homeless] have serious and chronic forms of mental illness" (8:88). The APA estimate was quickly accepted as authoritative despite its questionable validity. The definition of "serious and chronic form of mental illness" was not specified. Also, the estimate was based on only 12 empirical studies, half of which used samples from clinical sites, which are an inappropriate basis for community prevalence estimates (9). Four of the studies used samples from Great Britain, which may have limited validity for estimating trends among homeless groups in the United States (10). Two of the studies were published more than 25 years ago and may not be relevant to an estimate of mental illness in contemporary homeless populations. In sum, only 4 of the 12 studies were recent community studies with U.S. samples. Of these, 3 were based on samples drawn from a single shelter, and one did not include specific rates by diagnostic categories. In view of these limitations, the APA estimate is difficult to defend on empirical grounds.

Several other national estimates are also difficult to defend. On the basis of a national survey of shelter operators in 1984, the U.S. Department of Housing and Urban Development (HUD) asserted that "many of the homeless are . . . mentally ill—22 percent of the shelter population according to the national survey" (11:24). In 1988, HUD surveyed a national probability sample of shelter managers, who estimated that 34 percent of their adult clients, on average, might have the problem of mental illness (12). The criteria used to determine who is mentally ill were not specified, and the validity or reliability of the shelter operators' reports of mental disorder among their clients was not addressed.

In 1984, the U.S. Department of Health and Human Services (HHS) estimated that "from 33 to 66 percent of the homeless in shelters are characterized principally by mental illness on an acute or chronic basis, and 25 to 35 percent are former patients of mental hospitals" (13:4). It is impossible to estimate the validity of this estimate, since neither the definition of mental illness nor the basis for the HHS estimate is specified. Furthermore, both the 1984 HUD (11) and HHS (13) reports state that people with mental illness are found with greater frequency in the "street" than in the "shelter" population, but provide no empirical support for this assumption.

Despite great interest in the question of mental disorder among homeless people, contradictory estimates of its prevalence such as those discussed above, which have little or no empirical basis, only contribute to confusion over the issue. A first step in assessing the prevalence is to review the recent empirical literature.

A Literature Review

To be included in the current overview, research reports had to include (a) the results of *quantitative* primary or secondary analysis of nonclinical, noninstitutional samples of the homeless population in the United States; (b) a complete description of the methodology used; (c) at least one indicator of mental disorder; and (d) a publication or release date in or since 1975. Altogether, 62 reports of original empirical research were identified which met these specific criteria (14–75). Thirty-seven distinct data bases were represented among them.

The primary source of the material was a computer-assisted search of nine bibliographic data bases in November 1987. In addition, reference lists published in recent literature reviews (1,6,8,76–79) were consulted. Despite an aggressive search, this literature review is not assumed to be exhaustive. The search was limited by time period (since 1975), geography (United States), and design (quantitative). Dissertations and theses were not reviewed, and many conference papers identified in the reference lists of reports were not accessible. The literature reviewed was selected for its relevance to questions concerning the relative prevalence and distribution of mental disorders among homeless people. Other important mental health aspects of homelessness, such as coping strategies, subsistence adaptation, social networks, and social supports, are not considered (80).

An examination of their design characteristics found all of the studies to be descriptive and cross-sectional, with most depending exclusively on self-report. They varied in definition of homelessness, sample selection method, size, site, and type of geographic location. Most used adults samples exclusively, although several included children with their mothers (17,75), or homeless and runaway youths (54,67). Few used representative samples (21,31,39,57,58,60), and in most instances, mental health assessment for the generation of prevalence estimates was not the primary goal of the study.

Various mental health indicators were used. Several studies reported on more than one mental health variable. Since the choice of mental health indicator was expected to affect reported prevalence rates (1,6,73,81–83), results from studies of homeless adults were divided for separate discussion into four categories on the basis of the indicator used: history of psychiatric hospitalization, measure of psychological distress, measures of psychotic symptoms, and specific psychiatric diagnoses. A brief discussion of the literature on children and adolescents is presented separately.

Mental Disorder among Homeless Adults

Psychiatric Hospitalization History

Thirty-nine studies reported rates of previous psychiatric hospitalization among homeless adults, and seven of these included hospitalization history as the principal factor in a composite mental health indicator (27,33,47,56,65,68). Samples were drawn from mixed sites in 51 percent of studies, from shelters or missions exclusively in 42 percent, or from other single sites in 8 percent (Table 5.1).

The rate of previous psychiatric hospitalization ranged from 5 percent to 42 percent, with 15–35 percent in most studies (Table 5.1). In five studies in which comparison figures were available, homeless people demonstrated a higher prevalence of previous hospitalization than did domiciled comparison groups (24,31,35,55,68). Many of those previously hospitalized reported a single episode of hospitalization. In eight studies, one-third to two-thirds of those previously hospitalized had been hospitalized only once (14,15,47,49,55,58, 60,70). It was reported in three studies that in some instances, initial psychiatric hospitalization had occurred after the onset of homelessness (47,51,55).

TABLE 5.1 SELF-REPORTED HISTORY OF PSYCHIATRIC HOSPITALIZATION AMONG HOMELESS ADULTS, 1975–1989

Authors, Year Published/ Released[a]	Data Collection Period	Location	Site(s)	Sample N	Males : Females (% : %)	Lifetime Psychiatric Hospitalization Total (%)	Male (%)	Female (%)	Comments
Arce et al., 1983 (14)	1982	Philadelphia	Shelter	193	78 : 22	35	—	—	Authors note that those admitted to shelters probably have greater overall psychiatric disability than do nonadmitted applicants
Bassuk et al., 1984 (16)	1983	Boston	Shelter	78	83 : 17	28	—	—	
Bassuk et al., 1986 (17)	1985	Massachusetts	Shelters	80	0 : 100	8	—	8	Mothers with children
Benda et al., 1986 (18)	1985–86	Richmond, Va.	Shelters, meal program, agencies, streets	345	89 : 11	30	—	—	
Breakey et al., 1989 (19)	—	Baltimore	Shelters, jail	204	61 : 39	—	23	42	
Brown et al., 1983 (20)	1982	Phoenix	Meal program	150	89 : 11	19	—	—	
Brown et al., 1983 (20)	1983	Phoenix	Shelters, meal programs, urban camps	195	86 : 14	11	—	—	
Burt and Cohen, 1989 (21)	1987	20 large cities nationally	Shelters, meal programs	1,552	67 : 33	18[b]	17[b]	19[b]	Rates varied for single men (19%), single women (27%), and women with children (8%)

Study	Year	City	Location	N	Ratio				Comments
Chicago, 1983 (22)	1983	Chicago	Shelters, streets	50	—	23	—	—	
Crystal et al., 1982 (26)	1981	New York City	Shelters	128	100:0	18	18	—	
Crystal et al., 1986 (27)	—	New York City	Shelters	1,508	—	20[c]	—	—	
Crystal and Goldstein, 1984 (24)	1982–83	New York City	Shelters	1,014	85:15	15	13	27	
Crystal and Goldstein, 1984 (25)	1982–83	New York City	Shelters	7,285	78:22	18	15	28	
Farr et al., 1986 (28)	—	Los Angeles (Inner city)	Shelters, meal programs, congregating areas	328	96:4	27	—	—	Authors note that figure is likely overestimated due to inclusion of respondents with alcohol- or drug-related hospitalization
Fischer and Breakey, 1987 (30)	1986	Baltimore	Shelters, jail	162	59:41	27	—	—	Inpatient treatment in state hospital
Fischer et al., 1986 (31)	1981–82	Baltimore	Shelters	51	94:6	33	—	—	Compared to 5% of male householders in Eastern Baltimore ECA[d] study
Gelberg et al., 1988 (33)	1985	Los Angeles County (West Side)	Shelters, food programs agencies, streets, other	529	73:27	29[e]	31[e]	22[e]	
Kahn et al., 1987 (34)	—	Tucson	Meal program	106	92:8	—	—	—	In previous three years, 25%
Knickman and Weitzman, 1989 (35)	1988	New York City	Shelter intake site	704[f]	4:96	5	—	—	Compared to 1.1% of comparison sample

(continued)

TABLE 5.1 (*Continued*)

Authors, Year Published/ Released[a]	Data Collection Period	Location	Site(s)	Sample N	Males : Females (% : %)	Lifetime Psychiatric Hospitalization Total (%)	Male (%)	Female (%)	Comments
Kroll et al., 1986 (42)	1984	Hennepin County, Minn.	Shelters	68	88 : 12	18	—	—	
McChesney, 1987 (44)	1987	Los Angeles (Inner city)	Shelters	181	93 : 7	12	—	—	
Morse, 1982 (45)	1981	St. Louis (Inner city)	Shelter	163	100 : 0	41	41	—	
Morse et al., 1985 (47)	1983–84	St. Louis	Shelters	248	51 : 49	25	25[e]	25[e]	Authors note that actual rate for sample is probably 3–5% higher; also, for 26% of cases, initial homelessness preceded mental hospitalization
Mulkern et al., 1985 (48)	—	Boston	Shelter, streets	327	81 : 19	39	—	—	Excludes subsample from a shelter for "mentally ill" homeless people
Multnomah County, 1983 (49)	1983	Portland, Oreg.	Shelters, streets	120	85 : 15	18	—	—	Institutionalized in a state mental hospital
Piliavin et al., 1989 (51)	1985–86	Minneapolis	Shelters, meal programs, drop-in programs	331	85 : 15	18	—	—	

Robertson et al., 1985 (55)	1983–84	Los Angeles County (Inner city and West Side)	Shelters, meal programs, streets	238	77:23	20	18	27	Compared to 2.9% of householders in the Los Angeles ECA study
Rosnow et al., 1985 (56)	1984–85	Milwaukee	Shelters, streets	237	87:13	42	—	—	Indicates combined psychiatric, alcohol, and drug hospitalizations
Rossi et al., 1986 (58)	1985–86	Chicago	Shelters, streets	717	73:27	23	—	—	
Roth et al., 1985 (60)	1984	Ohio	Shelters, streets, hotel, motel, other	979	81:19	30	—	—	
Segal et al., 1977 (66)	1973	Berkeley, Calif.	Meal program	295	—	22	—	—	
Snow et al., 1986 (68)	1984	Austin, Tex.	Shelter, food program	767	99:1	11	—	—	Compared to 0.26% of adult male population in Texas
Snow et al., 1986 (68)	1985	Austin, Tex.	Shelters, meal program, streets, other	164	86:14	7	—	—	Compared to 0.26% of the adult male population in Texas
Solarz, 1985 (69)	—	Detroit	Shelter	125	63:37	32[d]	30[d]	35[d]	Combination of self-report and state department of mental health records
Solarz and Mowbray, 1985 (70)	1983	Detroit	Shelters	75	72:28	26	22[d]	35[d]	Combination of self-report and state department of mental health records
Sosin et al., 1988 (71)	—	Chicago	Shelters, meal programs, treatment programs	178	63:37	20[b]	—	—	

(continued)

TABLE 5.1 (*Continued*)

Authors, Year Published/ Released[a]	Data Collection Period	Location	Sample			Lifetime Psychiatric Hospitalization			Comments
			Site(s)	N	Males:Females (%:%)	Total (%)	Male (%)	Female (%)	
Susser et al., 1989 (72)	1985	New York City	Shelters	918[b]	100:0	12[b]	12[b]	—	New admissions (15%); other clients (12%)
Toro and Wall, 1989 (73)	1987–88	Eastern city	Shelter, meal program, streets	76	79:21	33	—	—	2% in previous six months
Vernez et al., 1988 (74)	1987	3 California counties	Shelters, streets	315	—	28	—	—	

[a]The number in parentheses is a reference citation.
[b]Estimated from data provided in article.
[c]Unpublished data, provided by second author, S. Ladner.
[d]ECA, Epidemiologic Catchment Area.
[e]Unpublished data, provided by first author.
[f]Family head of household, with family including at least one child or a pregnant woman.

MEASURES OF PSYCHOLOGICAL DISTRESS
AND OTHER SYMPTOM SCALES

Standardized symptom scales were used in 18 studies. Nearly two-thirds of these studies used samples drawn from mixed sites, and one-third used samples from shelters only. In general, when compared on standardized indicators of psychological distress, homeless samples scored higher than did the general population (Table 5.2).

Homeless adults also reported elevated rates of suicidal ideation and suicide attempts. Robertson et al. (55) found that 6.7 percent of respondents in their Los Angeles sample had attempted suicide in the preceding 12 months, compared to 0.2 percent for the non-Hispanic sample of the Los Angeles Epidemiologic Catchment Area (ECA) (53). In other studies, the rate of suicidal ideation during the preceding year was 25 percent (33), and the lifetime rate of attempted suicide was 22 percent (33) and 16 percent (57). Burt and Cohen (21) found that about 20 percent of respondents in their national homeless sample had attempted suicide at some point in their lives, compared to the national ECA estimated lifetime prevalence rate of 3 percent. Men sampled in New York City shelters had the following rates: suicide attempts, 19 percent; multiple attempts, 6 percent; and current suicidal thoughts, 7 percent (72).

PSYCHOTIC SYMPTOMS

Three studies used a short list of psychotic symptoms adapted from the National Institute of Mental Health (NIMH) Diagnostic Interview Schedule (DIS) (33,50) or the Psychiatric Epidemiology Research Interview (PERI) (44,58). Gelberg et al. (33) reported that 40 percent of their respondents had experienced at least one of six psychotic symptoms during the previous two weeks. Mc-Chesney (44) reported that 38 percent of her shelter respondents had experienced at least one of four psychotic symptoms during the previous year. Rossi et al. (58) reported that 23 percent of their respondents had experienced two or more of five psychotic symptoms during the past year, and that the average score on each of five symptoms was higher in their homeless sample than in a domiciled inner-city sample in New York City.

PSYCHIATRIC DIAGNOSIS

Rates of specific psychiatric disorders were reported in eight studies that varied widely in geographic area, source and composition of sample, and diagnostic method. Samples were derived only from shelters or missions in five studies and from mixed sites in three studies. Seven studies used direct interviews, and one used shelter records that included clinical evaluations. Three methods were used to arrive at psychiatric diagnoses: structured clinical interviews; structured

TABLE 5.2 MENTAL HEALTH STATUS (AS MEASURED WITH SYMPTOM SCALES) AMONG HOMELESS ADULTS, 1975–1989

Author, Year Published/ Released[a]	Symptom Scale	Sample Location	Sample Sites	N	Percentage Meeting Criteria for Symptoms	Comments
Bassuk et al., 1986 (17)	BPRS[b]	Massachusetts	Shelters	80	NA	Majority described by moderate to extremely severe symptoms of anxiety (72%), depression (67%), and tension (58%)
Morse, 1982 (45)	BSI	St. Louis	Shelter	163	40	Two standard deviations above the mean for nonpatients
Solarz and Mowbray, 1985 (70)	BSI	Detroit	Shelters	75	NA	Women scored in 90th percentile and men in 95th percentile; no significant gender differences on subscale or global score
Morse and Calsyn, 1986 (46)	BSI, Global Severity Index	St. Louis	Shelters	248	47	Higher on all subscales compared to nonpatient population
Toro and Wall, 1989 (73)	BSI, Global Severity Index	Eastern city	Shelter, meal program, streets	76	41	Above 90th percentile; sample scored midway between psychiatric inpatients and nonpatients
Sosin et al., 1988 (71)	BSI, Global Severity Index	Chicago	Shelters, meal programs, treatment programs	174	45[c]	Above 90th percentile
Burt and Cohen, 1989 (21)	CES-D (modified)	20 large cities nationally	Shelters, meal programs	1,552	50	Used 6 of 20 CES-D items; no gender differences;[c] single women (46%) lower than women with children (59%)

Study	Instrument	Location	Sample source	N	%	Findings
Farr et al., 1986 (28)	CES-D	Los Angeles	Shelters, meal programs, congregating areas	328	72	High compared to 9.8% for Los Angeles ECA study
LaGory et al., 1990 (43)	CES-D	Birmingham	Shelters, streets	150	75	Age 16 and above; 59% scored 20+; this was high compared to <20% in general population
Robertson et al., 1985 (55)	CES-D	Los Angeles	Shelters, meal programs	65	49	Age 16 and above; high compared to 20% for Los Angeles community sample; no gender differences
Rossi et al., 1986 (58)	CES-D (modified)	Chicago	Shelters, streets	717	47	Used 6 of 20 CES-D items; no gender differences
Susser et al., 1989 (72)	CES-D (modified)	New York City	Shelters	223	69	Score of 16+ among new shelter admissions
Fischer and Breakey, 1987 (30)	GHQ	Baltimore	Shelters, jail	162	53	Women higher than men (61% v. 49%)
Fischer et al., 1986 (31)	GHQ	Baltimore	Shelters	51	34	High compared to Eastern Baltimore ECA study for males under age 65 (12%)
Gelberg and Linn, 1989 (32)	General Health Survey	Los Angeles County (West Side)	Shelters, food programs, agencies, streets	529	27	Felt symptoms of distress at least a good part of the time, compared to 39% of general population
Kahn et al., 1987 (34)	MMPI	Tucson	Meal program	106	—	Three standard deviations above the mean (i.e., T-score of 80 or above): schizophrenia (35%), psychopathic deviance (26%), depression (22%), mania (26%), and paranoia (27%)

(continued)

TABLE 5.2 (*Continued*)

Author, Year Published/ Released[a]	Symptom Scale	Sample			Percentage Meeting Criteria for Symptoms	Comments
		Location	Sites	N		
Susser et al., 1989 (72)	PERI (modified)	New York City	Shelters	695	36[c]	Score 11+
Roth et al., 1985 (60)	PSS	Ohio	Shelters, streets, hotels, motels, other	979	31	Less than 5% required structured, protective environment

Source: Adapted from Table 2 in Robertson M, Mental disorder among homeless persons in the United States: An overview of recent empirical literature. *Administration in Mental Health 14*:14–27, 1986.

[a]The number in parentheses is a reference citation.

[b]BPRS, Brief Psychiatric Rating Schedule; NA, data not available; BSI, Brief Symptom Inventory; CES-D, Center for Epidemiological Studies Depression Scale; ECA, Epidemiologic Catchment Area; GHQ, General Health Questionnaire; MMPI, Minnesota Multiphasic Personality Inventory; PERI, Psychiatric Epidemiology Research Interview; PSS, Psychiatric Status Schedule.

[c]Estimated from data provided in report.

survey-type interviews, with the DIS, usually done by nonclinicians; and secondary analysis of shelter records to retrieve psychiatric diagnoses that had usually been made by clinicians. DSM-III or DSM-III-R (72) criteria were used in all studies. Furthermore, three studies reported rates of primary diagnosis (14,16,17), and two reported rates of disorder without exclusion (i.e., primary and other diagnoses) (31,39). The temporal bases for prevalence estimates are noteworthy, since presenting disorders or point prevalence estimates were reported in some studies (14) and one-month, six-month, or lifetime prevalence rates in others (31,39).

Not surprisingly, the rates of principal diagnostic categories did not converge (Table 5.3). For example, the rates of schizophrenia range from 2 percent to 34 percent and the rates of affective disorders from 6 percent to 24 percent. As noted by others (6,9,78), results cannot be validly compared across such methodologically distinct studies. In addition to the psychiatric diagnoses summarized in Table 5.3, four studies reported rates of mental retardation between 1 percent and 5 percent (14,16,17,49).

OVERLAP BETWEEN MENTAL DISORDER AND ABUSE OF ALCOHOL OR OTHER DRUGS

The prevalence of the dual diagnosis of mental illness and alcohol or other drug abuse (DSM-III criteria) varied across three California counties from 14 percent to 37 percent (74). Prevalences reported in other studies were 12 percent in Los Angeles's Skid Row (28), 10 percent in Tucson (34), and 26 percent in Boston (65). In Saint Louis, Morse and Calsyn (46) reported that their chronic group (defined by multiple or extended psychiatric hospitalizations) had significantly increased drinking problems—61 percent v. 29 percent for other homeless groups—although there were no differences in other drug use. In contrast, Crystal et al. (27) reported in their New York study that the psychiatric subgroup was only minimally more likely to have substance abuse problems—including problems with the past or present use of alcohol or the use of heroin or other substances—than were other homeless populations (43% v. 32%).

VARIATION ACROSS SAMPLE SITES

SHELTERS. Rates of psychiatric hospitalization varied widely across shelters within individual studies. For example, the prevalence of previous hospitalization among residents of 13 shelters in Saint Louis varied from 0 percent to 42 percent (47). The potential impact of shelter admission criteria on prevalence rates is underscored by Mulkern et al. (48), who reported that residents of a Boston shelter intended for homeless people with mental illness had a psychiatric hospitalization rate of 80 percent, compared to 38 percent in the study's other shelters.

TABLE 5.3 THE PREVALENCE OF PSYCHIATRIC DISORDERS (AS MEASURED USING DSM-III OR DSM-III-R CRITERIA) AMONG HOMELESS ADULTS, 1975–1989

| Author, Year[a] | Location | Sample | | | | Percentage in Diagnostic Categories | | | | |
		Sites	Selection	N	Males : Females (% : %)	Schizophrenia (%)	Affective Disorder (%)	Personality Disorder (%)	Organic Brain Syndrome (%)	Substance Abuse Disorder (Secondary) (%)
CLINICAL INTERVIEW										
Bassuk et al., 1984 (16)	Boston	Shelter	Census	74[b]	82 : 18	29.0	9.0	21.0	—	29.0[c]
Bassuk et al., 1986 (17)	Massachusetts	Shelters	Census	80	0 : 100	2.5	10.0	70.0	—	8.8 (3.7)[d]
Breakey et al., 1989 (19)	Baltimore	Shelters	Random	125	100 : 0	12.1	18.6	46.5	—	75.4
Breakey et al., 1989 (19)		Jail	Random	78	0 : 100	17.1	23.7	45.3	—	38.2
Susser et al., 1989 (72)	New York City	Shelters	Census	177[e]	100 : 0	8.0[f]	—	—	—	—
INTERVIEW WITH DIAGNOSTIC INTERVIEW SCHEDULE[g,h]										
Fischer et al., 1986 (31)	Baltimore	Shelters	Random	51	94 : 6	2.0	23.6[i]	11.8[j]	7.8[k]	31.4
Koegel et al., 1988 (36)	Los Angeles	Shelters, meal programs, congregating areas	Probability	328	96 : 4	11.5[l]	20.9[m]	17.4[n]	3.4[k]	31.2

Toro and Wall, 1989 (73)	Eastern city	Shelter, meal program, streets	Mixed	76	79:21	1.4	13.7	25.7[o]	—	34.2
SHELTER RECORDS, SECONDARY ANALYSIS										
Arce et al., 1983 (14)	Philadelphia	Shelter	Census	179[p]	78:22	34.4	5.6	6.7	5.0	24.6

Source: Adapted from Table 3 in Robertson M, Mental disorder among homeless persons in the United States: An overview of recent empirical literature. *Administration in Mental Health* 14:14–27, 1986.

[a]The number in parentheses is a reference citation.
[b]Original sample included four children.
[c]Alcohol only.
[d]Personal communication with first author.
[e]New arrivals at shelter only.
[f]Prevalence (likely underestimated per first author) includes 14 with a definite diagnosis of schizophrenia and 3 with schizoaffective bipolar disorder. In addition, 4 others had a definite psychotic history but diagnosis could not be made.
[g]Figures may not be added across categories; diagnoses are not based on exclusions.
[h]Six-month prevalence.
[i]Figure included 2% affective disorder; 21.6% anxiety somatoform disorder.
[j]Antisocial personality disorder only.
[k]Cognitive impairment as measured by the Mini–Mental State Exam, an accepted measure of organic brain syndrome; however, mental retardation, anxiety, or low education cannot be ruled out.
[l]Experienced symptoms in previous three years.
[m]Broad summary figure. Excludes persons with a single episode, with no symptoms in previous three years, with episode explained by grief, or with dysthymia as only affective disorder.
[n]Antisocial personality adapted to exclude adult conduct disorder symptoms that are characteristic of the homeless experience (e.g., not having a place to live for 30 days or more) (22).
[o]Three symptoms "confounded" with circumstances of homeless were dropped from the computer scoring program.
[p]Authors note that those admitted to shelters probably reflect greater overall psychiatric disability compared to nonadmitted applicants.

SHELTER VERSUS STREET SAMPLES. Despite the widely reported assumption that homeless people outside of shelters are more mentally disabled as a group than are those who use shelters or other structured services (11,13), no consistent differences in psychiatric hospitalization rates have been found between the street and shelters or other sample sites (48,56,60). Further, three studies revealed no differences in composite indicators of mental health (inclusive of psychiatric hospitalization rates) as a function of the time spent by respondents in "the street" versus other homeless or marginal settings (46,65), or of the frequency of the use of free food or lodging facilities (68). In singular contrast, in a Los Angeles study those previously hospitalized for psychiatric problems or alcohol or other drug problems were the least likely to have spent the previous night in a shelter (33).

With other mental health indicators, results were more mixed. Respondents in a Chicago street sample had a higher level of depressive symptoms than did those in the shelter sample (58). In a Los Angeles Skid Row study, hotel voucher recipients had higher rates of current depressive symptoms or demoralization than did respondents in more traditional settings (41). Other studies reported no variation in measures of psychological distress by sample site (32). In the statewide Ohio study, there were similar rates of disorder (as measured by the Psychiatric Severity Index of the Psychiatric Status Schedule [PSS] scale) among street (32%), shelter (34%), and other homeless (28%) subsamples, although the street sample tended to be more behaviorally dysfunctional than the sheltered one (60). These relatively minor differences between sites appear to be incompatible with the suggestion (84) that the relatively broad definition of homelessness in the Ohio study was responsible for its low rate of mental disorder.

Results obtained with psychiatric diagnostic criteria were also mixed. In the California counties study, higher rates of schizophrenia or major affective disorders were found in shelters than in street sites (74), while in a Baltimore study, a higher rate of schizophrenia was found in jails than in shelters or missions (19), a finding that is consistent with concerns about the criminalization of mental illness in homeless persons (85–87).

THE DISTRIBUTION OF MENTAL HEALTH INDICATORS

GENDER. Gender comparisons were infrequently reported in the literature reviewed. However, with notable exceptions (33,47,60,61), women were generally found to report higher rates of psychiatric hospitalization (Table 5.1) (19,23–25,55,69,70), or of composite indicators in which psychiatric hospitalization was the dominant factor (47,65), than did men. The higher rates of psychiatric hospitalization of homeless single women occurred in all age groups, in a study of New York City shelters (23). Women also had a somewhat

THE PREVALENCE OF MENTAL DISORDER

higher prevalence of major mental illness (including major affective disorders and schizophrenia), according to studies from three California counties (74) and Baltimore (19). However, a subgroup that differed markedly in this respect consisted of homeless women with dependent children. In a study with samples from 20 cities, women with dependent children had lower hospitalization rates (8%) than did either homeless men (19%) or homeless women without children (27%) (21).

No gender-related difference in psychological distress was found in four studies with standardized instruments (21,53,59,70). In the Ohio study, women showed higher rates of psychiatric symptomatology, while men had higher rates of behavioral disturbances (60). In a Los Angeles study, the rate of suicide attempts during the past 12 months was higher in women (13.3%) than in men (4.9%) (55). Again, women who were homeless with their children had a lower rate (14%) of lifetime suicide attempts than did women who were homeless without children (26%) (21).

AGE. Relationships between mental health indicators and age were mixed. Several studies showed higher rates of mental health problems among younger people (39,58,61,68), while others found no age difference (74).

ETHNICITY. Most of the few available studies reported little or no difference across racial or ethnic groups (74), whether they used psychiatric hospitalization (29,58,61), current depressive symptoms (58), or current psychiatric diagnoses (59). However, in the Ohio statewide survey, blacks had slightly less psychiatric symptomatology but somewhat more behavioral disturbances as assessed by the PSS (29,61); and in a Chicago study, American Indians, blacks, and Hispanics had higher symptom rates and were more likely to report recent psychiatric hospitalizations than were whites (58).

MOBILITY. There is evidence that homeless people as a group are relatively stable geographically, although they often report frequent movement between residential settings within a community (17,55,78,88). Homeless people who have mental disorders have been reported to be more mobile than other homeless people in some studies but not in others (15,60,68,78).

Mental Disorder among
Homeless Children and Adolescents

Little empirical work has been done on homeless children and adolescents. In general, the evidence suggests that they have seriously elevated levels of mental health problems by comparison with the general population.

Homeless Children with Their Parent(s)

In a study of children residing with their mothers in 14 shelters for homeless families in Massachusetts, Bassuk et al. (16,17) found that 47 percent of the children aged five years or younger had at least one developmental delay on the Denver Developmental Screening Test, and one-third had two or more delays. Among children aged 5 to 18, half scored over nine on the Achenbach Child Behavior Checklist and were referred for further psychiatric examination, while about one-third scored above 13.8 on Beck's Childhood Depression Scale, strongly suggesting clinical depression. According to their parents, 43 percent of the children had repeated a grade in school.

Similar findings were reported by Wood et al. (89), who found that 28 percent of the homeless children in their Los Angeles sample had been placed in remedial classes and 30 percent had repeated a grade; and by Miller and Lin (90), who found that of the children sampled from emergency shelters in King County, Washington, 9 percent had showed "mental health problems" during clinical examination and 5 percent had had psychiatric visits during the preceding six months.

Runaway and Homeless Youths in New York

Shaffer and Caton (67) reported on diagnostic interviews of 117 youths in New York City shelters that excluded applicants who were psychotic, intoxicated, violent, or suicidal, or who had serious substance abuse problems. At least one suicide attempt was reported by 24 percent of the sample (33% for females, 15% for males). This is higher than the 10–12 percent rate Shaffer and Caton found in adolescent psychiatric outpatients. The suggested cutoff score for psychiatric disability, 40 on the Achenbach Child Behavior Checklist, was exceeded by 82 percent of the sample. There was a history of psychiatric hospitalization in 9 percent of cases (14% for females, 3% for males), which was attributed by the authors to suicide attempts. The shelter users were described as having a psychiatric profile indistinguishable from that of adolescents attending a child psychiatric clinic.

Runaway and Homeless Youths in Hollywood

Robertson (54) systematically sampled 96 homeless adolescents, aged 13 to 17, from 30 service and "street" sites in the Hollywood area of Los Angeles County. Using DSM-III criteria, as operationalized in the DIS, she found an elevated lifetime and 12-month prevalence of major depression (26% and 24%, respectively), alcohol abuse and/or dependence (48% and 38%), and drug abuse and/or dependence (39% and 20%). Anxiety, measured with the Revised Children's Manifest Anxiety Scale, was twice as prevalent as in age- and sex-matched comparison groups. About 29 percent had attempted suicide in the preceding 12 months, with young women reporting a greater attempt rate than young men. The sample had a 24-percent rate of hospitalization for psychotic problems. Four or more psychotic symptoms were reported by 29 percent of the sample (50).

Limitations of the Literature

DIFFICULTIES IN ESTIMATING PREVALENCE RATES OF MENTAL DISORDER

The broad range of estimates suggested by the empirical literature (91) reflects the difficulty of characterizing the mental health status of homeless people and the inadequacy of current empirical research. The limited definitions and tools used to evaluate mental health status in the general population (66) also affect the assessment of homeless adults and children (83,92). Reported rates of mental disorder vary dramatically depending on whether psychiatric diagnosis, current symptoms, or treatment history is used to define mental disorder (1,73,83). Some estimates include alcohol and drug abuse with mental disorders, while others report substance abuse and mental disorder separately (6,28,46).

Furthermore, the operationalized definition of "homelessness" has not been standardized. Neither the size nor the composition of the homeless population seems to be static. Population characteristics such as high mobility, the lack of an address, diffusion through communities, and movement in and out of "homelessness" prohibit accurate estimates or a census of the homeless population (1) and render certain traditional research methods inadequate (83,93). Prevalence rates might also be affected by changes in the social and economic climate (9)—for instance, periods of high unemployment and housing scarcity are expected to affect the relative number of "newly," or "episodically" homeless people who might be less likely to demonstrate chronic disability (8).

Prevalence rates are further affected by design characteristics and project execution that may result in systematic undercounting or overcounting. For example, several authors suggest that recent empirical studies systematically *underestimate* mental disorder in the homeless population owing to

• Sampling from shelters or other service facility populations that are not representative of the larger homeless population, assuming *greater* disability among those who do *not* use services (28,94,95);
• Self-selection of healthier people in samples at study sites (20);
• Mental health assessment resulting from short-term observations, ignoring the history of symptoms or behaviors not currently visible (8);
• Failure to provide multiple diagnoses (8); and

• Broad definitions of homelessness which "dilute" estimates of the prevalence of disorder (84).

In contrast, others suggest that recent studies systematically *overestimate* mental disorder among the homeless population owing to

• Sampling from shelters or other service facility populations that are not representative of the larger homeless population, assuming *greater* disability among those who use services, since those who are more intact psychologically may use alternative resources (28);
• Sampling from service sites during the day, which excludes those working or looking for work;
• The inaccuracy of mental health assessments of persons whose subsistence needs are not being met (68,76,96)—for instance, symptoms may vary as a function of the time between "coming out from the streets" and the psychiatric evaluation (76);
• The interpretation of symptoms of physical disease or malnutrition as symptoms of mental health problems (97,98);
• The use of assessment tools that either are inappropriate for a nontraditional population (60,97,99) or may not appropriately distinguish mental health problems from environment-specific behaviors (e.g., limited hygiene, bizarre behavior and appearance) (50,68,96,99,100);
• The use of assessment tools that may not distinguish traditional symptoms of pathology from inadvertent consequences of the homeless condition (101); and
• The use of "point prevalence" estimates, which are likely to overstate the characteristics of those with longer histories of homelessness or long-term residents of shelters, who might include more disabled individuals (83). This final point is supported by studies showing that the prevalence of various indicators of mental health problems is higher among those with longer-term histories of homelessness (40,43,72). However, other studies show little or no difference in mental health status as a function of the duration of homelessness (34), or show higher prevalence among more recently homeless people (72).

DIFFICULTIES IN ASSESSING MENTAL HEALTH STATUS:
PSYCHIATRIC HOSPITALIZATION HISTORY

CONSTRUCT VALIDITY. Previous psychiatric hospitalization was the most consistently used mental health indicator in the studies reviewed. Although it is often interpreted as a proxy for serious mental disorder, its validity as an indicator of either major mental disorder or current service needs remains unclear. Breakey et al. (102) called psychiatric hospitalization an "imperfect index" of psychiatric morbidity because, in their Baltimore sample, 10–20 percent of respondents *without* a diagnosis admitted prior psychiatric hospitalization (false positives), while 35 percent of women and 50 percent of men *with* diagnoses of major mental illness reported no previous hospitalization (false negatives).

A confounding factor is suggested by Ball and Havassey (103), who describe the use of psychiatric facilities as "a safe place to sleep" and state that homeless people find ways to get picked up by the police and taken to the psychiatric emergency room or to jail. Rose et al. (104) report that the decision to admit homeless veterans to a Veterans' Administration (VA) facility was often determined in part by the individuals' "social situation" (i.e., lack of a home).

Another confounding factor is introduced when one considers the reason for admission to a hospital. For example, of those who had records of admission to psychiatric hospitals, 62 percent had been admitted primarily for substance abuse problems in the study by Snow et al. (68), and 41 percent had been admitted for alcohol-related problems in the study by Piliavin et al. (51).

Lovell and Barrow warn that the "use of treatment characteristics should not be confused with a measurement of [current] need" (83:5), since several studies show that people with treatment histories are not necessarily those in need of services. For example, Roth et al. (60) report that 47 percent of those with previous psychiatric hospitalization had minimal or no current psychiatric symptoms.

THE RELIABILITY OF SELF-REPORT.   Self-reported information has been called a "questionable measure" because one cannot be sure that the information provided is reliable. An underreporting bias might be assumed, given the stigma attached to mental illness, and homeless mentally ill people's fears about treatment (83).

However, Solarz (69) and Solarz and Mowbray (70) concluded that self-report was a reliable indicator of the presence or absence of psychiatric hospitalization histories, although self-report was less accurate with respect to history of involvement with the mental health system (e.g., total number of hospitalizations, particularly among persons with extensive and complicated psychiatric histories). Similarly, Robertson et al. (55) compared the research interview responses of 24 women residents of a shelter with that shelter's intake records. There was 92 percent agreement on 15 specific items, one of which was psychiatric hospitalization history. Whenever a difference was noted, research interviews revealed sensitive information that was missing from the respondent's shelter record. Garrett and Schutt (105) also found self-reports of mental health problems to be more accurate than aggregate estimates by shelter staff. However, self-report was not equivalent to clinical assessment, and self-reported mental health difficulties were thought to be underreported.

MARJORIE J. ROBERTSON

DIFFICULTIES IN ASSESSING MENTAL HEALTH STATUS: MEASURES OF CURRENT DISTRESS

Although current distress may be related to subsequent mental disorders (106,107) symptom scales measuring distress are more often used to evaluate current function or level of disability, rather than specific diagnosis. The assessment of current mental health status often draws from a broader conceptualization of mental health. Symptom scales are useful because they facilitate comparison studies; they are also useful for modeling change in mental health status over time; furthermore, they may be administered by lay interviewers, thereby reducing research costs. However, as observed by Lovell and Barrow (83) and Lovell et al. (chapter 24), current symptoms may not be sufficiently specific, since they may reflect not only ongoing psychiatric conditions but also reactions to a stressful environment, strategies of adaptation, or behavior perpetuated by an institutional environment (chapters 8 and 24).

DIFFICULTIES IN ASSESSING MENTAL HEALTH STATUS: PSYCHOTIC SYMPTOM SCALES

The reliability and validity of psychotic symptom scales are discussed extensively by Lovell et al. in chapter 24. Their analysis, as well as that of others (44,58,101), shows that several queries (e.g., "Have you ever felt that there were people who wanted to harm or hurt you?") may not necessarily test for paranoid ideation or other "psychotic symptoms" because the study conditions fail to control even minimally for possible ecological or environmental explanations of the symptoms (101,102).

As discussed in detail in chapter 24, the most problematic aspect of the use of isolated psychotic symptoms is the questionable meaning of particular items for homeless persons. Three studies (33,44,58) that used a short list of psychotic symptoms isolated from an original standardized instrument included a question to assess paranoid ideation (e.g., "Have you ever felt that there were people who wanted to harm or hurt you?" (44,58). Because the "fear harm" item had the highest score relative to a domiciled comparison group, Rossi et al. concluded that "paranoid delusions among the Chicago homeless occur in superabundance . . . [although it] may well be that the fear of harm reported by some of the homeless is not delusional, but reflects the greater risk of theft, assault and robbery that the homeless face" (58). Similarly, McChesney concluded that the symptom "appeared to elicit not paranoid ideation but an accurate assessment of the realities of life on the street" (44). McChesney subsequently dropped the item from her symptom scale; Rossi et al. did not.

Koegel and Burnam (101), who applied the DIS, which includes a section on psychotic symptomatology, noted that one-quarter of the individuals *without* a diagnosis of schizophrenia in their study reported the belief that they were being

78

watched; a similar number reported the belief that they were being followed or plotted against. Upon probing, such beliefs had seemed plausible enough to interviewers to indicate that although the symptoms were present, they probably were not psychiatrically relevant. The authors concluded that "studies which rely on gross measures of psychotic symptoms as evidence of chronic mental illness may not distinguish such cases from those which truly reflect psychosis" (101). Estimates of disorder based on symptom scales fail to control even minimally for competing etiologic explanations of the symptom (102).

DIFFICULTIES IN ASSESSING MENTAL HEALTH STATUS: PSYCHIATRIC DIAGNOSIS

RELIABILITY. Psychiatric diagnosis may be the most unreliable of the three methods unless carefully standardized (79). The issue is only partially addressed by the application of standardized instruments such as the DIS, as shown by Lovell et al. (chapter 24).

VALIDITY. The validity of DSM-III symptoms for homeless adults remains unclear, since symptoms of some disorders are characteristic of the homeless experience (chapter 24). This may lead to overdiagnosis of some psychiatric disorders, such as antisocial personality, among homeless adults (101). Also, in response to the low reported rate of major mental disorder in their sample, Fischer and Breakey note that there may be some problem in the sensitivity of the DIS in identifying illnesses such as schizophrenia, affective disorders, or cognitive impairment in the population (78).

An Assessment of Findings

To draw this review to a close, I return to the original three questions about the prevalence of mental disorder among homeless people.

THE PREVALENCE OF MENTAL DISORDER AMONG HOMELESS PEOPLE

Efforts to estimate the prevalence of mental disorder among homeless people must be informed by the existing studies, most of which are local. However, the literature has serious limitations. As pointed out in chapter 4, there is an apparent overrepresentation of studies of single adult individuals, particularly males, sampled from traditional missions or shelters. Clearly underrepresented subpopulations include single women, homeless families with and without children, homeless and runaway youths, and elderly people. Also underrepresented are people in street sites, improvised shelters (e.g., vehicles and abandoned buildings), small shelter settings (e.g., a church with a few people per night), or odd places (e.g., hospital emergency rooms).

There has been little agreement on the definition or operationalization of the concepts of "homelessness" and "mental disorder" across studies. The validity of the mental health indicators and assessment tools used has been largely untested in homeless populations (chapter 24). Depending on the indicator used to assess mental health status, estimated prevalence rates vary widely.

All studies have been cross-sectional. Few have drawn random or representative samples. Many drew convenience samples from a single shelter or mission (chapter 4). Perhaps most importantly, few were designed as epidemiologic studies (6).

Because of these serious limitations, the empirical literature reviewed here forms an inadequate basis for estimating the prevalence of mental health problems among homeless people. Any credible estimate of the prevalence of disorder in the homeless population in general, or even in subpopulations (e.g., single males) is still premature (1,6).

RELATIVE PREVALENCE

In all cases where comparisons were made, homeless adults, adolescents, and children demonstrated higher rates of mental health problems than did the domiciled comparison groups. This tendency was seen with the three types of mental health indicators. This apparently significant excess in mental disorder among homeless people is not surprising when we consider the broader mental health literature, in which the frequency of mental disorder is inversely related to socioeconomic status (81).

DISTRIBUTION

Detail on subgroup variation is sparse. Most studies lacked adequate sample size or demographic diversity. Some simply failed to describe subgroup differences. The most significant findings were those related to gender. As noted above, the available evidence suggests that there are higher rates of psychiatric hospitalization, suicide attempts, and serious mental disorders among women. This is compatible with the general mental health literature, which documents a consistent excess of mental health problems in women (90). However, men appeared to have higher rates of substance abuse. Women with children had lower rates of psychiatric hospitalization or suicide attempts than did other women (4,75,79).

It also appears that most of the evidence contradicts the notion that homeless people on the street manifest greater disability than do those in sheltered settings.

FACTORS AFFECTING PREVALENCE RATES

As suggested by the current review, and others (6,78,107), there are significant gaps in our knowledge about homeless people and their mental health status. More carefully designed and executed epidemiologic research is needed. As discussed throughout this chapter, multiple factors appear to affect the rates of mental disorder reported in individual studies. These include geographic area; the local social, economic, and political context; the definition of the target population; the sample site(s); the sample selection; the definition of mental disorder; mental health indicators or assessment tools; and the circumstances under which mental health evaluations are conducted. Researchers are cautioned to consider these factors in the design and execution of research on the mental health status of homeless people.

References

1. General Accounting Office. *Homeless Mentally Ill: Problems and Options in Estimating Numbers and Trends.* Report to the Chairman, Senate Committee on Labor and Human Resources, GAO/PEMD-88-24. Washington, D.C.: General Accounting Office, 1988.

2. Wright J. The mentally ill homeless: What is myth and what is fact? *Social Problems 35:*182–191, 1988.

3. Piliavin I, Westerfelt H, Elliott E. Estimating mental health among the homeless: The effects of choice-based sampling. *Social Problems 36:*525–531, 1989.

4. Fischer P. Estimating prevalence of alcohol, drug, and mental health problems in the contemporary homeless population: A review of the literature. Paper presented at the National Conference on Homelessness, Alcohol and Other Drugs, San Diego, Calif., 1989.

5. Snow D, Baker S, Anderson L. On the precariousness of measuring insanity in insane contexts. *Social Problems 35:*192–196, 1988.

6. Robertson MJ. Mental disorder among homeless persons in the United States: An overview of the empirical literature. *Administration in Mental Health 14:*14–27, 1986.

7. Morrissey JP, Dennis DL. *NIMH Funded Research Concerning Mentally Ill Persons: Implications for Policy and Practice.* Washington, D.C.: Alcohol, Drug, and Mental Health Administration (ADAMHA), U.S. Department of Health and Human Services, 1986.

8. Arce AA, Vergare MJ. Identifying and characterizing the mentally ill among the homeless. In Lamb HR (ed.), *The Homeless Mentally Ill.* Task Force Report to the American Psychiatric Association. Washington, D.C.: American Psychiatric Association, 1984, pp. 75–90.

9. Priest RG. The epidemiology of mental illness: Illustrations from the single homeless population. *Psychiatric Journal of the University of Ottawa 3:*27–32, 1978.

10. Priest RG. A USA-UK comparison. *Royal Society of Medicine, London: Proceedings 63:*441–445, 1970.

11. U.S. Department of Housing and Urban Development. *A Report to the Secretary on the Homeless and Emergency Shelters.* Washington, D.C.: HUD, Office of Policy Development and Research, 1984.

12. U.S. Department of Housing and Urban Development. *A Report on the 1988 National Survey of Shelters for the Homeless.* Washington, D.C.: HUD, Office of Policy Development and Research, Division of Policy Studies, 1989.

13. U.S. Department of Health and Human Services. *The Homeless: Background, Analysis, and Options*. Washington, D.C.: HHS, 1984.

14. Arce AA, et al. A psychiatric profile of street people admitted to an emergency shelter. *Hospital and Community Psychiatry 34:*812–817, 1983.

15. Bachrach LL, et al. The homeless mentally ill in Tucson: Implications of early findings. *American Journal of Psychiatry 145:* 112–113, 1988.

16. Bassuk EL, Rubin L, Lauriat A. Is homelessness a mental health problem? *American Journal of Psychiatry 141:*1546–1550, 1984.

17. Bassuk EL, Rubin L, Lauriat A. The characteristics of sheltered homeless families. *American Journal of Public Health 76:*1097–1101, 1986.

18. Benda B, Crowley S, Erickson P. *The Homeless of Richmond*. Richmond, Va.: Richmond Community Service Board, 1986.

19. Breakey W, et al. Health and mental health problems of homeless men and women in Baltimore. *JAMA 262:*1352–1356, 1989.

20. Brown C, et al. *The Homeless of Phoenix: Who Are They? And What Do They Want?* Phoenix: South Community Mental Health Center, 1983.

21. Burt M, Cohen B. Differences among homeless single women, women with children, and single men. *Social Problems 36:*508–524, 1989.

22. City of Chicago. *Homelessness in Chicago*. Chicago: Chicago Department of Human Services, Social Services Task Force, 1983.

23. Crystal S. Homeless men and homeless women: The gender gap. *Urban and Social Change Review 17(2):*2–6, 1984.

24. Crystal S, Goldstein M. *Correlates of Shelter Utilization: One-Day Study.* New York: City of New York, Human Resources Administration, Family and Adult Services, 1984.

25. Crystal S, Goldstein M. *The Homeless in New York City Shelters*. New York: City of New York, Human Resources Administration, Family and Adult Services, 1984.

26. Crystal S, Goldstein M, Levitt R. *Chronic and Situational Dependency: Long-Term Residents in a Shelter for Men*. New York: City of New York, Human Resources Administration, Family and Adult Services, 1982.

27. Crystal S, Ladner S, Towber R. Multiple impairment patterns in the mentally ill homeless. *International Journal of Mental Health 14(4):*61–73, 1986.

28. Farr RK, Koegel P, Burnam A. *A Study of Homelessness and Mental Illness in the Skid Row Area of Los Angeles*. Los Angeles: Los Angeles County Department of Mental Health, 1986.

29. First RJ, Roth D, Arewa BK. Homelessness: Understanding the dimensions of the problem for minorities. *Social Work 33:*120–121, 1988.

30. Fischer PJ, Breakey WR. Profile of the Baltimore homeless with alcohol problems. *Alcohol Health and Research World 11(3):*36–37, 61, 1987.

31. Fischer PJ, et al. Mental health and social characteristics of the homeless: A survey of mission users. *American Journal of Public Health 76:*519–524, 1986.

32. Gelberg L, Linn L. Psychological distress among homeless adults. *Journal of Nervous and Mental Diseases 177:*291–295, 1989.

33. Gelberg L, Linn LS, Leake BD. Mental health, alcohol and drug use, and criminal history among homeless adults. *American Journal of Psychiatry 145:*191–196, 1988.

34. Kahn M, et al. Psychopathology on the streets: Psychological assessment of the homeless. *Professional Psychology: Research and Practice 18:*580–586, 1987.

35. Knickman J, Weitzman B. *A Study of Homeless Families in New York City: Risk Assessment Models and Strategies for Prevention*. Final Report, vol. 1. New York: New York University, Health Research Program, 1989.

36. Koegel P, Burnam MA. Alcoholism among homeless adults in the inner city of Los Angeles. *Archives of General Psychiatry 45:*1011–1018, 1988.

37. Koegel P, Burnam MA. *The Epidemiology of Alcohol Abuse and Dependence among Homeless Individuals: Findings from the Inner City of Los Angeles.* Report prepared for the National Institute of Alcohol Abuse and Alcoholism, Rockville, Md., 1987.

38. Koegel P, Burnam MA. Traditional and non-traditional homeless alcoholics. *Alcohol, Health, and Research World 2(3):*28–35, 1987.

39. Koegel P, Burnam MA, Farr R. The prevalence of specific psychiatric disorders among homeless adults in the inner-city of Los Angeles. Manuscript, 1986.

40. Koegel P, Burnam MA, Farr R. The prevalence of specific psychiatric disorders among homeless individuals in the inner-city of Los Angeles. *Archives of General Psychiatry 45:*1085–1092, 1988.

41. Koegel P, Farr RK, Burnam MA. Heterogeneity in an inner-city homeless population: A comparison between individuals surveyed in traditional Skid Row locations and in voucher hotel rooms. *Psychosocial Rehabilitation Journal 10(2):* 31–45, 1986.

42. Kroll J, et al. A survey of homeless adults in urban emergency shelters. *Hospital and Community Psychiatry 37:*283–286, 1986.

43. LaGory M, Ritchey FJ, Mollis J. Depression among the homeless. *Journal of Health and Social Behavior 31:*87–101, 1990.

44. McChesney KY. *Characteristics of the Residents of Two Inner-City Emergency Shelters for the Homeless.* Los Angeles: Los Angeles Office of the City Attorney, 1987.

45. Morse G. *Homeless Men: A Study of Service Needs, Predictor Variables, and Subpopulations.* St. Louis: University of Missouri–St. Louis, Department of Psychology, 1982.

46. Morse G, Calsyn RJ. Mentally disturbed homeless people in St. Louis: Needy, willing, but underserved. *International Journal of Mental Health 14(4):*74–94, 1986.

47. Morse G, et al. *Homeless People in St. Louis: A Mental Health Program Evaluation, Field Study, and Follow-up Investigation,* vol. 1, *Text of Report.* St. Louis: Missouri Department of Mental Health, 1985.

48. Mulkern V, et al. *The Homelessness Needs Assessment Study: Findings and Recommendations for the Massachusetts Department of Mental Health.* Boston: Human Services Research Institute, 1985.

49. Multnomah County. *The Homeless Poor.* Portland, Oreg.: Multnomah County Social Services Division, 1983.

50. Mundy P, et al. The prevalence of psychotic symptoms in homeless adolescents. *Journal of the American Academy of Child and Adolescent Psychiatry 29:*724–731, 1990.

51. Piliavin I, Sosin M, Westerfelt H. *Conditions Contributing to Long-term Homelessness: An Exploratory Study.* Madison: University of Wisconsin–Madison, Institute for Research on Poverty, 1989.

52. Robertson MJ. Homeless veterans: An emerging problem: In Bingham R, Green RE, White SB (eds.), *The Homeless in Contemporary Society.* Newbury Park, Calif.: Sage Publications, 1987.

53. Robertson MJ, Boyer R. Assault and recent injury as predictors of suicide ideation and attempts among homeless adults. Paper presented at the annual meeting of the American Public Health Association, 1984.

54. Robertson MJ. *Alcohol Use and Abuse Patterns among Homeless Adolescents in the Hollywood Area: A Report to the National Institute on Alcohol Abuse and Alcoholism.* Berkeley, Calif.: Alcohol Research Group, 1989.

55. Robertson MJ, Ropers RH, Boyer R. *The Homeless in Los Angeles County: An Empirical Assessment.* Los Angeles: University of California–Los Angeles, School of Public Health, 1985.

56. Rosnow MJ, Shaw T, Concord CS. *Listening to the Homeless: A Study of Homeless Mentally Ill Persons in Milwaukee.* Milwaukee: Wisconsin Office of Mental Health, 1985.

57. Rossi PH. The condition of the homeless in Chicago. Internal Research Report.

Amherst, Mass.: University of Massachusetts, Social and Demographic Research Institute, 1987.

58. Rossi PH, Fisher GA, Willis G. *The Condition of the Homeless in Chicago: A Report Based on Surveys Conducted in 1985 and 1986.* Amherst, Mass.: University of Massachusetts, Social and Demographic Research Institute, 1986.

59. Roth D. Homeless veterans: Comparisons with other homeless men. In Robertson M, Greenblatt M (eds.), *Homelessness: The National Perspective.* New York: Plenum, in press.

60. Roth D, et al. *Homelessness in Ohio: A Study of People in Need.* Columbus: Ohio Department of Mental Health, Office of Program Evaluation and Research, 1985.

61. Roth D, Toomey BG, First RJ. Gender, racial, and age variations among homeless adults. In Robertson, Greenblatt (eds.), *Homelessness.* See ref. 59.

62. Sachs-Ericsson N, et al. *Report of Research on the Homeless Mentally Ill in Colorado, Study 1: Survey of Denver Areas Sample.* Denver: Colorado Division of Mental Health, 1987.

63. Schutt RK. A short report on homeless veterans. Manuscript, 1986. A Supplement to Schutt RK, *Homelessness in Boston: The View from Long Island.* Boston: University of Massachusetts, 1986.

64. Schutt RK. *Boston's Homeless: Their Backgrounds, Problems, and Needs.* Boston: University of Massachusetts, 1985.

65. Schutt RK, Garrett GR. *Homeless in Boston in 1985: The View from Long Island.* Boston: University of Massachusetts, 1986.

66. Segal SP, Baumohl J, Johnson E. Falling through the cracks: Mental disorder and social margin in a young vagrant population. *Social Problems 24:*387–400, 1977.

67. Shaffer D, Caton C. *Runaway and Homeless Youth in New York City.* New York: Ittleson Foundation, 1984.

68. Snow DA, Baker SG, Anderson L. The myth of pervasive mental illness among the homeless. *Social Problems 33:*301–317, 1986.

69. Solarz A. Social supports among the homeless. Paper presented at the annual meeting of the American Public Health Association, 1985.

70. Solarz A, Mowbray C. An examination of physical and mental health problems of the homeless. Paper presented at the annual meeting of the American Public Health Association, 1985.

71. Sosin M, Colson P, Grossman S. *Homelessness in Chicago: Poverty and Pathology, Social Institutions and Social Change.* Chicago: University of Chicago, School of Social Service Administration, 1988.

72. Susser E, Struening E, Conver S. Psychiatric problems in homeless men. *Archives of General Psychiatry 46:*845–850, 1989.

73. Toro P, Wall D. Assessing the impact of some sampling and measurement methods in research on the homeless. Manuscript, 1989.

74. Vernez G, et al. *Review of California's Program for the Mentally Disabled.* Santa Monica, Calif.: Rand Corporation, 1988.

75. Weitzman B, Shinn M, Knickman J. Mental health problems as risk factors for homelessness. Paper presented at the annual meeting of the American Public Health Association, 1989.

76. Milburn NG, Watts RJ. Methodological issues in research on the homeless and the homeless mentally ill. *International Journal of Mental Health 14(4):*42–60, 1986.

77. Bachrach LL. The homeless mentally ill and mental health services: An analytical review of the literature. In Lamb (ed.), *The Homeless Mentally Ill,* pp. 11–53. See ref. 8.

78. Fischer PJ, Breakey WR. Homelessness and mental health. *International Journal of Mental Health 14(4):*6–42, 1986.

79. Breakey WR. Recent empirical research on the homeless mentally ill. Paper presented at Alcohol, Drug, and Mental Health Administration (ADAMHA) meeting on research meth-

odologies, concerning homeless persons with serious mental illness and/or related substance abuse disorders, Bethesda, Md., July 23, 1987.

80. Rivlin A. Making a difference: Concern for the homeless. Invited address before the annual meeting of the American Psychological Association, 1985.

81. Lovell A. Classification and its risks: An analysis of psychiatric categorization in homelessness research. In Rosenblatt A (ed.), *A Critique of American Health and Welfare Policy: Making Sure the Solution Isn't the Problem*, vol. 3, *Homelessness*. Albany, N.Y.: Nelson A. Rockefeller Institute of Government, in press.

82. Lovell A, Barrow S, Struening E. Between relevance and rigor: Methodological issues in studying mental health and homelessness. Manuscript (early draft of chapter 24 of this book), 1985.

83. Lovell AM, Barrow SM. Measurement issues in services research on the homeless mentally ill. In *Proceedings of the 8th Annual MSIS National Users Conference*. Orangeburg, N.Y.: Nathan Kline Institute for Psychiatric Research, Information and Sciences Division, 1984.

84. Frazier SH. Responding to the needs of the homeless mentally ill. *Public Health Reports 100:*462–469, 1985.

85. Fischer P, Breakey W, Ross A. Criminal activity among the homeless. Paper presented at the 68th annual meeting of the American Anthropological Association, Washington, D.C., 1989.

86. Snow D, Baker S, Anderson L. Criminality and homeless men: An empirical assessment. *Social Problems 36:*532–541, 1989.

87. Fischer PJ. Criminalization of homelessness. In Robertson, Greenblatt (eds.), *Homelessness*. See ref. 59.

88. Appleby L, Slagg N, Desai PN. The urban nomad: A psychiatric problem? *Current Psychiatric Therapies 2:*253–262, 1982.

89. Wood D, et al. *California Children, California Families over the Brink: Homeless Families in Los Angeles*. Sacramento: California Assembly Office of Research, 1989.

90. Miller D, Lin E. Children in sheltered homeless families: Reported health status and use of health services. *Pediatrics 81:*668–673, 1988.

91. Goldman HH, Gaitozi AA, Taube CA. Defining and counting the chronically mentally ill. *Hospital and Community Psychiatry 32:*21–27, 1981.

92. Bachrach L. Interpreting research on the chronically mentally ill: Some caveats. *Hospital and Community Psychiatry 35:*914–917, 1984.

93. Koegel P, Burnam A. A design for drawing a probability sample of homeless individuals. Paper presented at the National Institute of Mental Health Conference on Mental Health Statistics, San Francisco, 1985.

94. Lovell AM, Barrow SM. Psychiatric disability and homelessness: A look at Manhattan's Upper West Side. Manuscript, 1981.

95. Baxter E, Hopper K. Shelter and housing for the homeless mentally ill. In Lamb (ed.), *The Homeless Mentally Ill*, pp. 109–139. See ref. 8.

96. Baxter E, Hopper K. The new mendicancy: Homeless in New York City. *American Journal of Orthopsychiatry 53:*393–408, 1982.

97. Kaufman CA. Implications of biological psychiatry for the severely mentally ill: A highly vulnerable population. In Lamb (ed.), *The Homeless Mentally Ill*, pp. 201–242. See ref. 8.

98. Wells JH, Strickland DK. Physiogenic bias as invalidity in psychiatric symptom scales. *Journal of Health and Social Behavior 23:*235–252, 1982.

99. Chafetz L, Goldfinger SM. Residential instability in a psychiatric emergency setting. *Psychiatric Quarterly 56:*20–34, 1984.

100. Barrow S, Lovell AM. *Evaluation of Programs for the Mentally Ill Homeless: Pro-*

MARJORIE J. ROBERTSON

gress Report. New York: New York State Psychiatric Institute, Community Support System Evaluation Program, 1984.

101. Koegel P, Burnam MA. Problems in the assessment of mental illness among the homeless: An empirical approach. In Robertson, Greenblatt (eds.), *Homelessness.* See ref. 59.

102. Breakey W, et al. Severe mental illness in the homeless. Paper presented at the 116th annual meeting of the American Public Health Association, Boston, Mass., November 16, 1988. Abstract, p. 244.

103. Ball FJ, Havassey BE. A survey of the problems and needs of homeless consumers of acute psychiatric services. *Hospital and Community Psychiatry 35:*917–921, 1984.

104. Rose SO, Hawkins J, Apodaca. Decision to admit: Criteria for admission and readmission to a Veterans Administration hospital. *Archives of General Psychiatry 34:*418–421, 1977.

105. Garrett G, Schutt R. Homelessness in the 1980s: Social services for a changing population. Paper presented at the meeting of the Eastern Sociological Society, New York, N.Y., 1986.

106. Aneshensel C. The natural history of depression symptoms: Implications for psychiatric epidemiology. In Greeley JR (ed.), *Research in Community Mental Health,* vol. 5. Greenwich, Conn.: JAL Press, 1985.

107. Bachrach LL. *Report and Analytic Summary of a Meeting of DHHS-Supported Researchers Studying the Homeless Mentally Ill.* Rockville, Md.: National Institute of Mental Health, Office of State and Community Liaison, 1984.

CHAPTER 6

Criminal Behavior and Victimization among Homeless People

Pamela J. Fischer, Ph.D.

The crime and violence once endemic to American Skid Rows appear to have survived the demise of Skid Row (1,2) to become a feature of the contemporary homeless lifestyle (3,4). The literature of the past decade documents high rates of criminal activity in homeless populations by presenting rates of arrests reported by homeless individuals sampled in shelters and streets as well rates of homeless episodes reported by incarcerated people (5–13). However, little effort has been expended to determine the prevalence, type, or function of criminal behavior in the contemporary homeless population.

It may be instructive to consider patterns of criminal activity among the mentally ill population in general because the high rates of mental illness found in the homeless population (14–16) suggest that the populations overlap. This is most apparent in certain subgroups of the mentally ill population, such as the "young chronics," who have been associated with high rates of criminal activity, arrest, and suicide as well as a tendency to be transient and at least occasionally homeless (7,17–21). The detection of substantial and possibly increasing (22,23) proportions of jail and prison inmates with histories of mental illness has prompted investigations into whether mental illness is being criminalized as a consequence of deinstitutionalization and the reforms in involuntary commitment laws (24–26). There is concern that control of the severely mentally ill may be shifting from the mental health system to the criminal justice system (9,10,27–31). Indeed, jails have been described as dumping grounds for the chronically mentally ill (32,33). It is likely that in the absence of other means of control, homelessness itself might also be criminalized (12,34,35). Consequently, it becomes a matter of importance to evaluate interactions between homelessness, mental illness, and criminal activity or risk of arrest.

It is also important to consider the criminal activity of homeless people from another perspective. Contemporary studies of the homeless population point to the important role of law enforcement personnel as providers of services, including general and mental health care, and to jails as service sites for large numbers of homeless people (36). The National Coalition for Jail Reform (37) estimates that as many as 20 percent of inmates of American jails, around 2 million people, are pseudooffenders (the developmentally or physically disabled, the mentally ill, or those charged with minor offenses such as loitering, disorderly conduct, and so forth), a category that easily accommodates homeless people. Thus, the jail may be "our most enduring asylum" (37:388).

Finally, it is essential to consider homeless people as victims as well as perpetrators of crime. The considerable trauma that results from victimization may translate into substantial needs for health and mental health services, as well as other specialized human services. In addition, the roles that victimization plays in both precipitating and perpetuating homelessness must be examined.

Criminal Activity among Homeless People

Differences in definitions of both homelessness and criminal activity make it difficult to compare or generalize findings of recent studies. It has been shown how definitional criteria affect both sampling and measurement, producing widely ranging prevalence estimates for other conditions of interest, such as mental disorders (14). By the same token, definitions of criminal activity vary in recent studies. For example, studies often fail to distinguish between arrest and conviction or between jailing and imprisonment, making it difficult to assess the magnitude of criminal activity in the homeless population.

Criminal activity among homeless populations is most often documented using two distinct but related sources of information. The first consists of indicators of current criminal activities derived largely from incidental findings concerning other aspects of the homeless lifestyle rather than criminal activity per se. For example, measures of socioeconomic status have produced information on illegal methods of income procurement such as panhandling, prostitution, and the like, and epidemiologic studies have determined the prevalence of illicit drug use. Information elicited specifically about crime-related behavior constitutes the second and more direct source. Typically, this includes reported rates of prior arrest and incarceration as well as less specific accounts of "trouble with the law."

ILLEGAL INCOME

Homeless people universally report high rates of unemployment (16,38–48). Although they report higher rates of public support than does the general population, the proportion enrolled in these programs appears to be low relative to their scant financial resources (43). Thus, many supplement their income through illegal means. For example, 13 percent of homeless respondents in Los Angeles (42) and 33 percent of those who reported occasional income in Chicago (49) reported panhandling. An additional 12 percent of the Chicago sample admitted to illegal activities, including prostitution, and two-fifths of the Los Angeles sample reported "other" sources of income, which the interviewers judged to include undisclosed illegal means of income supplementation. In a Baltimore study, 34 percent of the men and 28 percent of the women in the sample had resorted to at least one illegal means of obtaining income, including panhandling, stealing, selling drugs, or prostitution (5,6). Around one-fifth of a sample of Detroit shelter residents reported benefiting from some source of illegal income during the prior six months (about 10% indicated that their main source of income was derived illegally); controlled substance traffic appeared to be the biggest contributor to illegal income. In addition, in almost one-fifth of cases there was evidence that respondents were engaged in abuse of welfare programs by failing to report income earned in addition to their public assistance allotments (12).

Although there is little contextual information surrounding these reports, there is some evidence of differential distribution of illegal income procurement among the homeless population. For example, among Baltimore homeless people, those with arrest histories were about twice as likely to report current illegal activities as were those without such histories (5,6). Homeless youths report illegal activities, particularly prostitution, at alarming rates compared to both nonhomeless age mates as well as homeless adults (50). Studies of homeless adolescents in Hollywood (51) and homeless adults in Baltimore (5,6) suggest that abusers of alcohol and other drugs are more likely to engage in prostitution and other illegal activities than are homeless individuals who are not substance abusers. In Detroit, men appeared to be more likely than women to be involved in current illegal activities (12).

DRUG USE AMONG HOMELESS PEOPLE

Drug trafficking, except on a small scale, is found relatively rarely among homeless people, perhaps because successful dealers can marshal sufficient resources to avoid homelessness. However, the use of street drugs often contributes to arrest and incarceration because it is itself an illegal activity and because crimes are committed under the influence of drugs as well as to support the drug habit (52). Although it is generally accepted that alcohol is the drug of choice, probably from economic necessity as well as from habit or preference, contemporary studies of homeless populations show as many as half of respondents reporting the use of illicit drugs (14,53,54). For example, in a Phoenix study, 5 percent of the homeless people surveyed reported regular drug use, and 16 percent revealed occasional use (40). In a Los Angeles study, 10 percent of the sample had used drugs within the last six months and 31 percent had used drugs at some point in their lives (42). Half of the residents in a Detroit shelter reported using marijuana, and 10 percent had used other illegal drugs during the previous month (12). More than one-fifth of respondents reported current drug use in studies in Chicago (49) and in Saint Louis (55), where two-fifths of the drug users reported more than one episode per week.

Although no significant differences in drug use were found between homeless men and women in studies in Baltimore (39) and Washington, D.C. (56), nearly twice as many men as women reported regular past or current use of drugs in a one-day shelter survey in New York. While women were less than half as likely as men to have been incarcerated, those with prison records were more likely to report drug use (57). Three-fifths of the homeless people sampled in a soup line in Tucson used street drugs, and two-thirds reported "difficulty with the police" as a result of alcohol or drug use (58). In a Baltimore study, three-quarters of homeless drug users but three-fifths of nonusers had experienced arrest (5). Schutt and Garrett (59) found that 30 percent of the homeless individuals surveyed in a Boston shelter took hard drugs and that drug users were almost three times as likely as people with neither drug nor mental health problems to have current legal problems.

ARRESTS AND INCARCERATIONS

Recent studies of homeless samples report rates of arrest and/or incarceration in the range of one-fifth to two-thirds (5,6,12,39,42,44,46,48,49,57,59,60–63). These studies suggest that rates of arrest in the homeless population exceed expected rates: in the general population, it is estimated that 22 percent of men and 6 percent of women have individual arrest histories (64).

The chronological precedence of homelessness vis-à-vis arrests is not clear. There is evidence that arrests and incarcerations are of recent occurrence: 22 percent of the homeless respondents in a Saint Louis study reported that they had been arrested after becoming homeless, and 10 percent had been convicted and imprisoned (61); more than three-quarters of a Los Angeles sample of homeless people with arrest histories reported such events within six months prior to interview (42). In a Detroit sample, nearly half reported an arrest within the previous year (12). In a Baltimore study, the majority of previously arrested homeless men and women reported an arrest within the year (5,6). Furthermore, the risk of arrest has been found to increase with the duration of homelessness (5,65). A Baltimore study found that 88 percent of men and 54 percent of women homeless longer than a year had been arrested, compared to 64 percent of men and 35 percent of women homeless less than a year, although only 15 percent of arrested people believed homelessness per se to have precipitated arrest, and 11 percent reported that they had tried to get arrested to have a place to stay for a while (5).

However, for some homeless people, arrests reflect a pattern established early in life. In a Detroit study (12), nearly three-fifths of homeless shelter residents had first been arrested before age 21, with the average age at first adult arrest being 22 years. In a Baltimore study, nearly two-fifths of homeless men and one-fifth of homeless women had first been arrested as juveniles (5,6,66).

In addition to high rates of arrest, recidivism appears to be frequent. In a Detroit (12) study, homeless shelter residents with arrest histories averaged 5.3 prior arrests. More than half of a Los Angeles homeless sample reported having been arrested as adults; of these, 64 percent had multiple arrests (46). In a Baltimore study, twice as many homeless individuals had been arrested as adults as had members of the domiciled comparison group, and four times as many homeless individuals had multiple arrests (44). In a study of all arrests in Baltimore in 1983, 53 percent of homeless arrestees had been arrested more than once—averaging 3.5 arrests for that year alone (34).

PATTERNS OF CRIMINAL ACTIVITY

Although recent studies frequently report rates of arrest or incarceration, there is little information on the type of criminal activity or its distribution in the homeless population. The ratio of jail to prison incarceration gives a good indicator of the seriousness of the offenses committed. In these recent studies, homeless respondents report having been jailed more frequently. For example, Baltimore homeless respondents were about twice as likely to have been in jails as in prisons (5,6). However, felonies account for perhaps one-third of convictions in recent reports (5,6,44,46,59,67).

Besides indicating the level of crime, the identification of jails as much more important facilities for the homeless than prisons has implications for the delivery of services (35,49,68,69). For example, in a Baltimore sample, about one-third of arrested homeless adults reported having received health and/or mental health services while in jail. Moreover, physical examinations revealed that the group with prior arrests had fewer health problems (5,6).

Solarz (12), in a study of 125 residents of a temporary shelter in Detroit, described their pattern of criminal activity as involving primarily nonviolent crimes against property, resulting in brief jail sentences. One-quarter of all homeless individuals surveyed had served one or more jail terms: two-fifths of all men in the study, compared with only 4 percent of all the women. More than half reported having been jailed sometime during the five or more years prior to survey; only 12 percent had been released during the past year. About half of the homeless individuals with jail histories had served only one sentence; 15 percent had served two or more. Two-thirds of the respondents with jail histories had served six months or less aggregated over all jail sentences. The largest category of offenses was burglary (52%), followed by miscellaneous offenses (39%), including disorderly conduct and contempt of court; fewer than one-fifth had been convicted of assaultive offenses. However, more serious offenses had also been committed, as reflected by the prior incarceration in prison reported by 14 percent of the study sample. All were men; thus, one-fifth of the homeless men surveyed had prison records. More than half had served more than one prison term, and nearly one-third had been released from prison within the year prior to the interview; one-fourth were currently on parole. About half of those with prison time had serviced sentences of five years or less, but two-fifths had served terms of more than 10 years. As with the jailed respondents, slightly more than half of those with prison histories had been convicted of property theft; however, the conviction records of respondents previously incarcerated in prison were more likely to contain convictions for crimes of violence. Nearly one-fourth of men with prison records had been convicted of murder (5% of all sampled men).

Differences in arrest patterns between homeless and domiciled adults were examined using Baltimore Police Department data on all arrests made during 1983 (34). Arrests of homeless persons were defined as those in which, at the time of arrest, the suspect reported no address or reported an address previously determined to be that of a mission, shelter, or soup kitchen. The study determined that the arrests of homeless suspects were mainly for relatively trivial crimes, with public order offenses being prominent. Offenses composing the crime index—serious and frequently occurring crimes monitored by the FBI (homicide, rape, robbery, aggravated assault, burglary, larceny, motor vehicle theft, and arson [70])—accounted for a smaller proportion of arrests among the homeless (25%) than among the general population (35%). Moreover, among the homeless arrestees, the more serious charges often resulted from relatively inoffensive actions, for instance, homeless people sleeping in vacant buildings were charged with burglary, and larceny arrests were generally for shoplifting. In 28 percent of the arresting officers' narratives, there was clear indication that the suspect was either mentally disturbed or intoxicated (34).

It appears that homeless people contribute little to overall crime rates (e.g., the study of Baltimore arrests for a single year determined that 1.3 percent of all arrests were attributed to homeless suspects [34]), and there is little evidence that the homeless population serves as a reservoir of dangerous criminals (5,12,52). Nevertheless, there is evidence that homeless people's criminal activity may have a substantial impact on a community. In Atlanta, an estimated 70–80 percent of 1982 arson was committed by vagrants occupying abandoned buildings, resulting in one death and eight injuries and property damage exceeding $100,000; the cost to the criminal justice system of crimes by homeless people was estimated to reach $3–4 million annually (69).

THE DISTRIBUTION OF CRIMINAL ACTIVITY. Descriptive studies provide evidence that criminal experience varies across homeless subgroups. Homeless men were found to be 1.3–5.7 times as likely as homeless women to engage in criminal activity (5,6,46,60,61,71,72). For example, in a Detroit shelter sample, men were twice as likely as women to have been arrested (12). Moreover, there are some indicators of sex differences in patterns of criminal activity. In New York City shelters, women with criminal histories were more likely to be felons than were men (57,60).

In Ohio, a greater likelihood of incarceration history was found among homeless individuals using shelters (64%) or living in the streets (58%) than among those using resources such as cheap hotels or temporary accommodations with friends or relatives (44%) (48). In a Baltimore sample, arrest rates were greater among those with high scores on an index of exposure to homelessness developed from interview items related to duration; chronicity; and "harshness" as measured by sleeping rough (i.e., sleeping without shelter), scavenging for food, and so forth (5).

Homeless adolescents frequently have been in trouble with the law, particularly as they may be detained as runaways (73,74). More than half of homeless youths in a Hollywood study had been in juvenile detention or jail, with one-third having become homeless upon discharge (51). Although it is not clear that homeless youths become homeless adults (50), early problem behaviors have been associated with later homelessness (75). In Baltimore, arrest rates were found to be higher among homeless men and women reporting childhood experiences of school expulsion, running away from home, or living outside their parental home, for instance, in foster care or juvenile detention centers (5).

Despite widespread decriminalization of public inebriation (76), recent studies suggest that alcohol abuse remains the greatest risk factor for arrest among the homeless population. For example, arrest rates were found to be twice as high among homeless alcoholics as among homeless nonalcoholics in Baltimore, with the magnitude of the difference being greater among women (63% v. 29%, or 2.2:1) than among men (91% v. 64%, or 1.4:1) (5,6). Robertson (77) found that 88 percent of homeless clients of a California alcohol treatment program had been incarcerated in jails or prisons; 69 percent claimed their offense had been alcohol-related. Recent studies of shelter populations in Boston found that more than half of the respondents with jail histories were alcohol abusers (67). Gelberg and colleagues (78) found that half of a California homeless sample had experienced alcohol-related arrests; and in a Minneapolis study the offenses for which homeless persons were incarcerated were related to alcohol abuse in nearly half of cases (79). In a Hollywood study, more than half of homeless adolescents were found to have been involved with the police because of drinking (51). Illicit drug use is also associated with arrest. Among New York City shelter clients with prison histories, 28 percent of men and 44 percent of women reported using drugs (57). Benda (80) found higher rates of arrest among Richmond, Virginia, homeless people who had abused alcohol or other drugs than among nonabusers. Studies of homeless people which have attempted to correlate arrests with psychiatric measures have found evidence of increased criminal activity among the mentally ill. Ladner et al. (81) found that nearly half of New York City shelter residents identified as mentally ill had jail histories. Schutt and Garrett (59) found that current legal problems were more frequent among mentally ill people (30%), drug abusers (26%), and alcohol abusers (17%). Moreover, 46 percent of mentally ill individuals who also abused alcohol had current legal problems, compared to less than 10 percent of those with neither mental illness nor substance abuse. Koegel and Farr (82) report that the chronically mentally ill adults in their Los Angeles homeless sample were about twice as likely as those who were not mentally ill to have been picked up by the police within the prior year, as well as to have spent time in jail. Among the homeless people in a Los Angeles County study, involvement with criminal activities was associated with previous mental hospitalizations (78). In a Minneapolis study, about 15 percent of incarcerations were related to mental illness (79). Arrest rates were found to be higher in the mentally ill among homeless adults in a Baltimore sample (5,6). In addition, diminished mental capacity may bring a greater risk of arrest (83). In Baltimore, homeless individuals with arrest histories were found to have lower levels of education, lower scores on IQ screening tests, and greater signs of cognitive impairment (5).

Victimization of Homeless People

There is considerable and growing evidence that homeless people fall victim to acts of violence at a rate that exceeds that of the general population. Homeless people are particularly vulnerable to street crime because of their lack of resources—both physical and social. Lacking shelter, they cannot escape to locked sanctuaries. Their appearance and bizarre behavior place them at the bottom of the social pecking order, where they become the natural prey of the young street bullies. Their disaffiliation makes it unlikely that they can marshal confederates for defense or retribution, thus increasing their appeal as victims. Moreover, homeless people may not avail themselves of lawful protection because they believe the police perceive them as less deserving than tax-paying citizens and thus fail to take their complaints as seriously as those of people judged to be socially "worthy." That society has tacitly branded homeless people as disposable increases their risk of abuse.

Indications of the excess prevalence of victimization in this population come primarily from two related sources: clinical studies, and surveys of homeless individuals in shelters and other sites. These reports suggest that the risk of attack is borne disproportionately by certain subgroups of the homeless population at large. In addition, surveys have examined violence, particularly domestic violence, as a causal factor in the etiology of homelessness.

CLINICAL STUDIES

Trauma has been cited as one of the leading causes of death and disability among contemporary homeless people (84). While it is not always possible to distinguish accidental trauma—which may result from the disorientation of the mentally ill or the incapacitation of the inebriated (85)—from trauma resulting from assault, the rates and types of injuries sustained by homeless populations are useful indicators of their victimization. Earlier studies of Skid Rows (86–90) called attention to the association of violence with the street life of alcoholic men, and recent clinical studies continue to report relatively high rates of trauma indicative of ongoing victimization of homeless people (91). About one-quarter of all adult clients seen in the national Health Care for the Homeless clinics sponsored by the Robert Wood Johnson Foundation and the Pew Trust presented with trauma (92). In New York, men of the Bowery— perhaps the archetypal Skid Row—were found to be victims of trauma at twice the rate of men living in single-room occupancy hotels (SROs) (93). This is impressive considering that residents of SROs appear to be at increased risk of violent acts relative to the general population. In a clinic located in a large SRO in New York City, trauma was found to be the presenting complaint in about one-fifth of cases (94). In another study, the "old guard" of the Bowery, men aged 50 years and older, had higher rates of fractures than did the general elderly population (95).

Nearly three-quarters of homeless adults examined by physicians in a California study reported having been victimized within the past year (96). More than two-thirds of a Baltimore clinical sample reported trauma as part of their medical histories (97). In a medical records review of homeless people treated at the Union Rescue Mission Infirmary in Nashville, one-fifth of cases were discovered to be injury-related (98). A survey of 487 homeless people in Dallas revealed that in the preceding year 34 percent had suffered fractures, 17 percent had suffered cuts or wound requiring stitches or hospitalization, and 2 percent had had eye injuries (99).

In the most detailed study to date of trauma to homeless individuals, the medical records of 340 homeless patients admitted to San Francisco General Hospital (SFGH) between January 1 and March 31, 1983, were reviewed (84). Of these patients, 15 percent were major trauma victims, and an additional 10 percent were admitted for cellulitis, a common sequela to trauma, so that trauma accounted for one-fourth of all homeless admissions:

Trauma victims . . . were typically males from twenty to thirty-nine years of age. They suffered a great variety of severe injuries, including stab wounds, head trauma, blunt trauma, multisystem trauma, gunshots, suicide attempts, burns, complex facial fractures, hip fractures, pneumothoraces, and lacerations of the neck, chest, liver, large and small bowel, and tendons of the hand. Stab wounds and fractures predominated and accounted for 65 percent of the major trauma injuries (84:84)

A six-month review of records at the SFGH emergency department revealed a similar rate of trauma presentation (30%), mostly for minor trauma resulting from assault (84). Moreover, the homeless patients were found to suffer alarmingly high rates of repeat trauma and hospitalization; nearly half had prior or subsequent hospitalizations at SFGH during the three-month study period.

In addition, the medical records of all patients treated at the Sexual Trauma Service of SFGH were reviewed over a nine-month period; 34 homeless patients were identified, representing nearly 10 percent of all patients seen. The incidence of treated sexual assault was estimated to be 20 times greater than in the general population. Three-quarters of homeless victims of sexual assault were female. The majority (41%) were victims of multiple-orifice assault, and half sustained injuries ranging from minor abrasions to major trauma, including skull fracture; all victims were judged to have experienced some degree of psychological trauma in addition. Moreover, 12 percent of the homeless victims of sexual assault had previously been treated by the Sexual Trauma Service (84).

SURVEYS OF HOMELESS POPULATIONS

Victimization of homeless people has been documented through surveys of homeless populations in three main forms: evidence of crime and violence within shelters; incidents of victimization reported by homeless individuals; and victimization as a precipitating event for homelessness.

EVIDENCE OF CRIME AND VIOLENCE WITHIN SHELTERS. It seems distressingly perverse that the very places where homeless people seek asylum, the shelters, are often, albeit by no means universally, the sites of greater risk than are the streets:

> For most men we talked to, [the shelter] conjured up three things: easily acquired wine, lots of "sick people—you know, psychos," and an ever present threat of violence . . . chronic fear is the rule, a low-grade apprehension that keeps them constant companion and intensifies as they get older. Those who prey on shelter clients—the "hawks" or "jackrollers"—are not stupid: older men are more likely to be on pension or getting VA checks and are sure to put up less of a fight. (100:399)

Theft in shelters is rife: retention of personal belongings is accomplished by guile or domination, as even the best-staffed facilities can provide little real security (100–102). Shelter clients may fear their fellows—some recently released from jail, prison, or mental hospital—who can be violent or exploitative; 34 percent of homeless people surveyed in Manhattan shelters and streets said they were afraid of being attacked in a shelter—a proportion similar to that of those who voiced fears of being attacked on the street (103). Lumsden (104) suggested that about 6 percent of clients of Dallas shelters could be classified as "troublemakers," a group of violence-prone young men who victimize the other shelter users. The proportion of men barred temporarily or permanently from the largest mission in Baltimore for causing problems, including violent behavior, arson, and stealing, increased from 5 percent in 1981, to 14 percent in 1986 (105). As the shelter-using population has become younger and more violent, physical danger has escalated to the point where the most vulnerable homeless people—such as the elderly—have been "crowded out" of the shelters (106).

However, the threat not only emanates from shelter clients but may occasionally issue from staff as well, although this appears to be the exception. Both intimidation and physical abuse, including the murder of clients, have been attributed to the staff of some of the immense public shelters in New York City (100,102,107,108).

THE INCIDENCE OF VICTIMIZATION.   Surveys of shelter users have produced substantial reports of recent victimization. More than one-third of people in a Detroit shelter had been crime victims within the year; nearly three-fifths had been victimized more than once, with one-fifth reporting four or more occasions (109). In Phoenix, nearly two-fifths of homeless people surveyed in soup lines had been robbed, assaulted, raped, or harassed at least once during the last six months (110). In Los Angeles (46), 36 percent of individuals in a homeless sample had been criminally victimized at least once during the previous six months, reporting an average of 2.24 episodes per person. Robbery or burglary were the most commonly reported offenses (33%), followed by assault (14%), and sexual assault (women only, 6%). In another Los Angeles study, 53 percent of the homeless people on Skid Row had been crime victims, half more than once; assault (67%) and robbery (59%) occurred most often (42). One of every 13 shelter users in a Saint Louis study reported sexual abuse, and more than one-fourth had been beaten or robbed (61). Half of the homeless people surveyed in New York had been physically assaulted, and one-fifth had been raped; three-quarters of the rape victims were women, accounting for nearly two-fifths of all the homeless women in the sample (103). In a Baltimore shelter sample, one-fifth of respondents indicated they had been mugged within the previous three months (6). In Anchorage (111), 65 percent of the homeless people studied had been assaulted, three-fifths on multiple occasions; the magnitude of the violence inflicted on the homeless people surveyed is indicated by the report that more than half required medical care, with two-fifths having been hospitalized. Respondents frequently reported multiple assailants (65%) and the use of weapons (44%). A survey of 695 men residing in New York City public shelters determined that 18–58 percent had been victims of one or more of four index crimes (simple and aggravated assaults, robbery, and theft) within the past year. Moreover, the homeless men had been victimized at rates 7–40 times as great as those reported for the general population (52).

Although street people attract the attention of bullies and often appear to be easy marks for robbers, there is evidence that they may also prey on each other (69,104). For example, in Chicago, 55 percent of the homeless people surveyed reported having been "hassled." Twenty-seven percent stated that these episodes were due to other homeless people; 12 percent responded that they were due specifically to street men; 10 percent counted other street people among their biggest problems (49). In a Detroit study, the assailant was known to the homeless victim in 79 percent of assaults and 39 percent of robberies (109).

VICTIMIZATION AS A PRECIPITATOR OF HOMELESSNESS. Recent personal crises, including dissolution of households after episodes of domestic violence, have been pointed to as precipitators of homelessness as well as criteria for dividing the homeless population into analytically meaningful subgroups (3,112–119). Domestic violence has been reported as the main reason a respondent was homeless in only a few studies (46,109,111,116). For example, family conflict was reported to have led to homelessness for one-quarter of the homeless mentally ill people surveyed in a Milwaukee study (47). In a follow-up study of patients discharged from state mental hospitals, Mowbray (personal communication, 1986) discovered that 9 percent were currently homeless; 17 percent of these stated that they had been forced into homelessness through being abused—beaten up or raped—at the places where they had resided after discharge. There is some evidence that rates of prior physical and sexual abuse may be higher in the mentally ill population than in the general population (120,121), which might affect the rates in the homeless population.

As might be expected, women are more likely to report victimization as the cause of homelessness than are men, who identify reasons related to unemployment, alcohol problems, and jail release (108,116). The issue is further complicated because battered women often have separate shelters, and surveys of homeless people may not include these specialized facilities within their sampling frames (48). However, victimization seems likely to be a hidden component where family or personal crises are cited as reasons for homelessness (42,48,49,119).

Evidence is emerging to link patterns of childhood abuse with homelessness. A number of studies have found high rates of childhood physical and sexual abuse in groups of homeless adults (5,66,122,123). Studies of homeless mothers and their children in Boston revealed that 42 percent of homeless mothers but only 5 percent of a comparison group of housed poor mothers had been abused as children, and twice as many of the homeless mothers (41%) as housed mothers (20%) had been battered in their adult relationships (122). Mothers who had been physically and sexually abused by their parents frequently repeated the pattern of abuse with their own children. These findings led Bassuk and colleagues to conclude that lifetime patterns of deprivation and violence foster a "newly emergent cycle of intergenerational homelessness [where] it is not only the economics of poverty that has created the new phenomenon of homeless families, but the combined effects of poverty, violence, and profound deprivation on a person's development and self-esteem" (124).

Similar findings are suggested for families in the Salvation Army Emergency Lodge in Saint Louis (125). In a Baltimore study, homeless women overall (41%) were twice as likely to report childhood physical or sexual abuse as were homeless men (21%); nearly half (48%) of the homeless women sampled from the jail reported such abuse (66). A comparison of homeless applicants for emergency housing and domiciled recipients of public assistance in New York City found that 11 percent of the homeless and 7 percent of the housed individuals reported childhood physical abuse; 10 percent of the homeless but only 4 percent of the housed clients had been sexually abused before age 18. Furthermore, the homeless clients were more likely to experience abuse as adults (26% v. 16%) (126). A survey of homeless adults in Manhattan shelters and streets also suggests association of early childhood trauma with later homelessness: among 158 young (63% under 40 years of age) homeless people, of whom about two-fifths were women, nearly one-quarter had been abused as children; almost half of those reporting child abuse indicated that the abuse had been sexual in nature (103). In addition, they had experienced other serious problems while they were growing up (e.g., 27% had had trouble getting along with their parents, and 35% had often played hooky), and they had failed to form expected social attachments as adults (e.g., 59 percent had never married, 43 percent had no contact with their relatives, and 49 percent had no one to turn to for help). Fifty-one percent had been homeless longer than one year (103).

A more direct association between abuse and homelessness has been described among runaway and throwaway youths (50). Three-fifths of teenagers in a San Francisco study had been sexually abused before leaving home (127). Half of shelter-using homeless youths in a New York study reported parental abuse "such that they had repeatedly sustained bruises, cuts or welts or else had had to receive treatment in a hospital on at least one occasion" (128:65). Robertson (129) found that among Hollywood street kids, 24 percent had become homeless at least once due to physical abuse in the home and 8 percent due to sexual abuse. Comparison of young runaway and nonrunaway users of Los Angeles outpatient medical clinics showed rates of physical and sexual abuse to be 4–8 times higher among the runaways. In this study, unlike many others, sexual abuse was reported more often than physical abuse (22% v. 16%, respectively) (130). These studies clearly establish abuse in the home as a significant contributing factor to homelessness among young people.

Victims of gentrification are easily precipitated into homelessness. This phenomenon has been well documented in New York City, where tenants of

SROs—primarily poor, elderly or disabled long-term residents—were found to be "standing in the way of the gentry" (131). Conversion of these SRO hotels into more profitable condominiums was dependent upon relocation of the existing tenants. Eviction was often accomplished through illegal tactics including threats and harassment, lockouts, withdrawal of essential services, arson, burglaries, and physical assault. One such removal campaign was likened to a "three-week reign of terror" (131:27). The majority of the former tenants of converted buildings could not be located, but evidence uncovered in the investigation of criminal proceedings against landlords suggests that many became homeless, having no recourse but to shelters or the street. Furthermore, studies of the New York shelter population indicate that up to half of shelter clients had lived in SROs immediately before coming to the shelter (106).

THE RISK OF VICTIMIZATION

While homeless people appear to be more vulnerable to attack than are members of the general population, recent reports indicate that certain homeless individuals are at even greater risk of victimization. Historically, the public inebriate has been the target for robbery and beating because "drunks" have been regarded as contemptible figures, and because, often being elderly, physically disabled, and stuporous, they offer little resistance (100). Higher risk appears to continue to attach to alcohol and drug use in the contemporary homeless population. Rates of injuries were found to be higher for the alcohol and drug abusers among the clients of the Johnson-Pew national Health Care for the Homeless clinics (92). Higher rate of assault, robbery, and theft were reported by homeless men in New York City shelters who had serious drinking problems as indicated by alcohol-related arrests (52). In Baltimore, the homeless respondents who were identified as alcohol and drug abusers were more likely to report being victims of crimes that had resulted in injuries within the past year (5). The Fulton County medical examiner determined that 70 percent of 40 deaths of homeless individuals were alcohol-related; 13 percent were due to homicide or suicide (85).

The unfit seem to have less chance to escape, if not survive. Brickner suggests that "bag-ladies on the street with massively swollen legs wrapped with rags are . . . more easily victimized and subject to assault" (132:9–10). Among New York homeless men, rates of assault and robbery were highest among those who reported poor health and physical disabilities (52). Women, more vulnerable in most respects than men (118), are also at greater risk of attack with sexual intent (5,38,49,66,110,133–135).

Living on the streets appears to increase the risk of victimization. For example, in a Baltimore study higher rates of recent victimization in men compared to women were attributed to a higher index of risk associated with men's greater likelihood of "sleeping rough" and being intoxicated (34). Gelberg and colleagues (78) found that three-quarters of street people but about half of shelter users reported victimization. High rates of victimization, particularly sexual assault, have been reported among homeless youths, whose risk status is increased by high rates of exposure to the streets, to alcohol and drug abuse, and to prostitution (50,128–130).

Homeless people with obvious disabilities, not only physical disabilities but also mental retardation and mental illness—particularly the "space cases"— also attract undue attention from the street predators (52,83,133,136). Farr and colleagues (42) found that the chronically mentally ill among the Los Angeles homeless people surveyed were more likely to have been victimized— particularly, assaulted—within the previous year and were more likely to report more than one type of victimization. Since there is evidence that homeless women may be more likely than homeless men to be mentally disturbed, their risk of attack may be compounded (81).

Criminal activity itself appears to increase the risk of victimization. A criminal record has been described as a factor that may either contribute to homelessness or create a barrier to recovery by adding to overall individual burden (63,80). An example of this effect can be seen in a Baltimore study in which homeless people with prior arrest histories were nearly twice as likely to have been crime victims and almost three times as likely to have been raped (5).

REACTIONS OF HOMELESS PEOPLE TO VICTIMIZATION

Homeless people may be thought, to some extent, to be passive victims. Nevertheless, they are by no means unaware of the constant threat of violence inherent in street life. They often report safety to be of major concern (71): 62 percent of those surveyed in Anchorage indicated a need for improved personal safety, including more police protection (111). Men on the Bowery were found to have a fear of crime significantly greater than that reported by New York City community men of similar age, although the fear of crime was equally pervasive among both street-dwelling and non-street-dwelling Bowery men (95). In a survey of 112 homeless users of acute psychiatric services at San Francisco General Hospital, Ball and Havassy (133) found that the problems most often mentioned were being robbed (25%); being assaulted, raped, or harassed (21%); or being the victim of specific interpersonal animosities (18%). In Toronto, 86 percent of 80 skid row inebriates questioned responded that they perceived an increase in muggings and beatings of street people—a perception corroborated by police and administrators of service programs for the homeless, who also noted an increase in brutal, injury-producing attacks (137). However, Muhlin (52) found that despite high rates of victimization, only 20 percent voiced a fear of being hurt—less than rates previously found in general community samples. This surprising finding was explained as due to the homeless respondents' denying or becoming enured to the brutality of their environment.

The relationship between homeless people and the law enforcement system, particularly the police, is unclear, as reports in the literature are mixed. On the one hand, researchers often report that homeless crime victims tend not to invoke formal justice: "Street people live outside the law in an environment where conflicts are often resolved by force or the threat of force. Arguments about property, women, sleeping space and the like are settled between complainants who muster friends as witnesses, seconds and potential retaliators" (136:361). On the other hand, the police and jails appear to be among the most frequent providers of services to the population (3,138): "the most common response [of the public] to homeless people is to invoke the formal justice system, to call the police" (49:53). For example, the public inebriate or vagrant formerly consumed a disproportionate amount of time from the law enforcement system (E. Eisenstadt, personal communication, 1984), and currently, substantial proportions of the homeless are brought into shelters and other programs by police (11,60,112). Homeless people occasionally report inviting arrest to gain shelter (5,68,69,139). However, providing services to homeless people is not always seen by police as falling in their bailiwick. Police and court officers may view time spent in dealing with individuals "whose legal transgressions are trivial in comparison [to their psychiatric problems]" (136:360) as time taken from their "proper" duties; thus they may eventually become less responsive to homeless people's needs.

Police intervention is sought in an estimated 16–60 percent of crimes against homeless individuals (42,109–11); the more serious or violent crimes are more likely to be reported (110). However, national data suggest that less than half of all violent crimes and only one-quarter of personal thefts are reported to the police (140). One reason that homeless people fail to report crimes to the police is that police may be regarded as enemies rather than champions. The proportion of those reporting police harassment ranges from 1 percent to 41 percent (40,42,46,49,133). Nearly half of the homeless people in a Los Angeles study said they went out of their way to avoid the police, although two-thirds in that same study had reported that they counted the police among the people they could turn to for help (42). In a Baltimore study, homeless adults with arrest histories were nearly four times more likely to report police harassment than those without arrest histories (5).

Consequently, homeless people adopt "street-smart" strategies for self-protection. The respondents in a Los Angeles study report avoiding unsafe places (89%), avoiding people (77%), seeking the companionship of a trusted person (53%), sleeping in the daytime (24%), and carrying weapons (24%) (42). Women have significant and warranted fears of attack and frequently report developing adaptive strategies, including reclusiveness and offensive dress and grooming, to reduce their risk of becoming victims (49,134, 135,141). Some homeless people appear to use arrest as a survival strategy, having learned that police can be maneuvered into placing them in the relative safety of a jail (68,134,139). This behavior may be reinforced by pervasive police beliefs that "they are saving the men's lives when they send them to jail to get 'built up'" (142:499). Women are perceived as using their vulnerability to advantage in gaining asylum via police: "They take women to jail just for sleeping in a doorway, whereas guys have to get violent if they want to get a place in jail" (133:920).

Discussion

Reports of substantial proportions of homeless people with histories of incarceration make it apparent that criminal activity is a prominent characteristic of the contemporary homeless population. However, little has been reported to date concerning the nature of their criminal behavior and its function in the etiology and maintenance of the homeless lifestyle. Information regarding criminal behavior comes mainly from reports of arrest and/or incarceration rates generated by recent studies of shelter-using homeless people, which seldom include sufficient data to reconstruct the pattern of criminal activity underlying the prevalence of arrest and incarceration. Where the offenses are reported, the results suggest that homeless people are most often arrested for relatively trivial and essentially victimless crimes arising more from the homeless condition than from deliberate criminal intent.

It is possible to interpret the role of criminal activity in the behavioral repertoire of homeless people in four different ways. First, it is likely that some habitual criminals accumulate in the homeless population through "downward drift" (80). Furthermore, histories of arrest and incarceration may be associated with chronic deviant behavior for some individuals, particularly those with antisocial personalities and drug disorders. Homelessness per se is not a causal factor in this pattern of crime; rather, homelessness may be a natural part of the life cycle of people whose livelihood drives principally from illegal sources, reflecting their need to go underground to evade arrest or to survive a period of waning fortune. Consequently, chronic criminal behavior of this magnitude probably will be relatively unaffected by services aimed at ameliorating homelessness.

Second, for many homeless individuals, criminal activity may be one of the few means available to augment their meager resources to meet subsistence needs. The majority of homeless people are currently unemployed; many have been so for a long time. Those who report current employment often indicate that it is part-time or temporary work, including casual labor as well as "jobs" such as selling blood. The homeless find it difficult to obtain gainful employment for a variety of reasons ranging from inability to "dress for success," or lack of education and training, to incapacitation. Yet substantial proportions of the homeless population are not enrolled in public support programs. Thus, many resort to illegal acts on a modest scale, such as petty pilfering, shoplifting, small-scale drug dealing, nonpayment of cab fares and restaurant tabs, prostitution, and so forth. Criminal activity of this ilk reflects necessity and might be substantially reduced by improving the flow of eligible homeless people into the social services net.

Third, behavior that is functionally adaptive in the homeless ecology may lead to arrest. The skills that enhance the survival prospects of the homeless person on the streets (e.g., breaking into an abandoned building or parked vehicle for shelter, trespassing, or sleeping on benches in violation of park laws), though lacking inherent criminal intent, are often illegal or readily criminalized. The extreme case of functional criminal behavior occurs when homeless people manipulate police into making arrests in order to obtain temporary asylum in jail. A homeless man in Baltimore reported that much of his extensive criminal history was due to his desire to have a safe home in the jail: his modus operandi for ensuring a speedy arrest had been to set a fire, but he later came to realize that his method was too destructive and now follows the more benign course of setting off a false alarm, with the same satisfactory result (W. R. Breakey, personal communication, 1987). Such people may be thought to be criminally homeless rather than homeless criminals (cf. 143).

Last, arrests may indicate diminished mental capacity, as in the case of offenders who exhibit ill-judged or bizarre behavior that lands them in correctional institutions rather than in more appropriate systems of social services, treatment, or institutionalization. Psychotic behavior—sometimes violent—or the disorientation associated with intoxication, mental illness, and mental retardation may call the police into play. Indeed, some homeless individuals' disheveled appearance alone may be alarming enough to induce citizen complaints. Since the options of the police are limited to informal dispositions (e.g., moving the person on), emergency detentions for psychiatric evaluation (found to be ineffective in the past), or arrest (perhaps regarded as an alternative to hospitalization) (36), there is reason to believe that homelessness, as well as mental illness, has been criminalized. This may have great impact on the criminal experience of the relatively large number of mentally ill and alcoholic individuals among the homeless population who become "police patients" (144).

It is difficult to discuss criminal behavior without considering its obverse, victimization. The most obvious impact of victimization is on people's health: the literature abounds with reports of trauma in homeless populations which far exceeds that experienced by the general population. The effect of such violence goes beyond the infliction of physical suffering and/or permanent disability, as it also leads to psychological demoralization and the ever-present fear and distrust of others frequently reported by homeless people.

Studies of the costs that the victimization of homeless people imposes on systems for health care and other human services need to be undertaken. It is likely that preventive measures to ensure adequate protection of vulnerable individuals—from more effective policing to the provision of safe housing, including residential treatment facilities for mentally ill and substance-abusing homeless people—would have benefits outweighing their costs.

It is important to consider the place in the life history of homelessness that victimization and, to some extent, crime occupy. While it is clear that certain patterns of both criminal behavior and victimization are caused or intensified by homelessness, there is insufficient longitudinal data to describe the role each plays in causing or maintaining homelessness in individuals. Recent reports indicate that criminal behavior is frequently cited as a pathway into homelessness. People report having been released from correctional institutions directly to the streets with few resources with which to achieve reassimilation into society. A criminal history presents a barrier to employment (41,47,80–81) that may prove to be virtually insurmountable and thus perpetuate both the cycle of crime and the homeless condition.

Victimization—most often domestic violence—is also blamed for precipitating people into homelessness. While men are sometimes affected, women appear to be the principal victims. However, evidence of the precipitating effect of victimization on other groups (e.g., runaway youths, children, and elderly people) is beginning to emerge (81,145). Bassuk (145) documents the critical need to intervene in the vicious cycle of abuse and neglect that enmeshes victim-mothers—who in turn victimize their children—to prevent the pattern of impairment and instability that can lead to homelessness from becoming entrenched through generations.

Although overall rates of both criminal activity and victimization are high in the samples of homeless people discussed here, individual risk appears to vary according to demographic and psychosocial characteristics. For example, men are arrested at greater rates and give evidence of involvement in more serious types of crimes than women. The duration and circumstances of homelessness appear to increase the risk of both arrest and victimization. The abuse of drugs, and particularly of alcohol, seems to be strongly associated with arrest. Alcohol and other drugs may increase the risk of arrest through their effects (e.g., drunk and disorderly offenses) or through illegal activities associated with procuring alcohol and drugs (e.g., theft to support drinking or other drug use, drug dealing). It appears that intoxicated or disoriented people also risk victimization disproportionately. More information is needed on differential distribution of risk among subgroups of the homeless population.

The movement of substantial proportions of the homeless population through the criminal justice system represents a significant public health problem. For many, if not most, arrest and incarceration represent failures of the appropriate human services systems to meet their needs. To a great extent, police and corrections personnel have supplanted the health and social services systems in providing services to this group of people in need of care. For some homeless people, this is not altogether a bad thing, as by circumstance of guile their interaction with the criminal justice system provides a gateway to other service systems. However, in the main, the criminal justice system is being burdened with a task that is not within its proper bailiwick, which raises critical questions related to the costs and benefits of such a diversion—questions that should be resolved not only in economic but also in humanitarian terms.

References

1. Bahr HM. The gradual disappearance of Skid Row. *Social Problems 15:*41–45, 1967.
2. Siegal HA, Inciardi JA. The demise of Skid Row. *Society 19(2):*39–45, 1982.
3. Fischer PJ, Breakey WR. Homelessness and mental health: An overview. *International Journal of Mental Health 14(4):*6–41, 1985.
4. Garrett GR. Alcohol problems and homelessness: History and research. *Contemporary Drug Problems 16(3):*301–332, 1989.
5. Fischer PJ, Breakey WR, Ross A. Criminal activity among the homeless. Paper presented at the 88th annual meeting of the American Anthropological Association, Washington, D.C., November 15–19, 1989.
6. Fischer PJ, Breakey WR, Ross A. Health, mental health, and criminal activity of the homeless. Paper presented at the 117th annual meeting of the American Public Health Association, Chicago, Ill., October 22–26, 1989.
7. Holcomb WR, Ahr PR. Arrest rates among young adult psychiatric patients treated in inpatient and outpatient settings. *Hospital and Community Psychiatry 39:*52–57, 1988.
8. James JF, et al. Psychiatric morbidity in prisons. *Hospital and Community Psychiatry 31:*674–677, 1980.
9. Lamb HR, Grant RW. The mentally ill in an urban county jail. *Archives of General Psychiatry 39:*17–22, 1982.
10. Lamb HR, Grant RW. Mentally ill women in a county jail. *Archives of General Psychiatry 40:*363–368, 1983.
11. Lipton FR, Sabatini A, Katz SE. Down and out in the city: The homeless mentally ill. *Hospital and Community Psychiatry 34:*817–821, 1983.
12. Solarz A. An examination of criminal behavior among the homeless. Paper presented at the annual meeting of the American Society of Criminology, San Diego, Calif., November 13–17, 1985.
13. Swank GE, Winer D. Occurrence of psychiatric disorder in a county jail population. *American Journal of Psychiatry 133:*1331–1333, 1976.
14. Fischer PJ. Estimating prevalence of alcohol, drug, and mental health problems in the contemporary homeless population. *Contemporary Drug Problems 16(3):*333–390, 1989.
15. Robertson MJ. Mental disorder among homeless persons in the United States: An overview of recent empirical literature. *Administration in Mental Health 14:*14–27, 1986.
16. Tessler RC, Dennis DL. *A Synthesis of NIMH-funded Research concerning People Who Are Homeless and Mentally Ill.* Rockville, Md.: Alcohol, Drug, and Mental Health Administration, 1989.
17. Appleby L, Slaff N, Desai P. The urban nomad: A psychiatric problem? *Current Psychiatric Therapies 2:*253–262, 1982.

18. Bachrach LL. Young adult chronic patients: An analytical review of the literature. *Hospital and Community Psychiatry 33:*189–197, 1982.

19. Caton CLM. The new chronic patients and the system of community care. *Hospital and Community Psychiatry 32:*475–478, 1981.

20. McFarland BH, et al. Chronic mental illness and the criminal justice system. *Hospital and Community Psychiatry 40:*718–723, 1989.

21. Sheets JL, Prevost JA, Reihman J. Young adult chronic patients: Three hypothesized subgroups. *Hospital and Community Psychiatry 33:*197–203, 1982.

22. Goldsmith MF. From mental hospitals to jails: The pendulum swings. *JAMA 250:*3017–3018, 1983.

23. McCarthy B. Mentally ill and mentally retarded offenders in corrections: A report of a national survey. In Coughlin TA, Tracy F (eds.), *Sourcebook on the Mentally Disordered Prisoner.* Washington, D.C.: National Institute of Corrections, 1985.

24. Bonovitz JC, Bonovitz JS. Diversion of the mentally ill into the criminal justice system: The police intervention perspective. *American Journal of Psychiatry 138:*973–976, 1981.

25. Cocozza JJ, Melick ME, Steadman HJ. Trends in violent crime among ex-mental patients. *Criminology 16:*317–324, 1978.

26. Steadman HJ, et al. The impact of state mental hospital deinstitutionalization on United States prison populations, 1968–1978. *Journal of Criminal Law and Criminology 75:*474–490, 1984.

27. Lamb HR. Alternatives to hospitals. In Talbott JA (ed.), *The Chronic Mental Patient: Five Years Later.* Orlando: Grune and Stratton, 1984.

28. Lamb HR. Deinstitutionalization and the homeless mentally ill. *Hospitals and Community Psychiatry 35:*899–907, 1984.

29. Teplin LA. The criminalization of the mentally ill: Speculations in search of data. *Psychological Bulletin 94(1):*54–67, 1983.

30. Whitmer GE. From hospitals to jails: The fate of California's deinstitutionalized mentally ill. *American Journal of Orthopsychiatry 50:*65–75, 1980.

31. Zitrin A, et al. Crime and violence among mental patients. *American Journal of Psychiatry 133:*142–149, 1976.

32. Johnson J, McKeown K, James R. Removing the chronically mentally ill from jail. In *Case Studies of Collaboration between Local Criminal Justice and Mental Health Systems.* Washington, D.C.: National Coalition for Jail Reform, 1984.

33. Monahan J, Steadman HJ. *Crime and Mental Disorder.* Washington, D.C.: National Institute of Justice Research in Brief, 1984.

34. Fischer PJ. Criminal activity among the homeless: A study of arrests in Baltimore. *Hospital and Community Psychiatry 39:*46–51, 1988.

35. Peele R, et al. The legal system and the homeless. In Lamb HR (ed.), *The Homeless Mentally Ill.* Washington, D.C.: American Psychiatric Association, 1984.

36. Murphy GR. *Special Care: Improving the Police Response to the Mentally Disabled.* Washington, D.C.: Police Executive Research Forum, 1986.

37. Briar KH. Jails: Neglected asylums. *Social Casework 64:*387–393, 1983.

38. Bassuk EL. The homelessness problem. *Scientific American 251(1):*40–45, 1984.

39. Breakey WR, et al. Health and mental health problems of homeless men and women in Baltimore. *JAMA 262:*1352–1357, 1989.

40. Brown C, et al. *The Homeless of Phoenix: Who Are They? And What Should Be Done?* Phoenix, Ariz.: Phoenix South Community Mental Health Center, 1983.

41. Crystal S, Ladner S, Towber R. Multiple impairment patterns in the mentally ill homeless. *International Journal of Mental Health 14(4):*61–73, 1985.

42. Farr RK, Koegel P, Burnam A. *A Study of Homelessness and Mental Health in the Skid*

Row Area of Los Angeles. Los Angeles: Los Angeles County Department of Mental Health, 1986.

43. Fischer PJ, et al. Baltimore mission users: Social networks, morbidity, and unemployment. *Psychosocial Rehabilitation Journal 9(4):51–63,* 1986.

44. Fischer PJ, et al. Mental health and social characteristics of the homeless: A survey of mission users. *American Journal of Public Health 76:519–524,* 1986.

45. Morse G, Calsyn R. Mentally disturbed homeless people in St. Louis: Needy, willing, but underserved. *International Journal of Mental Health 14(4):74–94,* 1985.

46. Robertson M, Ropers RH, Boyer R. *The Homeless of Los Angeles County: An Empirical Assessment.* Los Angeles: University of California–Los Angeles, School of Public Health, 1985.

47. Rosnow MJ, Shaw T, Concord CS. Listening to the homeless: A study of homeless mentally ill persons in Milwaukee. *Psychosocial Rehabilitation Journal 9(4):64–77,* 1986.

48. Roth D, et al. *Homelessness in Ohio: A Study of People in Need.* Columbus: Ohio Department of Mental Health, 1985.

49. Task Force on Emergency Shelter. *Homelessness in Chicago.* Chicago: Chicago Department of Human Services, 1983.

50. Solarz A. Homelessness: Implications for children and youths. *Social Policy Report 3(4):1–15,* 1988.

51. Robertson MJ, Koegel P, Ferguson L. Alcohol use and abuse among homeless adolescents in Hollywood. *Contemporary Drug Problems 16(3):415–452,* 1989.

52. Muhlin GL. Pack of wolves or flock of sheep? Crime and victimization among the New York City public shelter users. Presented at the annual meeting of the American Society of Criminology, Atlanta, Ga., October 29–November 1, 1986.

53. Milburn NG. Drug abuse: Is it a serious problem among homeless people? In Schaub JB, Newman MA (eds.), *Research and Statistics: Improving the Quality of Decisions.* Proceedings of the 28th National Workshop on Welfare, Research and Statistics. Austin: Texas Department of Human Services, 1988.

54. Mulkern VM. *Illicit Drug Use among Homeless Persons: A Review of the Literature.* Report to the Committee on Health Care for Homeless People, National Academy of Sciences. Washington, D.C.: Institute of Medicine, 1987.

55. Morse G. Homelessness: A multilevel assessment and intervention strategy. Manuscript, 1984.

56. Milburn NG, Booth J. Drug abuse among sheltered homeless people: Preliminary findings from a Washington, D.C., sample. Paper presented at the 116th annual meeting of the American Public Health Association, Boston, Mass., November 13–17, 1989.

57. Crystal S, Goldstein M. *Correlates of Shelter Utilization: One-Day Study.* New York: City of New York, Human Resources Administration, 1984.

58. Kahn MW, et al. Psychopathology on the streets: Psychological assessment of the homeless. *Professional Psychology: Research and Practice 18:580–586,* 1987.

59. Schutt RK, Garrett GR. *Homeless in Boston in 1985: The View from Long Island.* Boston: University of Massachusetts, 1986.

60. Crystal S, Goldstein M. *The Homeless in New York City Shelters.* New York: City of New York, Human Resources Administration, 1984.

61. Morse G, et al. *Homeless People in St. Louis: A Mental Health Program Evaluation, Field Study, and Follow-up Investigation,* vol 1. Jefferson City: Missouri Department of Mental Health, 1985.

62. Rosenheck R, Phil PGM, Leda C. *Reaching Out: The Second Progress Report on the Veterans Administration Chronically Mentally Ill Veterans Program.* West Haven, Conn.: West Haven Veterans Administration Medical Center, 1988.

63. Rosnow MJ, Shaw T, Concord CS. *Listening to the Homeless: A Study of Homeless*

Mentally Ill Persons in Milwaukee. Madison: Wisconsin Office of Mental Health, 1985.

64. McGarrell E, Flanagan T. *Sourcebook of Criminal Justice Statistics—1984.* Washington, D.C.: U.S. Department of Justice, Bureau of Justice Statistics, 1985.

65. Schutt RK. *Boston's Homeless: Report to the Long Island Shelter.* Boston: University of Massachusetts at Boston, 1988.

66. Fischer PJ, et al. Homeless mentally ill: The Baltimore study. Paper presented at the 116th annual meeting of the American Public Health Association, Boston, Mass., November 13–17, 1988.

67. Bassuk EL, Rubin L, Lauriat AS. Is homelessness a mental health problem? *American Journal of Psychiatry 141:*1546, 1984.

68. McGerigle P, Lauriat AS. *More Than Shelter: A Community Response to Homelessness.* Boston: United Community Planning Corporation, 1983.

69. Town K, Marchetti AG. *The Impact of Homelessness on Atlanta.* Atlanta, Ga.: Research Atlanta, 1984.

70. Federal Bureau of Investigation. *Uniform Crime Reporting Handbook.* Washington, D.C.: U.S. Department of Justice, 1980.

71. Calsyn RJ, Morse G. Homeless women and men: Commonalities and a service gender gap. *American Journal of Community Psychology 18(4):*597–608, 1990.

72. Rossi PH, Fisher GA, Willis G. *The Condition of the Homeless in Chicago.* Amherst: University of Massachusetts, Social and Demographic Research Institute, 1986.

73. Kufeldt K, Nimmo M. Youth on the street: Abuse and neglect in the eighties. *Child Abuse and Neglect 11:*531–543, 1987.

74. Robertson JM. Homeless adolescents: A hidden crisis. *Hospital and Community Psychiatry 39:*475, 1988.

75. Susser E, Struening EL, Conover S. Childhood experiences of homeless men. *American Journal of Psychiatry 144:*1599–1601, 1987.

76. Finn P. Decriminalization of public drunkenness: Response of the health care system. *Journal of Studies on Alcohol 46:*7–23, 1985.

77. Robertson MJ. Homeless adults in a county alcohol treatment program. Paper presented at the 117th annual meeting of the American Public Health Association, Chicago, Ill., October 22–26, 1989.

78. Gelberg L, Linn LS, Leake BD. Mental health, alcohol and drug use, and criminal history among homeless adults. *American Journal of Psychiatry 145:*191–196, 1988.

79. Kroll J, et al. A survey of homeless adults in urban emergency shelters. *Hospital and Community Psychiatry 37:*283–286, 1986.

80. Benda BB. Crime, drug abuse, mental illness, and homelessness. *Deviant Behavior 8:*361–375, 1987.

81. Ladner S, et al. *Project Future: Focusing, Understanding, Targeting, and Utilizing Resources for the Homeless Mentally Ill, Elderly, Youth, Substance Abusers, and Employables.* New York: City of New York, Department of Health and Human Services, 1986.

82. Koegel P, Farr R. Los Angeles mentally ill project. Paper presented at the Conference on NIMH-funded Research on the Homeless Mentally Ill: Implications for Policy and Practice, Bethesda, Md., Alcohol, Drug Abuse, and Mental Health Administration, July 24–25, 1986.

83. French L. The victimization of the mentally deficient: A latent function of deinstitutionalization. Paper presented at the annual meeting of the Society of Criminology, Atlanta, Ga., October 29–November 1, 1986.

84. Kelly JT. Trauma: With the example of San Francisco's shelter programs. In Brickner PW, et al. (eds.), *Health Care of Homeless People.* New York: Springer, 1985.

85. Hanzlick R. Deaths among the homeless: Atlanta, Georgia. *Morbidity and Mortality Weekly Report 36:*297–299, 1984.

86. Blumberg LU, Shipley TE, Barsky SF. *Liquor and Poverty: Skid Row as a Human Condition.* New Brunswick, N.J.: Rutgers Center of Alcohol Studies, 1978.

87. Bogue GJ. *Skid Row in American Cities.* Chicago: University of Chicago, Community and Family Study Center, 1963.

88. Olin JS. "Skid Row" syndrome: A medical profile of the chronic drunkenness offender. *Canadian Medical Association Journal 95:*205–214, 1966.

89. Pittman DJ, Gordon CW. *Revolving Door: A Study of the Chronic Police Case Inebriate.* Glencoe, Ill.: Free Press, 1958.

90. Wiseman J. *Stations of the Lost.* Chicago: University of Chicago Press, 1970.

91. Brickner PW, et al. Medical aspects of homelessness. In Lamb (ed.), *The Homeless Mentally Ill,* pp. 243–259. See ref. 35.

92. Wright JD, Weber E. *Homelessness and Health.* New York: McGraw-Hill, 1987.

93. Cohen CI, Sokolovsky J. Toward a concept of homelessness among aged men. *Journal of Gerontology 38:*81–89, 1983.

94. Buff DD, Kenny JF, Light D. Health problems of residents of single-room-occupancy hotels. *New York State Journal of Medicine 80:*2000–2005, 1980.

95. Cohen CI. The aging men of skid row: A target for research and service intervention. Manuscript, 1985.

96. Gelberg L, Linn LS. Assessing the physical health of homeless adults. *JAMA 262:*1973–1979, 1989.

97. Stine OC, Fischer PJ, Breakey WR. Co-morbid physical problems of homeless mentally ill persons in Baltimore. Presented at the 116th annual meeting of the American Public Health Association, Boston, Mass., November 13–19, 1988.

98. Couto RA, Lawrence RP, Lee BA. Health care and the homeless of Nashville: Dealing with a problem without a definition. *Urban Resources 2(2):*17–24, 1985.

99. Lumsden GH. *Report on the Health Status of the Homeless.* Dallas, Tex.: City of Dallas, Department of Health and Human Services, 1984.

100. Baxter E, Hopper K. The new mendicancy: Homeless in New York City. *American Journal of Orthopsychiatry 52:*393–408, 1982.

101. Archdeacon S. A homeless woman's story. *New York Magazine,* July 29, 1985.

102. Coleman JR. Diary of a homeless man. *New York Magazine,* February 26, 1983.

103. Jones BE, Gray BA, Goldstein DB. Psychosocial profiles of the urban homeless. In Jones BE (ed.), *Treating the Homeless: Urban Psychiatry's Challenge.* Washington, D.C.: American Psychiatric Association, 1986.

104. Lumsden GH. Housing the indigent and evaluation research: Issues associated with the Salvation Army sit-up shelter program. Paper presented at the Southwestern Social Science Association Meeting, Fort Worth, Tex., March 21–24, 1984.

105. Holt R. *Report of the Baltimore Rescue Mission.* Baltimore: Baltimore Rescue Mission, 1987.

106. Coalition for the Homeless. *Crowded Out: Homelessness and the Elderly Poor in New York City.* New York: CFH and Gray Panthers of New York City, 1984.

107. Nix C. City criticized for way it selects shelter guards. *New York Times,* November 1, 1986, p. 33.

108. Nix C. Guards held in two shelter killings. *New York Times,* October 31, 1986, p. A-20.

109. Solarz A. Criminal victimization among the homeless. Paper presented at the annual meeting of the American Society of Criminology, Atlanta, Ga., October 29–November 1, 1986.

110. Stark L. Victimization of the homeless in Phoenix. Manuscript, 1986.

111. Huelsman M. Violence on Anchorage's 4th Avenue from the perspective of street people. *Alaska Medicine 25(2):*39–44, 1983.

112. Arce AA, et al. A psychiatric profile of street people admitted to an emergency shelter. *Hospital and Community Psychiatry 34:*812–817, 1983.

113. Bassuk EL. The feminization of homelessness: Homeless families in Boston's shelters. Keynote address given at Shelter, Inc., Boston, Mass., June 11, 1985.

114. Bassuk E, Hopper K. *Private Lives/Public Spaces: Homeless Adults in New York City.* New York: Community Service Society, 1981.

115. Bobo BF. *A Report to the Secretary on the Homeless and Emergency Shelters.* Washington, D.C.: U.S. Department of Housing and Urban Development, 1984.

116. Hagen JL. The heterogeneity of homelessness. *Social Casework 68:*451–457, 1987.

117. McChesney KY. Absent or estranged kin: A crucial variable in explaining family homelessness. Paper presented at the 114th annual meeting of the American Public Health Association, Las Vegas, Nev., September 28–October 2, 1986.

118. Mowbray CT. Mental health and homelessness in Detroit: A research study. Paper presented at the Conference on NIMH-funded Research on the Homeless Mentally Ill: Implications for Policy and Practice, Bethesda, Md., Alcohol, Drug Abuse, and Mental Health Administration, July 24, 1986.

119. Solarz A, Mowbray C, Dupuis S. *Life in Transit: Homelessness in Michigan.* Lansing: Michigan Department of Mental Health, 1986.

120. Jacobson A. Physical and sexual assault histories among psychiatric outpatients. *American Journal of Psychiatry 146:*755–758, 1989.

121. Jacobson A, Richardson B. Assault experience of 100 psychiatric inpatients: Evidence of the need for routine enquiry. *American Journal of Psychiatry 144:*908–913, 1987.

122. Bassuk EL, Rosenberg L. Why does family homelessness occur? A case-control study. *American Journal of Public Health 78:*783–788, 1988.

123. Feldstein A. Health care for the homeless: Portland, Oregon. Paper presented at the 114th annual meeting of the American Public Health Association, Las Vegas, Nev., September 28–October 2, 1986.

124. Bassuk EL, Rubin L, Lauriat A. Characteristics of sheltered homeless families. *American Journal of Public Health 76:*1097–1101, 1986.

125. Whitman BY, et al. Children of the homeless: A high risk population for developmental delay. Paper presented at the 2nd meeting of the Homelessness Study Group, American Public Health Association, Washington, D.C., 1985.

126. Knickman JR, Weitzman BC. A study of homeless families in New York City: Risk assessment models and strategies for prevention. Presented at the 117th annual meeting of the American Public Health Association, Chicago, Ill., October 22–26, 1989.

127. Herrmann R. Center provides approach to major social ill: Homeless urban runaways, "throwaways." *JAMA 260:*311–312, 1988.

128. Shaffer D, Caton CLM. *Runaway and Homeless Youth in New York City.* New York City: Ittleson Foundation, 1984.

129. Robertson MJ. *Homeless Youth in Hollywood: Patterns of Alcohol Abuse.* Berkeley, Calif.: Alcohol Research Group, 1989.

130. Yates GL, et al. A risk profile comparison of runaway and non-runaway youth. *American Journal of Public Health 78:*620–821, 1988.

131. Coalition for the Homeless. *Single-Room Occupancy Hotels: Standing in the Way of the Gentry.* New York City: CFH and SRO Tenants Rights Association, 1985.

132. Brickner PW. Health issues in the care of the homeless. In Brickner PW, et al. (eds.), *Health Care of Homeless People.* New York: Springer, 1985.

133. Ball FLJ, Havassy BE. A survey of the problems and needs of homeless consumers of acute psychiatric services. *Hospital and Community Psychiatry 35:*917–921, 1984.

134. Strasser JA. Urban transient women. *American Journal of Nursing (December):* 2076–2079, 1978.

135. Valade RM. Homeless women and the role of the women's shelter. Manuscript, 1982.
136. Segal SP, Baumohl J. Engaging the disengaged: Proposals on madness and vagrancy. *Social Work 25:*358–365, 1980.
137. Giesbrecht NA, et al. Changes in the social control of skid row inebriates in Toronto: Assessments by skid row informants. *Canadian Journal of Public Health 72:*101–106, 1981.
138. Winograd E. *Street People and Other Homeless: A Pittsburgh Study.* Pittsburgh, Pa.: Emergency Shelter Task Force, 1983.
139. Larew BI. Strange strangers: Serving transients. *Social Casework 61:*107–113, 1980.
140. Timrots A, DeBerry M. *Criminal Victimization in the United States, 1984.* Washington, D.C.: U.S. Department of Justice, 1986.
141. Beck AM, Marden P. Street dwellers. *Natural History 86(9):*78–85, 1978.
142. Cumming E. Prisons, shelters, and homeless men. *Psychiatric Quarterly 48:* 496–504, 1974.
143. Pollak B. The vagrant alcoholic. *Proceedings of the Royal Society of Medicine 68:* 13–16, 1975.
144. Liberman R. Police as a community mental health resource. *Community Mental Health Journal 5(2):*111–116, 1969.
145. Bassuk EL. Homeless families: Single mothers and their children in Boston shelters. In Bassuk EL (ed.), *The Homeless Mentally Ill.* San Francisco: Jossey-Bass, 1986.

CHAPTER 7

Homeless Families and Their Children: Health, Developmental, and Educational Needs

Barbara Y. Whitman, Ph.D., Pasquale Accardo, M.D.,
Jane M. Sprankel, M.S.W.

Today, families with children are the fastest-growing segment of the homeless population (1,2). In New York City, for example, the number of homeless families in temporary shelter has increased from an average of 600 per month in the 1960s and 1970s to over 5,000 per month in the late 1980s (3). Nationwide, homeless families with children now account for about one-third of the homeless population. Most of them are headed by single mothers with dependent children, and more than half of these children are four years of age or younger (4–7).

The developmental impact of homelessness on children has been described as pervasive, severe, and cumulative (8,9). As one aspect of the cycle of poverty, the cycle of homelessness has become an interactive system. Homelessness breeds at-risk, frail, or damaged children; and at-risk, frail, or damaged adults are more vulnerable to the forces that bring about homelessness.

Thus, from a social epidemiological perspective, one must view the causes and outcomes of homelessness within the broader framework of a complex web of causation. This chapter approaches that nexus from a life-span perspective. After a brief discussion of the family, the impact of homelessness on pregnant mothers, newborns and infants, preschoolers, and school-age children will be examined. Research on the short- and long-term effects of homelessness on children has only recently been initiated. No reports of long-term effects are as yet available, and few reports of short-term follow-ups have been done with sophisticated methods (e.g., case control, longitudinal studies, ethnographic studies). Therefore, rather than waiting till more extensive research literature is available, we have used the currently available knowledge of developmental needs and of the homeless situation to project the effects homelessness is expected to have on children.

The Family

A family can be described as a small social system comprising a household or cluster of households which exists over time and is held together primarily by reciprocal affectional bonds. Membership in a family, once conferred, is permanent, with members entering by adoption, birth, or marriage and leaving only by death, if then (10). While a systems-theory definition of family does not require a permanent residence, nonetheless it is very difficult for a coherent family structure to be maintained over a long period of time in the absence of a family abode.

Carter and McGoldrick identified two sources of strain on family systems. External stresses are due to outside events over which a family has no control (e.g., unemployment, wars, some homelessness). Internal stresses are generated by the genetic, psychological, behavioral, and social dynamic baggage that is carried from one generation to another in any family system (11). The external stressor "homelessness" is often related to a variety of internal family stresses that complicate the family system as well as its response to homelessness. Some of the more frequently observed internal stressors are alcohol or other substance abuse, family discord, and family violence. Parental internal stressors often overlooked include mental retardation, learning disabilities, communication disorders, primary psychiatric diagnosis, borderline intelligence, extreme lack of education, and cultural incompatibility with the environment. For instance, in a study of 47 mentally retarded parents (IQ range, 35–69), 45 percent became temporarily homeless during a three-year period (12).

Pregnancy

Homeless women have a pregnancy rate about double the national average, pregnant homeless women have high perinatal and infant mortality rates, and their surviving babies show an excess of low birthweight (13). For homeless pregnant women in the 1980s, access to good-quality prenatal care has been even more limited than for other low-income women, in part because of inadequate transportation to medical facilities and failure to qualify for care for financial or other reasons (14). Exposure to infectious diseases in shelter settings and the high proportion of inadequately immunized children and adults contribute to the rapid spread of these diseases (15). Nutritional compromises occur: homeless pregnant women must often eat soup kitchen offerings that are high in salt and carbohydrates and too limited in flexibility to meet the needs of required dietary regimens. These risk factors are associated with or complicate the management of miscarriage, prematurity, preeclampsia or eclampsia, urinary tract infection, gestational diabetes, placental insufficiency, low birthweight for gestational age, and intrauterine infection.

Biological stresses during pregnancy tend to interact with each other. For example, women who enter pregnancy at 15 percent or more below ideal body weight are at increased risk of intrauterine growth retardation (16). Furthermore, chronic undernutrition makes pregnant women more susceptible to chronic or recurrent urinary tract infections or other infections, increasing the risk of premature delivery and mental retardation in the offspring (17).

Pregnancy often triggers the onset of diabetes mellitus or of hypertension, or aggravates the course of these conditions. Their successful management depends on the careful manipulation of environmental, behavioral, and nutritional variables throughout pregnancy. In homeless women, their management is complicated by the women's lack of access to care, as well as by inability to refrigerate medications such as insulin in shelters or welfare hotels, and by the danger created by the presence of syringes or medications, which can be stolen and sold by other shelter residents.

Drug addiction, alcoholism, and other substance abuse (including that due to poor medical supervision of prescribed pharmaceutical agents such as anticonvulsants or major tranquilizers), which often coexist with pregnancy in homeless women, can have teratogenic effects on developing fetuses. Fetal alcohol syndrome is one of the more common causes of mental retardation and other developmental disabilities (18). Similarly, "crack-addicted babies," who are being born at an alarmingly increasing rate, are at high risk of developmental disabilities.

Poverty, overcrowding, the lack of privacy, and the high incidence of rape and other sexual abuse of homeless women (chapter 6) increase the risk of infection with the organisms of syphilis and toxoplasmosis, with cytomegalovirus, and with herpes viruses. The transmission of these microorganisms to the fetus causes abortion, stillbirth, prematurity, intrauterine growth retardation, lethargy, poor feeding, microcephaly, mental retardation, hearing loss, chorioretinitis and visual impairment, and heart disease (19). It is also likely that homeless women are at increased risk of infection with the human immunodeficiency virus (HIV).

Thus, while the results of adequately controlled comparative studies of perinatal morbidity and/or mortality in homeless and domiciled pregnant women are only beginning to supplement clinical knowledge (20), a substantial amount is already known about the fetal risks associated with pregnancy in homeless women. Programs to bring preventive obstetrics, adequate nutrition, and environmental protection to homeless pregnant women must be implemented without delay.

115

Throughout the following discussion, the concept of *double vulnerability* must be kept in mind. The home and family environment into which the mother and child are discharged assumes a paramount importance in determining whether infants who have been stressed during pregnancy, labor, or delivery, and who may have some degree of central nervous system damage, will develop appropriately. Even a mild degree of brain damage, when compounded by a significantly suboptimal environment, yields a poor developmental outcome (21).

Infancy

PHYSIOLOGICAL IMMATURITY AND NUTRITION

Infancy is a period of great vulnerability, especially when the infant is born prematurely. For instance, the smaller the infant, the greater the damage inflicted by the extremes of temperature to which homeless families are often exposed, since such infants have increased problems with thermoregulation.

Immune mechanisms are immature at birth. This makes infants, especially premature ones, highly susceptible to infectious agents in the crowded and unhygienic environment of many shelters and hotels. Inadequate immunization has been well documented in homeless infants (22).

Poor nutrition is another factor that further increases homeless infants' susceptibility to infection. The nutritional intake of infants must meet both static needs (e.g., constant tissue repair, temperature maintenance, and activity) and dynamic needs (a growth rate that approaches the exponential in the first year of life, when most babies triple or quadruple their weight). Caloric restriction produces a rapid drop in weight, slower growth in height, and minimal slowing of the incremental growth of head circumference. With adequate realimentation, growth parameters return to normal at a rate depending on the duration of malnutrition. The most common specific nutritional deficiency in infants is iron deficiency, which is associated with lower Bailey Mental Development indices, attentional deficit, and increased solemnity and fretfulness (23).

DEPRIVATIONAL SYNDROMES

Deprivation in infancy and childhood significantly increases the risk of language delay and language disorders, which form the basis of a later, language-based learning disability. If the early deprivation is prolonged, children may fail to form an attitude of basic trust and may be vulnerable to decompensation in adolescence. Three conditions that are usually not discussed in the literature on homelessness but would be expected to occur with increased frequency as a consequence of homelessness will be described in some detail.

FAILURE TO THRIVE (FTT). FTT accounts for up to 5 percent of pediatric hospital admissions (24). Since many of its causal and contributing factors are the same as the factors associated with homelessness, its incidence can be expected to increase in the homeless population. The chief characteristics of FTT include poor physical growth, developmental delay, and behavioral peculiarities. FTT can be organic or nonorganic. Almost any chronic disease can produce organic FTT. With poor medical care, inadequate shelter, insufficient immunization, malnutrition, and increased exposure to infectious agents, homeless infants are prone to develop diseases that will present as FTT.

NONORGANIC FTT. Nonorganic FTT (Table 7.1) remains a mixed and somewhat confusing subclass. A synonym for it is "reactive attachment disorder of infancy," diagnosis number 313.89 in the *Diagnostic and Statistical Manual of Mental Disorders*, third edition (DSM-III) (25). This diagnostic phrase indicates a disorder of parenting secondary to failure of maternal-infant bonding. Homeless mothers are at risk of almost all the factors contributing to such failure (Table 7.2). While much of the intervention needed here is psychosocial rather than medical, two medical contributions to prevention should be entertained: adequate early diagnosis and treatment of postpartum depression; and lengthening the homeless mother and child's initial newborn hospital stay so as to use this time to foster bonding and organize service support systems in anticipation of discharge.

Nonorganic FTT has always carried a pejorative connotation that places it in the spectrum of child abuse and neglect. But in homeless infants, FTT can also result from inadequate food or poor parental education with regard to infant

TABLE 7.1   BEHAVIORAL CHARACTERISTICS OF NONORGANIC FAILURE TO THRIVE

Child	Mother
Developmental delay	Poor self-esteem
Apathy, lethargy, withdrawal	Depression
Floppiness or plastic rigidity	Anger
Wide-eyed gaze	Anxiety
Difficulty with change in routine	Poor eye contact
Decreased vocalization	Tendency to hold child clumsily or away from herself
Sad or apprehensive facies	Poor perception of child's needs
Decreased anxiety with strangers	View of child as overly demanding
Indiscriminate affection	Little show of affection
Tactile defensiveness	Negative perception of mothering and child-rearing
Abnormal sleep pattern	
Irritability and antisocial behavior	
Self-stimulatory behavior	

TABLE 7.2 FACTORS ASSOCIATED WITH DISORDERS OF MATERNAL BONDING

Previous experience of the mother (caregiver)
    Deprivation early in life
    Loss of parent figures early in life
    Illness during childhood
    Death or illness of prior children

Events during pregnancy
    Lack of prenatal and/or obstetric care
    Emotional or physical illness
    Death or major illness of key family figure
    Other loss of significant relationship

Perinatal events
    Complications causing prolonged separation of mother and infant
    Acute illness in mother or infant
    Prematurity
    Congenital defects
    Other diseases or disturbances

Current life events
    Homelessness
    Marital stress
    Drug or alcohol abuse
    Financial crisis
    Mental or medical illness causing mother to be unavailable

feeding. Even when these are accompanied by some degree of maternal deprivation, the further contribution of hidden organic disease or mild central nervous system dysfunction to the infant's feeding behavior must not be ignored. Finally, professionals working with homeless families must be careful not to misinterpret the defensiveness of parents of children hospitalized with FTT as automatic evidence of an attachment disorder.

PSYCHOSOCIAL DWARFISM. When deprivation leads to poor growth and development in children over two years of age, it tends to produce the syndrome of psychosocial dwarfism, with its striking behavioral and biological abnormalities—disorders of eating and drinking (polydipsia; polyphagia alternating with refusal to eat; drinking from the toilet bowl; eating from garbage cans; and roaming and foraging); eccentric sleep pattern; enuresis and encopresis; social distancing; pain agnosia and self-injurious behavior; delayed puberty; mental retardation and language delay; pathogenic family relationships; and neuroendocrine changes with low levels of growth hormone and dwarfism. The behavior and symptoms are reversible with a change in domicile (26).

ABUSE. The biological and emotional stresses of homelessness during pregnancy and the perinatal period can produce neurologically impaired infants who later contribute by their limitations to the family's problem of adapting to a difficult if not impossible situation. The stress of homelessness might be expected to significantly increase the incidence of child abuse (whether as physical abuse, neglect, or sexual abuse) from within the family or from those outside it. Indeed, homelessness itself is a form of societal abuse of children.

Toddlers and Preschool Children

Middle childhood is a relatively healthy period compared to infancy and adolescence, yet homeless children of this age group remain vulnerable. As they become ambulatory and independent, they incur an increased risk of accident, injury, and environmentally induced illness, as well as cognitive, language, social, and emotional delays and deviances.

ENVIRONMENTAL HAZARDS. Many homeless families take refuge in condemned buildings, and some live in markedly deficient public or private shelters, where children are at increased risk of rodent bites, rodent-borne infections, and lead intoxication from exposed, old, lead-containing paint (27). The building conditions (no banisters on stairs, no screens on windows, unprotected wiring) contribute to physical injury.

Motor problems emerge as a major area of concern in this age group. Preexisting prenatal or birth influences on motor development become manifest. Mothers, in their efforts to protect children from the hazards of the environment, often overrestrict and overconfine them. Muscular weakness due to nutritional causes, combined with underuse due to restriction, leads to a lack of motor experience and a motor clumsiness that may contribute to accidents and difficulties in coordination.

THE EFFECT OF DEPRIVATIONAL ENVIRONMENTS. In other pediatric populations, it has been noted that deprivational environments are significantly correlated with language and cognitive delays. Indeed, the federal program Head Start was launched because of such observations. Thus, it is predictable that children of families stressed by homelessness will exhibit such delays. Considerable evidence has already been advanced for such delays in preschool homeless children (chapter 5). For instance, in a series of 75 children of homeless families in Saint Louis, 15 percent of boys and 3 percent of girls tested in the mentally retarded range, while an additional 39 percent of boys and 29 percent of girls scored in the borderline slow-learners range; language delay was found in 69 percent of boys and 76 percent of girls (28). Since language delays are the largest predictor of later learning disabilities and school problems, one can predict a difficult time ahead for such children.

Some caution in interpreting data of this kind is in order. Testing children of homeless families is not a straightforward task for several reasons. First, the families are in a state of crisis. Thus the child's capacity to sit and attend to the testing situation, to process and recall information, and to give answers to the tester may be impaired by the emotional and transitional nature of the crisis situation.

Second, testing itself is an added stress on the parents. It is an additional demand of a program that also requires them to look for housing and for jobs and to attend General Education and Development (GED) classes (to earn high-school equivalency certificates), parenting classes, budget seminars, and other program components. These demands are time consuming and require of the parents a level of organization and schedule keeping that would be a challenge to anyone and may not be part of their behavioral repertoire.

Finally, the demand for testing raises in the parents the fear that their children will not test adequately, that they themselves will be accused of inadequate, neglectful, or abusive parenting, and that their children will be removed by the authorities. For many, this fear is not without a basis in reality. Thus the demand for testing often puts parents in a psychological double-bind. However, once the parents have participated in the testing program, they are usually grateful for the information and the direction and guidance in helping their children that they are given.

PSYCHOSOCIAL ISSUES. Many homeless children, even those with developmental delays, have attended preschool programs such as Head Start, or day care. Often these experiences are sporadic, lack consistency in teaching strategies or teaching content from one place to another, and place performance stress on the children rather than addressing and filling the needs for which the children entered the preschool program. As the children negotiate the preschool years with deficiencies in social-interactive skills, they are often emotionally overwhelmed and adaptively taxed.

The School-Age Child

Children who successfully negotiate the toddler and preschool stage without undue external stress usually reach school age with a fund of social, emotional, and cognitive resources. Most of them make the transition to school successfully, so that the school world can become a place of learning, fun, and positive social interaction. The child whose family has entered the cycle of homelessness often lacks such resources.

The more intelligent homeless child will enter school with a set of competencies that are directed toward survival. These competencies and survival skills are often in striking opposition to the prevailing social norms of the school. Children who have been bright enough to learn these survival skills often find themselves in disciplinary trouble at school and experience emotional and cognitive confusion as their hard-won survival skills are confronted as "inappropriate." For instance, they may steal pencils, crayons, or paper from their classmates or hoard food from the cafeteria. On the streets, such behavior may be adaptive and keep them alive, while in the classroom it is judged to be socially deviant behavior.

DISCONTINUOUS SCHOOL ATTENDANCE. Frequent moves by the family require multiple school transfers, with school advancement and learning lost each time. Homeless children are often not enrolled in school while the family resides in a shelter because, as shelter stays are supposed to be temporary, the families or the authorities wait to enroll the children (29,30). Yet such temporary stays often last several months. The cumulative effect of these losses results in academic underachievement, multiple retentions, and gaps in learning and knowledge.

HUNGER, PRIVACY, AND LEARNING. In an effort to keep children in their "schools of origin," children are often bussed long distances. As a side effect, breakfast is frequently missed both at school and at the shelter. Thus, the youngster arrives at school hungry (31). Nutritional deficiencies make learning more difficult, and hungry children have a hard time paying attention and concentrating.

Moreover, teachers' performance and study expectations often cannot be met in the shelter or hotel setting. Survival needs and the shelter environment often preclude adequate study space and time. Study skills are not learned.

STEREOTYPING AND LABELING. Stereotyping and labeling by teachers or peers is a common phenomenon. Behavior difficulties, learning problems, and emotional reactivity are attributed to "homelessness," with the result that underlying, treatable attention problems or learning disabilities go unattended. Often, children are isolated by a repetitious cycle of labeling, reaction, more labeling, and so on.

Parental attempts to negotiate with school authorities are often met with similar stereotyping and labeling. The parents are viewed as personally incompetent because of their homelessness, rather than as people in situational distress. This perceived "incompetence" pervades their interactions and negotiations with school staff, often adding to the parents' frustration in trying to meet their children's needs.

THE EFFECTS OF FREQUENT SCHOOL CHANGES. In some cases, a child may have such obvious problems that he or she is referred for detailed testing; but before the testing is done or the results are available, the family may have to move. Each move brings a new school, a new referral, and further delays. Ultimately, the child may never be appropriately tested and/or identified as needing special education. Even for those children whose learning problems are correctly identified, each school transfer represents time lost. Children with attention deficits or learning disabilities are placed in regular classrooms until their records arrive or until they can be reidentified and retested. Thus, those vulnerable homeless children who most need optimal teaching in a special-education setting in order to maximize their potential receive a double insult from their school experience.

Parents Are Also People in Crisis

In working with homeless families, a number of observations concerning the parents emerge. Whether they are newly homeless or *again* homeless, they are, first and foremost, people in crisis. Thus, it can be expected that their behavior, emotional status, personal interactions, and decision-making capacities reflect their crisis status. If, in addition, they are uneducated, retarded, mentally ill, or substance abusers, they come to this situation with an already less-than-optimal functional status, which can be only further impaired in the crisis. It would be a mistake to try to assess the adequacy of their parenting until the stress of the immediate crisis is alleviated and some steps have been made toward remediating the long-term situation.

On the one hand, after several weeks in a shelter with adequate food, heat, and sleep, parenting strengths not previously noted often begin to emerge. When parents are under the stress of meeting physical survival needs, their children's developmental issues and needs may take a second place in their priorities. After the survival needs have been met, many homeless parents have their first opportunity to express their concerns for their children and to ask for help with the children's routine and special needs.

On the other hand, another phenomenon often emerges in the shelter situation. We term this the *developmental hierarchy*. Many homeless parents are in their late teens and early twenties. It is often the first time in years, if ever, that they have had adequate shelter and food and some help in meeting their own developmental needs for education, vocation, and basic relationships. Often, this personal opportunity takes a hierarchical priority over their parenting duties and their children's needs. When this is brought to their attention, and their obligation to be responsible for their children is underscored, they will usually make a successful attempt to once again attend to their children. Again, it would be a mistake to judge these parents and their parenting skills at this point.

Support services to address the adults' needs as people, as parents, and as children themselves may better serve to interrupt the cycle of homelessness.

Professional Attitudes

It was previously noted that when homeless parents interact with school staff concerning their children, they are often dismissed as "inadequate people" due to their homeless status. This attitude is not limited to school personnel. We have found it among protective service and/or foster care workers, medical and mental health professionals, clergy, and other representatives of the helping professions. All too often, homeless families find themselves put under greater stress by those from whom they have sought help. They are at risk of losing their children to state authorities owing to uninformed and hasty professional decisions, or of being labeled and abused in a medical and mental health system that does not adequately understand the concept of crisis. Thus, homeless parents may become wary, withdrawn, and less likely to seek and use professional help. By a perverse Pygmalion principle, they seemingly justify, by their reticent and recalcitrant behavior, these mistaken professional attitudes and therefore continue the isolation associated with the vicious cycle of homelessness.

Remedies Needed

Homeless families, nationwide, represent a rapidly growing population of parents and children. The solutions are not simple, nor is "homelessness" the only issue. Clearly, housing is a major component of intervention for these families. Despite the well-documented need for more low-income permanent housing units, the likelihood of a major change in housing availability in the very near future is small (32). Thus, the first issue is to provide an adequate supply of decent temporary shelter. Families and children should not have to spend their lives on the street; in cars, condemned buildings, or welfare offices; or in dangerous, crowded, substandard shelters or hotel rooms. Since the average length of stay of families in emergency shelters is extended—6.2 months in New York City—these housing units must meet appropriate standards and be monitored to assure compliance with the standards. The Stuart B. McKinney Homeless Assistance Act (PL 100-77) reflects a beginning federal recognition of this need, but even this act encouraged the delivery of shelter services to the exclusion of permanent housing initiatives until the amendments of 1989, when a modest effort to provide temporary and permanent housing was legislated.

Access to appropriate sheltering and housing for families overwhelmed by the crisis of homelessness needs to be simplified and publicized. Further, the special needs of families with young children must be considered in developing accessibility criteria. Networking among service providers to assure this access is vital (chapter 14). The provision of temporary shelter or even permanent housing is doomed to failure if unaccompanied by educational, vocational, medical and emotional support, as well as support in parenting.

Homeless pregnant women should be provided with safe and hygienic housing as well as adequate nutrition early in pregnancy, and with access to good primary prenatal care and secondary and tertiary perinatal care. It is very important that homeless postpartum women and their infants not be discharged precipitously or prematurely. Indeed, they need to be kept longer than other postpartum women because discharge to the street, shelter, or poor-quality hotel is considerably more hazardous than discharge to an intact home. Hospital social workers should make every effort to obtain permanent housing for homeless postpartum women, their new infants, and the rest of their families. There should be close follow-up of homeless postpartum women and their infants by visiting nurses. Social workers have an important role in assuring that these families are tracked.

Economic and other barriers to preventive prenatal and postnatal care and to infant and child health care must be overcome by making adjustments in reimbursement policies at the governmental and institutional levels, as well as in agency and professional practices and attitudes, and by establishing outreach programs in shelters and other sites where families congregate. At the least, these programs should include prenatal care; infant services; complete immunization of infants and children; early diagnosis; detection and treatment of otitis media and of hearing and vision defects; early detection and therapy of children's urinary tract infections; rheumatic fever prevention; early identification and habilitation of physical and mental developmental disabilities; early detection of and intervention with abuse, neglect, or psychological problems; and appropriate medical care of acute and chronic illnesses.

In the educational area, it is of paramount importance to ameliorate the fragmentation, interruption, and inferior quality of the education available to homeless children, and to counteract the bureaucratic processes and the attitudes among educational and other staff which impact on the education and mental development of homeless children. An integrated inter–school district educational record system for homeless children, the education of teachers and other staff about homelessness and homeless families, and the individualization of remedial efforts would represent initial steps in that direction, as would the provision of adequate nutrition and an adapted shelter environment suitable for homework. Title VII-B of the McKinney Act mandates these services, yet the funding remains unrealistic.

Homeless families must have services that help them overcome the problems that interfere with their ability to maintain themselves in their homes. They need educational supplements, vocational training, and practical, publicly funded employment opportunities to get them started toward improved family functioning. In their role as parents, homeless mothers and fathers need economic and emotional support. Training in parenting skills and knowledge of how to access and use existing services for their children are important components of this support. In many ways, these families need the services that state child protection agencies were created to give. Perhaps a better expenditure of funds would place monies into existing agencies to free specialized personnel to work with these families, rather than create another level of bureaucracy.

To break the cycle of homelessness, services are needed not only for the families but also for the professionals who contribute to the repetitious cycle of labeling, stigmatizing, and blaming the victim. It is inappropriate to refer a mother to talk to the child's teacher when the teacher may be a major source of the problem. Adequate provision of services requires training and sensitization of involved professionals. One night spent in a shelter by a professional may be worth six months of traditional professional training. Training for professionals is provided by the McKinney Act, but it awaits funding.

Small, well-intentioned private groups have built or rehabilitated one or two housing units, placed families in these units, and then "adopted" the families. While this one-to-one caring is often positive for all concerned, these projects often fail because of lack of understanding of the nature of the "rehabilitation process" for homeless families, many of whom have never had other basic needs met. Perhaps program monies would be better spent to provide such private efforts with a centralized coordinative and consultative support and training unit to give these smaller, more personal efforts a better chance at success.

References

1. Congress. *Homeless Families: A Neglected Crisis*. 63d Report of the Committee on Government Operations. Washington, D.C.: Government Printing Office, October 9, 1986.

2. Waxman LD, Reyes LM. *A Status Report on Homeless Families in America's Cities: A 29 City Survey.* Washington, D.C.: United States Conference of Mayors, 1987.

3. Alperstein G, Rappaport C, Flanigan J. Health problems of homeless children in New York City. *American Journal of Public Health 78:*1232–1233, 1988.

4. Hutchison W, et al. Multidimensional networking: A social response to the complex needs of homeless families and their children. A case study of the Salvation Army Emergency Lodge in the city of St. Louis. Unpublished monograph, St. Louis, Mo., 1985.

5. Bassuk E, Rubin L, Lauriat L. Characteristics of sheltered homeless families. *American Journal of Public Health 76:*1097–1101, 1986.

6. McChesney KY. New findings on homeless families. *Family Professional 1(2),* 1986.

7. Towber RI. *Characteristics and Housing Histories of Families Seeking Shelter from HRA.* New York: City of New York, Human Resources Administration, 1986.

8. Whitman BY, Stretch J, Accardo P. Children of the homeless. Written testimony. In House Select Committee on Children, Youth, and Families, *The Crisis in Homelessness: Ef-*

fects on Children and Families. Hearings before the Select Committee, February 24, 1987, p. 125.

9. Bass J, et al. Pediatric problems in a suburban shelter for homeless families. Pediatrics 85:33–38, 1990.

10. Terkelsen K. Toward a theory of the family life cycle. In Carter E, McGoldrick M (eds.), The Family Life Cycle: A Framework for Family Therapy. New York: Gardner Press, 1980, pp. 21–52.

11. Carter, McGoldrick (eds.). Family Life Cycle. See ref. 10.

12. Whitman B, Graves B, Accardo P. Parents learning together: Training parenting skills for retarded adults. Social Work 34:431–434, 1989.

13. Alperstein G, Arnstein E. Homeless children—A challenge for pediatricians. Pediatric Clinics of North America 35:1413–1425, 1988.

14. Arnstein E, Alperstein G. Homeless children and families: Health concerns. Feelings and Their Medical Significance 30(1):1–4, 1988.

15. Miller D, Lin E. Children in sheltered homeless families: Reported health status and use of health services. Pediatrics 81:668–673, 1988.

16. Harrigan J. Prenatal and obstetrical factors in mental retardation. In McCormack MK (ed.), Prevention of Mental Retardation and Other Developmental Disabilities. New York: Marcel Dekker, 1981, pp. 291–304.

17. Broman S, et al. Retardation in Young Children: A Developmental Study of Cognitive Deficit. Hillsdale, N.J.: Lawrence Erlbaum Associates, 1987, p. 279.

18. Abel E. Fetal Alcohol Syndrome and Fetal Alcohol Effects. New York: Plenum, 1984.

19. Papageorgiou P. Infectious diseases in the intrauterine period of development. In McCormack (ed.), Prevention of Mental Retardation, pp. 385–445. See ref. 16.

20. Chavkin W, et al. The reproductive experience of women living in hotels for the homeless in New York City. New York State Journal of Medicine 87:10–13, 1987.

21. Werner E, Smith R. Kauai's Children Come of Age. Honolulu: University Press of Hawaii, 1977.

22. Wright J. Poverty, homelessness, health, nutrition, and children. In papers of conference entitled Homeless Children and Youth: Coping with a National Tragedy, held at Johns Hopkins University, Institute for Policy Studies, Baltimore, Md., April 25–28, 1989.

23. Honig AS, Osler FA. Solemnity: A clinical risk index for iron deficient infants. Early Childhood Development and Care 16:69–84, 1984.

24. Accardo, P, Morrow J, Whitman B. Failure to thrive. In Conn RB (ed.), Current Diagnosis, 8th ed. Philadelphia: W. B. Saunders, in press.

25. American Psychiatric Association. Diagnostic and Statistical Manual of Mental Disorders, 3d ed. Washington, D.C.: APA, 1980.

26. Derivan A. Disorders of bonding. In Accardo PJ (ed.), Failure to Thrive in Infancy and Early Childhood: A Multidisciplinary Team Approach. Baltimore: University Park Press, 1982, pp. 91–103.

27. Mihaly L. Beyond the numbers: Homeless families with children. In papers of a conference entitled Homeless Children and Youth: Coping with a National Tragedy, held at Johns Hopkins University, Institute for Policy Studies, Baltimore, Md., April 25–28, 1989.

28. Whitman P, et al. Families and children of the homeless. Paper presented at the 2d meeting of the Homelessness Study Group, at the annual meeting of the American Public Health Association, Washington, D.C., 1985.

29. Seven Thousand Homeless Children: The Crisis Continues. New York: Citizens Committee for Children of New York, October 1984.

30. Meeting the Educational Needs of Missouri's Homeless Children. State Plan and Survey Report. St. Louis: Missouri Department of Education, June 1989.

31. Safety Network. New York: Coalition for the Homeless, March–April 1986.

32. Reamer FG. The affordable housing crisis and social work. Social Work 34:5–9, 1989.

CHAPTER 8

Understanding Homelessness:
An Ethnographic Approach

Paul Koegel, Ph.D.

W hile much of value has emerged from recent efforts to understand contemporary homelessness, our understanding of the homeless people who populate our streets and shelters remains superficial at best. Indeed, while there is now a body of evidence regarding their sociodemographic characteristics, prevalence of chronic disorder, and rates of service utilization, we have yet to arrive at any real sense of the human beings whose experience and characteristics underlie the percentages offered in study after study. We know little, for instance, about how homeless people actually live their day-to-day lives—the varied strategies they use to meet their needs, for instance, or the actual (rather than reported) nature of their relationships with others. We know even less about how they perceive their experiences, and how these perceptions combine with their beliefs and values to affect their behavior and choices in a given situation. And we know almost nothing about issues that demand a processual perspective—how people make it from one day to the next, the kinds of situational factors that act to perpetuate their condition, the oscillations in their life circumstances, and the causal relationships among the many strands that make up the fabric of their lives.

These gaps in our understanding are very much tied up with the way in which we have pursued information on homeless people. To date, cross-sectional designs featuring structured interviews with individuals at one point in time have overwhelmingly dominated the field. During the 1980s, widely publicized surveys of homeless populations were undertaken in virtually every major American city, including New York (1–4), Boston (5–7), Philadelphia (8), Baltimore (9,10), Washington, D.C. (11,12), Chicago (13,14), Milwaukee (15), Saint Louis (16), Detroit (17), Minneapolis (18), Phoenix (19), and Los Angeles (20,21); and in several states (22,23). Exceptions notwithstanding— most notably the work of researchers in New York City (24–29) but also studies done in Phoenix (30), Austin (31), Saint Louis (32), Los Angeles (33,34),

Connecticut (35), and Santa Barbara (36)—the effort expended in ethnographic research pales by comparison.

Strikingly absent have been the kinds of qualitative and naturalistic approaches to the study of human behavior which rely on ongoing observation of individuals within and across the varied contexts in which they may be found—approaches that are uniquely capable of achieving the longitudinal, contextual, and attitudinal understanding we currently lack. The reasons for this are many and cannot be adequately addressed here. Suffice it to say that lingering debates over whether such methods are sufficiently "scientific," in spite of their increasing acceptance in many fields (37–39), and an entrenched bias against such methods on the part of funding institutions, have acted to discourage research of this kind.

The result is a distressing paucity of careful ethnographic research on contemporary homelessness, and a continued ignorance of critical aspects of the lives of homeless people. This is somewhat surprising given the longstanding commitment to qualitative perspectives which is evident in the past literature on homelessness. Survey efforts such as Solenberger's study of 1,000 homeless men (40), and Sutherland and Locke's *Twenty Thousand Homeless Men* (41), for instance, were accompanied by the pioneer ethnographic studies of Anderson (42,43), just as later cross-sectional studies of a quantitative nature (44–47) were balanced by the insights provided by a strong ethnographic tradition (48–51).

This chapter uses the few available ethnographic studies of the contemporary homeless population to explore three ways in which our understanding of homelessness has been limited by a reliance on cross-sectional studies of a quantitative nature. Doing so should clarify how ethnography can enrich our understanding of who homeless people are, why they behave as they do, and by extension, why more ethnographic research is desperately needed.

Existing Distortions and the Ethnographic Corrective

1. *Individual characteristics, not the ecology in which homeless individuals find themselves, have been the almost exclusive focus of the attention of those concerned with homeless people.*

One of the primary tenets of the ethnographic approach is that behavior is most meaningfully understood when examined in context. This is because behavior is multiply determined and will vary depending not only on the characteristics of the individuals whose behavior we are interested in explaining but also on the settings in which they find themselves and the "others" with whom they interact. Therefore, to the extent that one focuses on individual characteristics alone, one leaves oneself open to flawed understandings of the phenomenon at hand.

While any number of issues could be used to exemplify how our failure to attend to the behavior of homeless individuals in ecological context has left us with misguided explanations of their behavior, one will have to suffice. A pervasive myth that surrounds homeless people is the notion that significant numbers of homeless individuals are unwilling to accept help. To a certain extent, this reflects the popular belief that people "choose" to be homeless, but more often it stems from the recognition that many individuals refuse services that are ostensibly available to them. In such cases, the assumption is invariably made that personal idiosyncrasies, orneriness, or mental illness prevents the individual from acting in his or her best interests. Such individuals, it is assumed, are "treatment resistant," a description most often applied to mentally ill homeless people.

But are individual characteristics sufficient to explain certain homeless individuals' unwillingness to use available services? Consider the following example. When a 200-bed facility for chronically mentally ill homeless men opened in New York City, significant numbers of beds remained empty, prompting the New York State Office of Mental Health to examine why the facility was so underutilized. Quantitative data, in the form of the number of referrals from the New York City shelter system and other selection points, supported the notion that chronically mentally ill homeless men were unwilling to avail themselves of this shelter and the long-term housing program into which it fed. However, qualitative data revealed that the procedures for accessing the shelter, and the organizational structure of the program in both the shelter and its associated mental health clinic, allowed only the best-functioning clients with the highest tolerance for traditional services to survive the obstacle course one had to navigate in order to receive services. More poorly functioning clients either were selected out by the service providers or selected themselves out, not necessarily because of their unwillingness to avail themselves of services but because of the formidable barriers that prevented them from doing so (52,53).

Consider a second example, again involving the mentally ill homeless population. A study aimed at determining what happens when mentally ill homeless individuals are referred to traditional mental health services included a regression analysis of data on clients who had received referrals. This analysis revealed that the presence of (a) a dual diagnosis of chronic mental illness and chronic substance abuse and (b) material need best predicted lack of acceptance into a mental health referral. However, qualitative interviews with service providers in each of the settings to which clients had been referred revealed a picture that went far beyond the characteristics of individual clients. According to Lovell (reported by Koegel [54:43]) and Plapinger (55), these interviews indicated that service providers believed not only that the presence of homeless individuals in their programs would adversely affect their other clients but also that it was impossible to manage homeless mentally ill clients because their needs were too overwhelming.

These examples suggest that if one looks past the quantifiable characteristics of homeless people which may lead them to seek or reject services, and focuses instead on the entire ecology of the service delivery arena, a very different picture emerges. Suddenly, the characteristics of service providers and service delivery settings become relevant, as does the nature of the interactions between service providers and clients within particular settings. Once these are attended to, conclusions highlighting "disorders of place" (chapter 24) and "treatment-resistant service providers" (54:44–46) emerge to compete with concepts such as "treatment-resistant clients."

The concept of "treatment-resistant providers" was clearly present in the comments of researchers during a colloquium on ethnographic approaches to the study of homeless women. Even while recognizing that differences among staff members exist, these researchers suggested that people who serve the homeless—particularly those who staff shelter programs—often lack the knowledge, skills, and attitudes that underlie the effective delivery of services. Their experience was that front-line staff members were poorly educated workers who were earning minimum wage in a job for which they had received little or no training. Often, their attitude toward homeless individuals was highly ambivalent. Many displayed a tremendous fear of homeless people. Others demonstrated a shocking ignorance and insensitivity, as demonstrated by one shelter worker's insistence that women live on the streets because they want sex. Still others, especially those who were acutely aware of their own low status or those who had previously been homeless themselves, betrayed a strong need to differentiate themselves from those they served, and reveled in the opportunity to set the rules for others. Most suffered from endemic burnout (54).

Whether as a result of being afraid, ignorant, status conscious, or merely petty, shelter workers sometimes acted out their feelings by trying to control clients in rigid and often arbitrary ways. Any hint of violence, whether verbal or physical, was consistently dealt with in exaggerated and inappropriate ways. A kick in an altercation between two women could easily lead to temporary banishment from a shelter, leaving the unfortunate perpetrator to face the greater violence of the streets. Even the hint of violence was sometimes enough to elicit a strong repressive action from staff. According to Liebow (reported by Koegel [54:45]), one woman was evicted from a shelter after it was reported to staff that she had kicked another woman on the bus during the day. So it was with alcohol intake as well. The merest hint of alcohol on a woman's breath was used to justify eviction from a shelter, even when the woman's conduct was otherwise exemplary. Staff members' concerns weighed heavily in determining staff-client interactions and shelter policies, contributing to the creation of an environment that, for good reason, was often rejected by homeless women (54:44–46).

All of this is to say that an ethnographic perspective allows us to see that the concept of "treatment resistance" is often used to dismiss or to ignore the legitimate concerns homeless people may have about how services are provided and about which services are provided. Services, for the most part, are utilized if they are valued, if they are offered with compassion and respect, and if accessing them does not involve costs that outweigh benefits (54:41–42,56). The most typical scenario provided by those involved in ethnographic research with homeless women was not one in which a homeless woman refused services. Rather, it was one in which a homeless woman recognized her need for services but either (a) could not find a reasonably accessible facility that offered the service in which she was interested; (b) encountered services that were inadequate, inappropriate, or dehumanizing; or (c) was asked to do something in exchange for the services which was unacceptable to her, such as to accept that she was chronically mentally ill or agree to take medication (54:42). A focus on ecological context, then, sensitizes us to the fact that the people we refer to as "treatment-resistant" are often people who want services but who, in seeking them, have failed to get what they want and have not returned, or have found that services are set up in such a way that accessing them is too difficult, too costly, or too frustrating.

2. *The research community's understandings of homelessness are based on static, rather than processual, perspectives.*

A second tenet of ethnographic approaches to the study of human behavior is that behavior must be studied *over time*. This is true not only because time allows one access to information and understanding that only a long-standing relationship can yield but also because time grants one a historical perspective that can allow the identification of issues that may otherwise be lost.

Perhaps the most obvious value of a diachronic perspective lies in its ability to highlight the effects of a homeless existence. Baxter and Hopper's example of Anne, one of many people whose experience they captured in their ethnographic research on homeless individuals in New York City, suggests how critically important it is to observe people over time, and how doing so raises questions about the etiology of their behavior:

I met Anne in the bus terminal in the Spring of 1980, days after she had begun residing there. She was friendly and articulate, clean, well-groomed, and wore a dress, stockings and a green coat, over which she expressed concern over having lost a button. I barely recognized her a few months later. Lice covered her eyebrows and the scratching made her manner appear frantic; her now-whispered voice was barely audible. She was dressed in multiple layers of dark, men's clothing with a hood pulled tightly over her head. She repeated elements of her story which I recalled from our earlier conversation, but this time in a broken and illogical fashion. I remembered how distastefully she had spoken of others who resorted to sleeping directly in view of the public, as she was motioned away from the entranceway by a tenant of the apartment building where she had sat down to rest. (25:401)

From the description that Baxter and Hopper give us, it is hard to tell whether Anne's deterioration is best understood as a function of chronic mental illness, the demoralizing effect of life on the streets, or some interaction of the two. Even so, this example underscores how behavior is not immutable—how it differs at different points in time—and how the long-term effects of homelessness can result in behaviors and appearances that are easily misinterpreted as signs of chronic mental illness (chapter 5) (57).

However, the value of a diachronic perspective goes beyond its ability to provide a corrective against erroneous impressions. A diachronic perspective also allows us to witness transition. When we interview a homeless person at one point in time, we are afforded a glimpse of an individual as he or she exists at the moment, living on the streets, in a shelter, or perhaps even in transitional housing. However, we do not get any sense of what happens when a homeless individual tries to leave the streets for the structure of a program, or what happens when a person "graduates" from a structured program into permanent housing. As a result, we have no sense of the process by which individuals leave each of these spheres for the others, in spite of the fact that attention to this process can help explain why so few individuals travel a linear path from street to program to housing, and why so many cycle continuously between these alternatives.

What do we learn when we attend to such issues of process? The ethnographic study of homeless women suggests that the movement from street to program, for instance, involves a complicated process of resocialization, the intricacies of which are rarely acknowledged. Over time, women who have spent long periods of time on the streets learn effective survival strategies for dealing with the rigors of street life; many of these strategies are inappropriate, ineffective, or even maladaptive in the radically different environment of the treatment program or shelter (27,39). The shift from a program to permanent housing is no less complicated. Many women who find in structured programs the opportunity to develop valued supportive ties, for instance, learn that departure from a program means losing those ties, since the new settings in which they find themselves often fail to provide the same opportunities to nurture these relationships (58). Unfortunately, many programs fail to hold clients because their staff are unaware of such issues and thus fail to deal with them.

There are countless other ways in which a diachronic perspective yields information inaccessible through more static perspectives—far more than can be elaborated here. One additional example is worth noting because it involves as fundamental an issue as the very pattern that contemporary homelessness assume. On the basis of data from cross-sectional surveys, which usually include some variation of the question "How long have you been homeless?"

we tend to think of homelessness as following two patterns. The first, "new" homelessness, is the experience of those who have lost their homes only recently, a group in which economically dispossessed people are thought to predominate. The second, "long-term" homelessness, is the experience of those for whom homelessness has become a way of life, a group thought to include a disproportionate number of individuals with chronic disorders.

For all its usefulness in capturing gross differences in the experiences of homeless people, such a typology ignores a third possibility: that over the course of their lives, individuals experience repeated episodes of homelessness. In fact, recent evidence suggests that a pattern of cyclical homelessness may be the experience of the vast majority of homeless people (14,59,60). Indeed, the distinguishing factor of contemporary homelessness may very well be the extent to which experiences in shelters, on the streets, or in welfare hotels are episodic facts of life on the margins (61).

Because we have relied primarily on the synchronic perspective embedded in cross-sectional surveys, we have failed to appreciate that homelessness is not necessarily something that one falls into and then either stays with or escapes from. Rather, it may be something that the marginal poor experience repeatedly as part of an existence characterized by limited resources and an only intermittent and tenuous grasp on stability. Equally important, we have failed to examine in a prospective way the *process* by which this movement into and out of homelessness occurs: the constellation of events that undermines the stability of those at risk of being homeless, and the constellation of events that precipitates a move toward greater stability. Thus, we have undermined our understanding of homelessness itself.

3. *The behavior of homeless people has been looked at almost exclusively from an outsider's perspective.*

If there is a third fundamental tenet of the ethnographic approach, it is that one must examine behavior from the point of view of the actor. This is not to say that an outsider's perspective, one that utilizes constructs foreign to the people at hand, is not essential to certain kinds of understanding. It is to say, however, that by attending to an insider's perspective—by looking at behavior in the context of the attitudes, beliefs, and constructs of the people exhibiting it—we can understand behavior in a very different light, and immeasurably enrich our understanding of the people in question.

When viewed through a middle-class lens—one that features certain assumptions regarding the nature of such things as employment, family relationships, and what one can expect from the future—the behavior of homeless people may make no apparent sense. However, the same behavior may be quite reasonable when viewed from an insider's point of view. From an outsider's perspective, for instance, it may seem inexplicable why a homeless person living on the streets would not jump at the chance to live in a single-room occupancy dwelling. An insider's view, on the other hand, might highlight that person's perception of a very real connection with the nameless people who pass by on the street, expectation that such people would provide help if needed, and fear that in the isolated world behind closed doors, one might die without even being noticed (27). From an outsider's perspective, it may seem that to reinstitutionalize homeless mentally ill individuals would be an act of kindness. However, an insider's perspective vividly underscores the dread with which homeless mentally ill individuals view institutional settings (62) and the fierce pride they take in making it on their own (63,64), however poor that adaptation may seem. Finally, because they employ an outsider's perspective, social workers in a shelter may arbitrarily define a homeless woman as single. However, an insider's perspective may reveal that the woman highly values the roles of wife and mother and does, in fact, have a partner; does have children who visit her in the shelter; and *does* see herself as filling these roles, even if economic factors have placed constraints on her which force her to cycle in and out of the shelter system and leave her unable to care for her children on an ongoing basis (26,65).

Perhaps the most vivid example of the way in which an insider's perspective can allow us to see behavior in a different light is its ability to inform our understanding of behavior that from an outsider's perspective appears pathological or symptomatic of psychiatric disorder (chapter 9). Earlier, the point was made, through the case of Anne, that environmental stresses associated with homelessness may produce symptoms that can be mistaken for those of chronic mental illness. It is also the case that in failing to attend to an insider's point of view, we sometimes mistakenly attribute psychiatric etiology to behavior that, if viewed in the context of a homeless person's daily life, may be considered adaptive (31,57). The paradigmatic case of this is the stereotypical "bag lady's" appearance, which may seem like prima facie evidence of schizophrenia and a concomitant obliviousness to hygienic care but from an insider's perspective can be seen as protection against the predatory intentions of others, particularly men (27,30,62). Similarly, ideation that from a clinical perspective may seem to reflect delusional thought processes may, in fact, be potent coping mechanisms employed in the effort to maintain a sense of dignity in a world that rarely acknowledges the legitimacy of one's claim to dignity (54:30;66).

A far more complex illustration can be drawn from ethnographic research with clients in an outreach program for homeless mentally ill people (29,67), which demonstrated how behaviors that social workers saw as bizarre and inappropriate could be appreciated, from an insider's point of view, as time-worn adaptations to poverty that mirrored practices commonly found among marginal and working-class poor people. Whereas social workers viewed their target population as a group of individuals who were incapable of eating properly or keeping clean without special training, a closer look at these individuals provided evidence that they were skillfully exploiting a harsh environment in order to meet these needs. Whereas social workers commented on their clients' inability to keep appointments or accurately assess what they could expect from various offices, observation revealed a well-developed ability to juggle the resources offered by a potpourri of unrelated public and private agencies, including the ability to be at a particular place at the appropriate time. And whereas social workers saw a devastating inability to manage money or to defer gratification, attention to an insider's viewpoint revealed a pattern of expenditures which reflected an investment in social relationships, a desire to take advantage of opportunities for enhancing one's dignity and self-esteem, and the recognition that immediate consumption was often the best defense against the threat of robbery. Murray (68) also makes several of these points in his discussion of how the cyclical time orientation of street dwellers affects their behavior. Preoccupation with pathology led these social workers to ignore the remarkable adaptive skills their clients possess. Even worse, it allowed them to mistake adaptation for pathology, a danger to which many people fall prey.

Conclusion

While ethnographic accounts of contemporary homelessness are scarce, enough material is available to demonstrate that approaches to the study of homeless people which examine their behavior in context, over time, and from their vantage point provide very different explanations of that behavior— explanations that cast homeless people in a far more positive light and reveal that they, like us, are merely trying, as artfully as possible, to use the resources available to them to meet their needs. For too long, we have been content to focus on what is "wrong" with homeless people, ignoring the fact that their adaptation in the face of adversity that few of us can imagine is often a testament to their strength and cleverness. While it is no one's wish to romanticize homelessness, we would do well to heed the message, embedded in ethnographic research, that homeless people display amazing adaptive skills, and that much of what they do makes sense if viewed from a perspective that takes into account the unique nature of their situation. Only then will we learn to understand homeless people and to more effectively meet their needs.

References

1. Crystal S. *Chronic and Situational Dependency: Long-Term Residents in a Shelter for Men.* New York: City of New York, Human Resources Administration, 1982.
2. Crystal S, Goldstein M. *Correlates of Shelter Utilization: One-Day Study.* New York: City of New York, Human Resources Administration, 1984.
3. Ladner S, et al. *Project Future.* New York: City of New York, Human Resources Administration, 1986.

4. Struening EL. *A Study of Residents of the New York City Shelter System.* New York: New York State Psychiatric Institute, 1986.

5. Bassuk EL, Rubin L, Lauriat A. Is homelessness a mental health problem? *American Journal of Psychiatry 141:*1546–1550, 1984.

6. Bassuk EL, Rubin L, Lauriat A. The characteristics of sheltered homeless families. *American Journal of Public Health 76:*1097–1101, 1986.

7. Mulkern V, et al. *Homelessness Needs Assessment Study: Findings and Recommendations for the Massachusetts Department of Mental Health.* Boston: Human Services Research Institute, 1985.

8. Arce AA, et al. A psychiatric profile of street people admitted to an emergency shelter. *Hospital and Community Psychiatry 34:*812–817, 1983.

9. Fischer P, et al. Mental health and social characteristics of the homeless: A survey of Baltimore shelter users. *American Journal of Public Health 76:*519–524, 1986.

10. Breakey WR, et al. Health and mental health problems of homeless men and women in Baltimore. *JAMA 262:*1352–1357, 1989.

11. Depp FC, Ackiss V. Assessing needs among sheltered homeless women. Paper presented at the conference entitled Homelessness: A Time for New Directions, Washington, D.C., July 19, 1983.

12. Milburn NG, Esselman M, Booth J. Drug abuse among homeless people. Paper presented at the 116th annual meeting of the American Public Health Association, Boston, Mass., November 13–17, 1988.

13. Rossi PH, et al. The urban homeless: Estimating composition and size. *Science 235:*1336–1341, 1987.

14. Sosin MR, Colson P, Grossman S. *Homelessness in Chicago: Poverty and Pathology, Social Institutions and Social Change.* Chicago: University of Chicago, School of Social Service Administration, 1988.

15. Rosnow MJ, Shaw T, Concord CS. *Listening to the Homeless.* Milwaukee: Human Service Triangle, 1985.

16. Morse G, et al. *Homeless People in St. Louis: A Mental Health Program Evaluation, Field Study, and Follow-up Investigation.* Jefferson City: Missouri Department of Mental Health, 1985.

17. Mowbray C, et al. *Mental Health and Homelessness in Detroit: A Research Study.* Lansing: Michigan Department of Mental Health, 1986.

18. Sosin M, Piliavin I, Westerfelt H. Toward a longitudinal analysis of homelessness. *Journal of Social Issues 46:*157–174, 1990.

19. Brown C, et al. *The Homeless of Phoenix: Who Are They? And What Should Be Done?* Phoenix: Phoenix South Community Mental Health Center, 1983.

20. Farr RK, Koegel P, Burnam MA. *A Study of Homelessness and Mental Illness in the Skid Row Area of Los Angeles.* Los Angeles: Los Angeles County, Department of Mental Health, 1986.

21. Robertson MJ, Ropers RH, Boyer MA. *The Homeless of Los Angeles County: An Empirical Evaluation.* Los Angeles: University of California–Los Angeles, School of Public Health, 1985.

22. Roth D, et al. *Homelessness in Ohio: A Study of People in Need.* Columbus: Ohio Department of Mental Health, 1985.

23. Vernez G, et al. *Review of California's Program for the Homeless Mentally Disabled.* Santa Monica: Rand Corporation, 1988.

24. Baxter E, Hopper K. *Private Lives, Public Spaces.* New York: Community Service Society, 1981.

25. Baxter E, Hopper K. The new mendicancy: Homelessness in New York City. *American Journal of Orthopsychiatry 53:*393–408, 1982.

26. Lovell AM. Social network and social support. Paper presented at the 116th annual meeting of the American Public Health Association, Boston, Mass., November 13–17, 1988.

27. Martin MA. Strategies of adaptation: Coping patterns of the urban transient female. Ph.D. diss., Columbia University, School of Social Work, 1982.

28. Morrissey J, et al. *The Development and Utilization of the Queens Men's Shelter.* Albany: New York State Office of Mental Health, 1985.

29. Schiller NG. Invisibility and compliance: Strategies of survival in a program for the homeless. Paper presented at the 83rd annual meeting of the American Anthropological Association, Denver, Colo., November 14–18, 1984.

30. Stark L. Strangers in a strange land: The chronically mentally ill. *International Journal of Mental Health 14:*95–111, 1986.

31. Snow DA, et al. The myth of pervasive mental illness among the homeless. *Social Problems 33:*301–317, 1986.

32. McCall GJ. Keeping track: What can ethnographers learn through tracking homeless individuals. Paper presented at the 88th annual meeting of the American Anthropological Association, Washington, D.C., November 15–19, 1989.

33. Koegel P. Ethnographic research with homeless mentally disabled adults: Issues and challenges. Paper presented at the 7th meeting of the Homelessness Study Group, at the 116th annual meeting of the American Public Health Association, Boston, Mass., November 13–17, 1988.

34. Koegel P. Ethnographic perspectives on the adaptation of homeless mentally ill adults. Paper presented at the 8th meeting of the Homelessness Study Group, at the 117th meeting of the American Public Health Association, Chicago, Ill., October 21–26, 1989.

35. Glasser I. *More Than Bread.* Tuscaloosa: University of Alabama Press, 1988.

36. Rosenthal R. Hanging out with homeless people: An alternative research strategy. Paper presented at the 88th annual meeting of the American Anthropological Association, Washington, D.C., November 15–19, 1989.

37. Agar MH. *Speaking of Ethnography.* Newbury Park, Calif.: Sage Publications, 1986.

38. Marshall C, Rossman GB. *Designing Qualitative Research.* Newbury Park, Calif.: Sage Publications, 1989.

39. Miles MB, Huberman AM. *Qualitative Data Analysis: A Sourcebook of New Methods.* Newbury Park, Calif.: Sage Publications, 1984.

40. Solenberger AW. *One Thousand Homeless Men.* New York: Russell Sage Foundation, 1911.

41. Sutherland EM, Locke HJ. *Twenty Thousand Homeless Men: A Study of Unemployed Men in the Chicago Shelters.* Chicago: J. B. Lippincott, 1936.

42. Anderson N. *The Hobo.* Chicago: University of Chicago Press, 1923.

43. Anderson N. *Men on the Move.* Chicago: University of Chicago Press, 1940.

44. Bahr HM, Caplow T. *Old Men Drunk and Sober.* New York: New York University Press, 1974.

45. Blumberg LV, et al. *The Men of Skid Row.* Philadelphia: Temple University Press, 1960.

46. Bogue D. *Skid Row in American Cities.* Chicago: University of Chicago Press, 1963.

47. Caplow T, Lovald BA, Wallace SE. *A General Report on the Population of the Lower Redevelopment Area.* Minneapolis: Minneapolis Housing and Redevelopment Authority, 1958.

48. Rooney JF. Group processes among skid row winos: A reevaluation of the undersocialization hypothesis. *Quarterly Journal of Studies on Alcohol 22:*441–460, 1961.

49. Rubington E. Variations in bottle-gang control. In Rubington E, Weinberg MS (eds.), *Deviance: The Interactionist Perspective.* New York: Macmillan, 1973.

50. Spradley J. *You Owe Yourself a Drink*. Boston: Little, Brown, 1970.

51. Wiseman J. *Stations of the Lost*. Chicago: University of Chicago Press, 1970.

52. Dennis D, et al. Sheltering the homeless mentally ill. *New York State Office of Mental Health Research Notes 2(4)*, 1987.

53. Dennis D, Gounis K, Morrisey J. Housing and the homeless mentally ill. *New York State Office of Mental Health Research Notes 2(5)*, 1987.

54. Koegel P. *Ethnographic Perspectives on Homeless and Homeless Mentally Ill Women*. Rockville, Md.: National Institute of Mental Health, 1987.

55. Plapinger J. *Program Service Goals: Service Needs, Service Feasibility, and Obstacles to Providing Services to the Mentally Ill Homeless*. New York: New York State Psychiatric Institute, Community Support Systems Evaluation Program, 1988.

56. Koegel P, Sherman D. Assisting and treating homeless mentally ill adults. In Wood D (ed.), *Delivering Health Care to Homeless Persons: A Guide to the Diagnosis and Management of Medical and Mental Health Conditions*. New York: Springer Publications, in press.

57. Koegel P, Burnam MA. Problems in the assessment of mental illness among the homeless: An empirical approach. In Robertson MJ, Greenblatt M (eds.), *Homelessness: The National Perspective*. New York: Plenum, in press.

58. Merves E. Conversations with homeless women: A sociological analysis. Ph.D. diss., Ohio State University, 1986.

59. Koegel P. Patterns of homelessness in the inner-city of Los Angeles. Paper presented at the 29th annual conference of the American Collegiate Schools of Planning, Los Angeles, Calif., November 5–8, 1987.

60. Piliavin I. Stayers and leavers among the homeless: Some recent findings. Paper presented at the conference sponsored by the National Institute of Alcohol Abuse and Alcoholism and entitled Homelessness, Alcohol, and Other Drugs, San Diego, Calif., February 2–4, 1989.

61. Hopper K, Susser E, Conover S. Economics of makeshift: Deindustrialization and homelessness in New York City. *Urban Anthropology 14:*183–236, 1985.

62. Rousseau AM. *Shopping Bag Ladies: Homeless Women Speak about Their Lives*. New York: Pilgrim Press, 1981.

63. Lowery M. Reaching out to the homeless: A model program. Paper presented at the Seeds of Change Conference, Chandler, Ariz., October 12–14, 1989.

64. Segal SP, Baumohl J, Johnson E. Falling through the cracks: Mental disorder and social margin in a young vagrant population. *Social Problems 24:*387–400, 1977.

65. Lovell AM. Marginality without isolation: Social networks and the new homeless. Paper presented at the 83d annual meeting of the American Anthropological Association, Denver, Colo., November 14–18, 1984.

66. Snow DA, Anderson L. Identity work among the homeless: The verbal construction and avowal of personal identity. *American Journal of Sociology 92:*1336–1371, 1987.

67. Schiller NG. The label of functional disability: A reproduction of ideology in a program to serve the homeless. Paper presented at the joint meeting of the Canadian Ethnology Society, the Canadian Association for Medical Anthropology, the Society for Applied Anthropology in Canada, and the American Ethnological Society, Toronto, Canada, May 9, 1985.

68. Murray H. Time in the streets. *Human Organization 43:*154–161, 1984.

CHAPTER 9

Understanding the Needs of Homeless and Near-Homeless People

Beverly Ovrebo, Dr.P.H.

> Social workers and other professionals working in our behalf, no
> matter how well-meaning, do not understand our needs.
>
> Leon Zecha, homeless man and organizer
> of the homeless in San Francisco, 1984

On becoming homeless, one enters a new world. One's main goal is to survive, while climbing out of homelessness. Homelessness is a nightmare world, apart from society, a world for which nothing in one's previous life could be adequate preparation.

This chapter offers a way of thinking about the worldview and actions of homeless and near-homeless people. The concepts and illustrations are derived from my field study of life in a near-homeless situation: the Century Hotel, a 96-room residential hotel in San Francisco's Tenderloin District (1). Residential hotels are strongly linked to homelessness because they are the bottom rung of the nation's housing ladder (2). Hotel dwellers who lose their dwellings are most likely to become homeless (3). This mobility is bidirectional, as residential hotels are often the places to which homeless people have climbed.

The Tenderloin is one of the most diverse and densely populated inner-city neighborhoods in the country. Squeezed into a few square blocks are dozens of low-class hotels and the shops and services that support the hotels' tenants. The Tenderloin is also "the street" on which many of San Francisco's homeless people struggle to survive.

This study uses as its analytic framework "social praxis," an application of Wittgenstein's theory of meaning to social inquiry (4–6). Social praxis endeavors to uncover shared meanings through the discovery of anomalies, those kinds of situations and practices that push meaning to its limits. Through the analysis of anomalies, one can more clearly see the ruling principles operative in highly normalized worlds such as the Century Hotel.

One of the major ways in which people use housing in this society is to promote their survival. Survival has three dimensions: economic survival (money concerns), functional survival (health concerns), and survival of the sense of self (identity concerns). These are the core concerns not only of the larger culture but also of hotel life, and the residential hotel can be examined in terms of these concerns. It is housing for the poorest of the poor according to market principles (money). Hotel residents must retain their functional independence (health) if they are to avoid the involuntary loss of their homes. Most hotel residents share a common entry path to hotel life and a common identity, that of stigmatized people marginal to society (the sense of self).

The Hotel Ethos

The many norms and practices of hotel life are organized around an ethos that consists of two basic principles: "Don't get into too much trouble," and "Don't hurt anyone." These two principles have specific meanings in relation to the three core concerns: money, health, and the sense of self. To manage one's finances poorly, that is, to prioritize money in such a way that survival items (rent and food) rank lower than amenities (drugs, alcohol, junk foods, and sex) could have dire consequences. Mismanagement often results in getting behind in one's rent and, eventually, being evicted. Losing one's ability to live independently makes it impossible to survive in the difficult living conditions of the hotel. Losing control of one's sense of self—that is, becoming unable to maintain an awareness of shared constructions of social reality—puts one at risk of not surviving. Not only does loss of control of one's sense of self threaten one's tenure at the hotel but it could result in one's becoming a burden and bother to other residents. Residents will not allow another resident to jeopardize their survival, no matter how close they are to each other. Any form of loss of control is viewed as "getting into trouble," against which there are strong sanctions.

Drawing boundaries is part of the second principle of the hotel ethos: "Don't hurt anyone." The main goal of hotel life is to survive, and to do so with as much pride and autonomy as possible. Residents will not tolerate interference with their right to pursue this goal. Therefore, the setting of limits posits the recognition that one person's survival cannot come at the price of another's. Violence and physical harm to other residents are rare in third-class hotels because the proscriptions against such behavior are strong. As far as money is concerned, residents are willing to help one another as long as their own economic survival is not at stake. Stealing and failing to repay loans are highly condemned. If stealing occurs, residents turn to the management, who in turn call the police. When loans are not repaid, the message is spread that one is "not good for the money," disallowing one from further borrowing while also causing one to lose status and belongingness in the hotel.

Losing one's sense of self is the greatest stigmatizer in the hotel. Residents use attacks on each other's sense of self as ways to control and sanction. This use of stigma as a weapon is a "taken for granted" part of living in the hotel. Spreading gossip against a resident who has violated hotel practices and norms is an important and effective way of sanctioning behavior. The resident who is gossiped about loses status, power, and belongingness.

The sense of self is, perhaps, the most central concern for residents, all of whom feel their marginalization and stigmatization by those in the larger society. Having entered the Century Hotel as marginalized individuals, what they have most in common is not what they have done (e.g., gone to prison as a consequence of illegal actions) but who they are to society. Thus, the management and protection of damaged identity is a prime value and a common activity of residents.

Money Concerns

Hotel residents refer to one another as being, to various degrees, "broke." Being broke is one of the common bonds among them. Being broke does not carry the stigma of being "poor." It is a struggle for most residents to avoid becoming "totally broke." The average monthly rent for the hotel room is at least half of each resident's monthly income. Once rent is paid, little is left for necessities such as food and the repayment of loans. Even less is available for the few amenities that make life bearable (newspapers, drugs, alcohol, cigarettes, sex, and getting one's possessions out of hock).

Residents generally do not trust one another around money, and fearing for one's money is taken for granted. Tenancy is an economic arrangement. Within the internal market of the hotel, almost anything can be bought—friends, errands, drugs, alcohol, sex, caring when sick. Yet as long as residents are on a money basis with one another, they neither trust nor respect each other. Residents value relationships in which money is not at issue or in which they can trust each other *even* with money, such trust being rare in the hotel.

Most residents do not receive enough money each month to pay for all their needs, and it is customary for them to run out of money. When this happens, they reduce the amount of food they eat and stop buying amenities. They hope for handouts. They also turn to others to lend them money, either residents, the management, or moneylenders. Those residents who have the most money and/or manage their money well are highly respected and are often asked to lend money. The rule followed by residents is either never to lend money, or to do so only for the closest of friends or for those they are sure will repay it. Making a practice of borrowing from the management (at 40% interest) or moneylenders (at 300% interest) is viewed as pathetic and foolish. Most residents adhere to a philosophy of "living light," having few worldly possessions that can be stolen or that make moving harder.

Health Concerns

Hotel residents are rarely healthy in the conventional sense. They define health in functional terms, as the ability to survive in one's room. All of them struggle with the same difficult environment, have very little money, and feel they are unable to help those at the point of being unable to survive. Professional help is seen as a direct path to institutionalization, which means the loss of one's room, one's worldly possessions, one's independence and autonomy, and one's self-respect. The professional helper is seen as one who is ultimately necessary but who takes from the resident more than the resident has to give.

A consequence of the unavailability of peer help when ill and of the high price of professional care is residents' great secrecy concerning health problems and their often elaborate cover-ups when health crises do occur. One resident tried to reassure me that he had never felt better in his life, all the while being unable to lift his head as he coughed and spit up blood.

Identity Concerns

Identity is a social construct, a map of the self which is negotiated within a culture and throughout a whole biography. Identity has two aspects: the public self—the self that is connected to society, culture, other people, and the outside world; and the private self—the center of autonomy and independence, of power and control for the individual. The norms of hotel residents serve to support both the public and private aspects of self.

THE PUBLIC SELF

THE NEED TO BE CONNECTED.   One resident told me that if I really wanted to help her mother, I should take her on a car trip, explaining, "Staying in one's room all day like she has, you can lose all track of time." Her basic need was to be reconnected to the world by way of the social meaning of time. The hotel room is often a private world, with idiosyncratic perceptions of space and time. One effect of isolation is disconnection from social space-time, often leading to personal disorientation. Part of being oriented is having a strong connection between one's sense of self and the social worlds of which one is a part. There are norms in the hotel against staying in one's room, darkening one's room, shutting off the world.

There is also a need to remain connected to the hotel space-time. The lobby serves an important orienting and connecting function for the residents, being a place where they can make the transition from their private to their public selves and connect with the hotel's world and the world outside the hotel. A core group of residents, the "old-timers," are the hotel's inner circle. This group has a strong sense of the ritualistic behaviors that provide not only stability and a sense of tradition for the hotel but also referents for norms and standards of behavior and sanctions for improprieties. They keep watch over the public world of the hotel and the outside news. Reading the paper every morning in the hotel lobby is another custom, a strategy to connect with society and the outside world. Newspapers usher in the world surrounding the hotel, with its disparate customs related to health and social needs.

THE NEED TO CARE AND BE CARED FOR.   There are many types of relationships among hotel residents, which meet some of the residents' needs for intimacy, as well serving pragmatic functions such as giving help, counsel, companionship, and entertainment. In hotels, it is common for social outsiders to become the objects of the residents' romantic fantasies. One reason for this is that romantic fantasy fulfills a need to have someone to care about but has minimum negative consequences.

THE PRIVATE SELF

THE NEED FOR FREEDOM.   A primary need of residents is to preserve their sense of freedom and dignity as consumers in an open market. As buyers, they receive the impersonal respect that is given to consumers, and the freedom to do with their money as they please. The ability to live on one's own in a difficult world is a prerequisite to remaining in the hotel. Independence, doing without help, increases one's status and respect. It is residents' greatest source of pride and self-control.

THE NEED FOR STATUS AND A STRONG SENSE OF SELF.   Pride is of prime value to residents—the pride of being independent, the pride of one's past, the pride of whom one knows. All this pervades residents' talk. Pride is often all that the residents have left when everything else is gone. In managing marginalized status, pride serves an important function. A belief in oneself, untarnished by what others may think, is a way to survive low social status. The preservation of pride explains many of the norms related to charity interactions and to the management and use of stigma. Strong norms about withholding judgment help to preserve residents' pride. Residents respect one another's pride and need for pride.

Subcultures emerge in the hotel as means of supporting pride and the sense of self. Artists praise one another's generosity, intelligence, and resourcefulness. Prostitutes are proud of their ability to survive economic hardships. One resident posited that hotel life was hardest for men, since "men are lost if they cannot work." Work is a major source of pride, yet few hotel residents have jobs. Pride is a way of managing the pain of severance from meaningful work. Work is also believed by the residents to be a way to redeem themselves and get their lives back together. Work, even if it does not pay, offers a way to reconnect oneself with the social sense of self, with a social role of which one can be proud.

THE NEED FOR POWER. Power is necessary to deal with the world and to support one's sense of self. Many norms and customs evolve in the hotel to provide power to residents and support their sense of control.

The main form of hotel power is social control, the power to sanction others' behavior. Residents gain power by using stigma as a weapon. Gossip, insults, and censure serve as offensive weapons, giving hotel insiders the greatest power to impose sanctions, since they have the clout of status and belongingness to back up attacks. Residents have considerable power. They can defend themselves from other residents and outsiders through the ability to socially or personally construct reality. Barriers to entrée to one's room provide defensive power, as do modes of managing charity and professional interactions via lying, refusal, and noncompliance.

The ultimate sanction among residents is the loss of entrée: to be rejected among outcasts is the greatest of all shames, and fear of this fuels social control within the hotel. When residents are uncontrollable, ignoring the hotel ethos by hurting others or getting into too much trouble, they are ostracized by other residents because they threaten the survival of the entire social world of the hotel. In this way, the residents have the power of maintaining the survival of their community.

Maintaining one's sense of being in control of one's life is highly valued. To lose control is shameful and may have serious consequences, such as the loss of entrée or even the loss of one's right and ability to stay in the hotel. Alcoholism and other addictions are strongly condemned because they represent a loss of control. Residents do and are expected to use drugs and alcohol, but if this takes precedence over paying the rent and taking care of oneself or causes one to break the hotel ethos, then one is out of control and subject to sanctions by the other residents.

Loss of control can be redeemed by following the norms for management of shame, that is, by taking responsibility for being out of control and by making amends for the damage caused. Blaming oneself is seen as a good sign, and taking total responsibility for one's actions is seen as indicating a strong sense of control.

THE NEED FOR A HOME. The hotel is not referred to as home by its residents. Home is where they were born or where their kin live and/or are buried. All human beings have a deep need for a home as that which sustains and nurtures humanness. This need for home is met by not viewing the hotel itself as home, because living in the hotel subjects the residents to stigma. To identify the hotel as a home would further tarnish an already compromised identity.

The need for something of one's own. No matter how poor, people want to have something of their own. One's room in the hotel is considered to be one's territory, and the residents are respectful of these boundaries. The management has the power to enter residents' rooms whenever necessary, a practice that is condemned by the residents. This puts the management and the residents at great odds over the issue of personal space.

The need to be connected to one's past. Residents also have a need to be connected to their past, although they often hide their past and cut off people in their past as a way of protecting their sense of self. They often emphasize their ancestral homes to increase their sense of pride. The custom of introducing residents to one another in terms of their ancestral homes is accepted in the hotel, protecting residents' identities and reinforcing their pride in their heritage. The lobby is perceived as the most homelike part of the hotel because the lobby is the home of the old-timers, who provide a sense of history and tradition in the hotel.

THE NEED FOR HOPE. The future facing residents is generally not a hopeful one. The exit paths for residents are usually involuntary (due to ill health or death, loss of control or ability to manage, or lack of funds) and downward (lower-class hotel, same-class hotel at higher rent, the street, or institutionalization). Residents have a need for hope. Construction of health and one's life circumstances (e.g., stating that one is healthy when ill, or has money when broke) serve to reinforce the notion that one is all right and provide an illusion that one's life will improve. Religious hopes are not common; the hotel tends to be secular. Residents seek something to live for on *this* earth, be it hope for functional independence of hope for romance. One resident talked of regaining hope through making a new friend: "It's just like coming alive again . . . after being in a dark room . . . when a man or woman finds something to live for." The first of the month offers residents their most reliable hope—the monthly check and the chance to live out the fantasies built by deprivation at the end of each month.

Apparent Anomalies of Hotel Life: The Functions of "Dysfunctional" Practices and Customs

The norms and customs of the hotel are basic to residents' survival, yet there are many hotel customs that appear dysfunctional to the outsider. These practices tend to reinforce views that hotel residents are less than human, and somewhat pathological, and that living in a hotel is somehow due to pathology. Some hotel customs that seem counter to the goal of individual residents' survival will be briefly reviewed before their actual function in the hotel world is discussed.

APPARENTLY DYSFUNCTIONAL PRACTICES OF HOTEL RESIDENTS

The absence of personal telephones in the hotel seems to be a liability. Residents have little access to phones, having to use the lobby phone to make calls. This means that they receive few calls and those they do receive are monitored by the management, severely limiting their privacy. Similarly, not having television also cuts residents off from mainstream society, eliminating a source of information and entertainment that could ease loneliness.

The common practice of sleeping all day and darkening one's room not only isolates residents from the world and from other residents but also greatly increases the risk of becoming disoriented and confused.

Alcoholism and drug addiction, which are also common, not only pose continual threats to residents' physical and mental health but also lead to loss of control, one of the greatest taboos of hotel life. Furthermore, the use of alcohol and drugs is expensive, and when their purchase takes precedence over paying rent or buying food, economic and functional survival is threatened.

The "hotel residents' appearance"—being old looking, wearing dirty clothes, and having uncombed hair, unshaven faces, and dirty nails and hair— identifies residents to the outside word, reinforcing their low status and their being viewed as untouchables. Being dirty creates distance among residents and threatens their self-image, particularly in an appearance-obsessed culture such as ours.

The way in which residents' health is constructed and defined, as well as their failure to seek help when sick, seems to lessen their ability to maintain functional independence and remain in the hotel. The health care of most residents is covered by MediCal, so that money is, in general, not an issue. Yet residents explain away the symptoms of life-threatening illnesses and avoid the health care system. This adds to the sense of isolation and increases the sense of powerlessness, the sense that there is nothing oneself or anyone else can do to prevent one's dying.

Living with vermin, raising them, or treating them like pets increases residents' risks of becoming ill. Cockroaches and mice compete with residents for food. Cockroaches damage hot plates and radios, and mice disturb sleep. Rat bites and diseases spread by rats or mice can be dangerous. Furthermore, the proliferation of vermin leads to conflicts not only with management, who may use it as an excuse to enter and clean the room, but also with neighbors.

Hoarding is a similar problem. The saving and storage of papers, junk, and mementos can create litter and odor and allow vermin to proliferate. In extreme instances, this can lead to one's no longer being able to enter the room.

Borrowing money from the management or moneylenders increasingly jeopardizes residents' control over their finances, and they become further in debt, having to borrow earlier and earlier in the month. They may owe so much money that their monthly checks are garnisheed to pay back loans, until there is not enough to pay the rent, and then they are evicted. The continual borrowing of money is symbolic of loss of control, and it is stigmatizing in the hotel, reducing one's status and sense of self. Borrowing from moneylenders also increases one's risk of bodily harm.

The "eviction game" is the practice of not paying one's rent for several months before the date when one will move. One waits for the manager to evict, meanwhile saving money. This practice forces one to move to a lower-class hotel, or as the word gets out in the neighborhood that one does not pay the rent, one may be barred from moving to another hotel, ultimately leading to homelessness.

FUNCTIONS OF THE ANOMALIES

How then can these anomalous customs be explained? While they appear to be dysfunctional, they serve certain basic interests and fill survival-related needs. Many of the anomalous customs lessen the pain of stigma, that pain experienced as a result of being a marginalized person. Living apart from those who have marginalized you, not having contact with people outside the hotel (e.g., not having a phone), avoiding scrutiny by avoiding medical examinations, not going to places outside of one's hotel or neighborhood where one would feel conspicuous and ashamed, all these practices serve to lessen the pain of a marginalized person. Darkening one's room, sleeping all day, and escaping through alcohol or drugs all serve to deaden the awareness of physical pain and the stigma and psychological pain that come from awareness of who one is and where one is in relation to the rest of society.

Having few possessions enables one to have a niche in a subculture that values freedom and "living light"—being adventurous and bohemian, and living a kind of frontier life. Thus, not having a phone or a television, not personalizing one's room, and having only a few clothes allows one to feel bohemian and also to feel that one is not really *in* the hotel. One is in transit; one's home and identity are not located in the hotel or in one's room.

Economic survival is served by keeping the number of possessions one relies on to a minimum. Not having a telephone, a television, or a refrigerator lessens one's expenses, as does not spending one's money on soap, haircuts, laundry, and new clothes. The "hotel residents' appearance" is the cheapest appearance to maintain and serves to lessen one's risk of being robbed, or asked to lend money. Darkening one's room and sleeping all day also reduces daily expenses. One's world shrinks to the size one can afford. This also increases one's sense of power. Residents cannot expand their power or money, but they do have the power to expand or contract their material needs.

The need for privacy is met as hotel residents make themselves inaccessible by staying in their rooms, not having phones, or avoiding medical examinations. The sense of control is increased by using the moneylender (having options such as where to borrow money when one needs it) and by playing the eviction game (temporarily stockpiling money, while having the advantage over the management).

Because residents have little money, the ability to borrow money, the feeling of living light and free, and the spending of money on pleasurable things (e.g., drugs, alcohol, and junk foods) rather than on life's necessities seem to them to sweeten life. Since they cannot afford to accumulate material goods of their own, they meet the need to have such goods by hoarding and collecting odds and ends. They adapt by giving value to whatever they can obtain and whatever is already in their lives, even if it is "trash" or vermin. If one cannot have what one values, one adapts by giving value to what one has.

What we see, then, is anomalous customs as survival paths, serving many functions for residents. However, they carry a price. Some anomalous practices tend strongly toward functionality, while others, such as addiction or hoarding, tend toward dysfunctionality. Accordingly, in the hotel there are norms and sanctions against the more dysfunctional customs, while the most functional anomalous customs (e.g., the absence of phones) are accepted and universally practiced. A custom such as sleeping all day tends to be common as a functional practice at certain times of the year (e.g., on cold days) and at the end of the month (to reduce the need for money and food), but when engaged in without such function, it tends to be looked down upon and gossiped about as a mode of losing control. Other practices, such as drinking and using drugs, are permitted and considered normal only as long as they are under control.

Residents in the hotel show a remarkable ability to adapt to difficult and degrading conditions and to evolve norms and rules that allow survival. There is also danger in this adaptation that who one is will become degraded, too. Living in trash, one can become "trash"; living with rats, one can become, as one resident put it, "a rat in a hole." Residents internalize their social valuelessness, and in spite of great pride, they may also come to internalize the belief found in the dominant culture that they are worth nothing and that those with whom they live are also worth nothing. That which is great within them, that which allows them to see and appreciate the greatness of others, is at risk of being extinguished. This is one of the great costs and tragedies of hotel life—the need to survive can extinguish the human spirit, forcing residents to focus all their talents, ingenuity, and skills on staying alive. One may stay alive, but what is sacrificed is that which nourishes one's full humanity.

Homelessness

Analyzing the meanings of life in the Century Hotel is instructive in understanding how much more unsurvivable homelessness is. Although it pushes residents to the limits of their ability to endure, the hotel is survivable. The hotel offers its residents a place to rest and to return to when tired; a shower and a toilet; a place to store possessions; running water; privacy and security; a place to orient themselves; and an address where they can receive checks every month. The hotel offers a normative world, a world of meaning that is shaped by the commonality of its residents' experiences, needs, and wants. The street is a nightmare world compared to the hotel. Living on the street means that one no longer belongs anywhere. Homelessness is typified by the absence of real choices. When one is offered two unacceptable options—spending the night in a shelter exposed to physical or mental abuse, or spending it on the street exposed to the cold of winter—one has no option at all. The homeless people who survive do so in the face of the greatest of odds.

Yet one finds in homeless people the same concerns for economic and functional survival and identity survival as in the hotel residents, though homeless people are more often pushed to the extreme. A few documents exist which describe homeless people's lives. These include both older (7) and more recent (8–10) monographs, accounts in the lay press (11,12), and ethnographic studies (chapter 8). A few illustrations will be given, with emphasis on identity survival.

Snow and Anderson reported on an ethnographic study of 168 homeless people in Austin, 70 of whom had made statements about self and identity. People who had been homeless less than six months tended to distance themselves from homeless people as a category and to fantasize in future-oriented terms, suggesting that they had retained an identity different from that of "a homeless person" and that they tried to keep a connection with a different future. People who had been homeless for more than two years accepted, at least outwardly, the identity of "a tramp," but they showed considerably more distancing from homeless institutions or some subgroups of homeless people (the power to reject), more ideological embracement (e.g., of religion), and a tendency to embellish their past or present situation (13).

The life history of April—a New York adolescent with a history of many losses in her family and of psychiatric hospitalizations, who found a home among the homeless in Grand Central Station and there took on a motherly role toward other homeless people, made many friends, and fell in love but eventually, after becoming addicted to crack, committed suicide—shows not only how the vitality of adolescence can create a social milieu within a homeless environment but also how vulnerable homeless adolescents are (12).

In the declining years of their lives, an elderly couple was for several years displaced from one Manhattan single-room occupancy hotel to another as the West Side was being gentrified. Eventually, they were each assigned to different hotels. The wife left the hotel and, becoming disoriented, established herself on a bench in Central Park. After a few days of searching, her husband found her and joined her there. They stayed there in the cold fall and early winter months until they could go together to a nursing home, having preserved their identity as a couple (14:38).

References

Epigraph. Zecha L. Statement of Leon Zecha, San Francisco Homeless Caucus, San Francisco, Calif. In House Committee on Banking, Finance, and Urban Affairs, *Homelessness in America—II.* Hearings before the Subcommittee on Housing and Urban Development, 98th Cong. 2d sess., January 25, 1984. Washington, D.C.: Government Printing Office, 1984, pp. 342–345.

1. Ovrebo B. A window on the world: Relationships between housing and health in a third class residential hotel. Ph.D. diss., University of California at Berkeley, School of Public Health, 1986.

2. Ovrebo B, Liljestrand P, Minkler M. *The Health and Social Needs of Elderly Residents of Single Room Occupancy (SRO) Hotels in the United States.* Policy Paper no. 7. San Francisco: University of California, Aging Health Policy Center, 1983.

3. Kasinitz P. Gentrification and homelessness. *Urban and Social Change Review 17:* 9–14, 1984.

4. Bloor D. *Wittgenstein: A Social Theory of Knowledge.* New York: Columbia University Press, 1983.

5. Pitken H. *Wittgenstein and Justice.* Berkeley: University of California Press, 1972.

6. Schurr EM. *The Politics of Deviance: Stigma Contests and the Uses of Power.* Englewood Cliffs, N.J.: Prentice-Hall, 1980.

7. Anderson N. *The Hobo: The Sociology of the Homeless Man.* Chicago: University of Chicago Press, 1923.

8. Hope M, Young J. *The Faces of Homelessness.* Lexington, Mass.: Lexington Books, D. C. Heath, 1986.

9. Brian K. *The Murder of a Shopping Bag Lady.* New York: Harcourt Brace Jovanovich, 1985.

10. Kozol J. *Rachel and Her Children.* New York: Crown, 1988.

11. Obst U. Anna's tangled destiny. *New York Woman 1(1):*118–124, 1986.

12. Hevesi D. Running away. *New York Times Magazine,* October 2, 1988.

13. Snow DA, Anderson L. Identity work among the homeless: The verbal construction and avowal of personal identities. *American Journal of Sociology 92:*1336–1371, 1987.

14. Coalition for the Homeless and SRO Tenants Rights Coalition. *Single Room Occupancy Hotels: Standing in the Way of the Gentry.* New York: CFH, 1985.

CHAPTER 10

Barriers to Health Care for Homeless People

Louisa R. Stark, Ph.D.

It is no secret that the U.S. system of delivering health care is in need of reform, especially as regards the availability of health care for the nation's poor. While the affluent of our society may receive the most up-to-date medical treatment for their ills, the poor are more likely to receive the crumbs from the table, if indeed they receive medical attention at all. This has been pointed out most graphically in a study of health care in Arizona, where in 1984 almost 7 percent of the members of low-income families who tried to obtain medical care were refused for financial reasons. Of those who were turned away, 31 percent had suffered serious illnesses or injuries, while 69 percent had been refused pediatric or prenatal care (1). This refusal of care has a twofold effect. On the one hand, poor people who need health care become reluctant to seek it, feeling that it may be denied them. On the other hand, health care is indeed denied to poor people. This is particularly true of the poorest of the poor—people who are homeless—who generally have had little or no access to any form of health care. In addition to this, because of their transient lifestyle on the streets or in shelters, often coupled with a lack of any kind of family or other support system, homeless people tend to meet barriers to obtaining health care which are more numerous and more difficult to overcome than those met by poor people who still have what is now a luxury—a roof over their heads.

In the past few years, there has begun to be an interest in the health problems of homeless people (2), as well as in examining the barriers that have precluded helping this segment of the population (3,4). However, their lack of access to health care has generally been approached from the viewpoint of the medical profession. The emphasis has been on examining those barriers that have come about because of problems in the structure of our health care system, or because of health care professionals' attitudes toward homeless people. We have little data on homeless people's attitudes toward health care and on the barriers to obtaining such care that these attitudes may pose. The purpose of this chapter is to examine some of these obstacles, those coming from the health profession and those generated by homeless people. To elucidate some of these barriers, we present the following case history from Phoenix, Arizona.

Excerpts from a Diary

March 14, 1984. This afternoon, as I was waiting by Library Park, an Indian named Tommy came running up to me and told me that his buddy Art was really sick. He asked me if I'd come and have a look at him. We found Art lying near the old library building, doubled up in pain. He was moaning as if going to die. I asked Art what was hurting him. "Nothing," he said. "It'll go away."

"What do you mean, it'll go away?" I asked. "It looks to me like you need some help. Maybe you should go to one of the hospital emergency rooms and have them take a look at you. You certainly don't look good to me."

"No. I'm fine," said Art. "And besides, there ain't any hospitals near here."

"Yes, there are. There are two. They are both right off Seventh Avenue. And you can get the bus to them easily," I answered. Of course, as soon as I spoke, I realized that (a) Art was too sick to take a bus anywhere—yet not sick enough to be transported by ambulance, and (b) he certainly did not have the 75 cents he would need for bus fare. So I suggested that I give him a ride to the nearest emergency room, some 10 blocks away. He was reluctant to accept my offer—still pleading, "No problem." He was also worried, it turned out, about what would happen to his shopping cart, which contained all of his worldly possessions. Finally, after enough insistence on my part that he had to get some sort of medical care, and then assurance on the part of his buddy Tommy that his possessions would be cared for, he reluctantly accepted my offer of transportation to the hospital.

Fortunately, when we arrived at the hospital's emergency entrance, I found a wheelchair parked by the door. And commandeering it, I managed to help Art out of the car and took him up to the front desk. Art was in such pain at that point that he was almost incoherent. Needless to say, he was unable to answer the admitting clerk's questions about his "condition." Finally, I took over and told her that it was obvious that he was very ill, and that that was the reason I had brought him to the emergency room. And that I would appreciate it if he could get some sort of help. That was fine, she said, but he would have to pay $25 to get in. And if he did not have the money, they would not be able to help him. "Let's go," said Art, suddenly somewhat more coherent. "There ain't no way I can pay that kind of money." At that point, a nurse walked by, saw Art and his condition, and whisked him into the emergency room. "Well," said the admitting clerk to me, "now YOU will have to pay the $25 for him."

So, I wrote out a check and settled back in the waiting room to wait for him.

In about 10 minutes, the same nurse came out and asked me to come with her. It turned out that she had been unable to persuade Art to take off his clothes. In as much pain as he was, he simply would not disrobe. As I entered the cubicle where he was lying, he turned to me and said: "Let's get out of here. I don't need no doctors or nurses poking at me." "Come on," I said. "They are not going to poke at you. They just need to examine you to find out just what is the problem. And you have to take off your clothes so they can do it." Then I realized the problem. Like many other homeless people that I have worked with, Art was embarrassed by his lack of cleanliness, both of his body and of his clothes. I asked the nurse for a bag in which he could put his clothes once he took them off—especially his underwear, which I KNEW must be in shreds and of great embarrassment to him. With a plastic bag, a hospital gown, and some privacy, he was finally persuaded to disrobe for an examination. I guess that the medical staff decided that Art was going to be a "difficult" patient because after the clothing problem, they asked me to stay on in the emergency room.

As I waited outside his cubicle in the emergency room, the admitting clerk entered and in a loud voice said to the doctor who was examining Art: "I've called the Indian Hospital, but they won't take him. They say that he has been off the reservation too long. So I guess we'll have to send him off to the county. I've called an ambulance and they'll be over shortly to transfer him. It's obvious that nobody's going to be willing to pay for him to stay here."

I couldn't believe my ears. Here were hospitals fighting NOT to care for a patient who was in serious condition. Needless to say, I was relieved to hear the doctor say that he would not allow Art to be transferred—that Art was seriously ill and would be admitted for inpatient care. "But you can't do that," said the clerk. "Who's going to pay for him? The Indians [Indian Health Service] aren't, and he obviously isn't enrolled in AHCCCS [the state insurance plan for the indigent]." I can just imagine how I would feel lying helpless on an examining table, with my finances and indigent state being discussed as a basis for whether to provide or deny me medical care. After a heated argument, the doctor demanded that the clerk cancel the ambulance and admitted Art to the hospital. His diagnosis is that Art has a serious gall bladder infection and will probably have to have surgery as soon as possible.

March 15, 1984. I visited Art today. He will be going into surgery tomorrow. The hospital staff has already taken a great liking to him. It's amazing what an equalizer a hospital gown can be. I can imagine that were most of them to have seen him homeless on the street, they probably would have tried every possible way to avoid him. Now he is being treated like everyone else, and even though he won't be operated on until tomorrow, he seems like a very different person from the one I have known on the streets. Much more relaxed and outgoing. And obviously enjoying the attention and care.

March 30, 1984.   Ran into Art at the Salvation Army Shelter today. Seems he was released from the hospital last week and told that he should spend six weeks at home "taking it easy." We both laugh at this one. But then I ask him, "What kind of arrangements did the hospital make for you when you were ready to leave."

"Oh," he answered, "they called the shelter and said that they were bringing me there. And that's about it."

"Weren't they concerned that you couldn't stay in the shelter during the day? That you'd have to spend the days on the street?"

"No," said Art. "If they was concerned, they never mentioned it."

So Art is back on the street again. He looks pale and has a terrible scar on his stomach which he showed me, remarking, "You'd think I survived a big knife fight, wouldn't you!" He was also subsisting on the one very starchy meal a day that he eats at the Saint Vincent de Paul Charity Dining Room. I can't imagine that this is really going to speed his recovery. I asked him if he is going to go back to the hospital for a check-up or another visit. He showed me an appointment slip for next Monday and also told me that the doctor felt that he might have something wrong with his heart and should have it examined.

June 22, 1984.   Saw Art this afternoon while he was waiting for the bus. He told me that he now has a job working as a welder. He is really happy with the work. And he's rented a room with Tommy, who is still unemployed but is "looking." Art said that he is feeling fine. When I asked him about his heart, he told me that he never did go back to the hospital after he was released. For one thing, he couldn't really afford it, he said. However, it seems that the hospital somehow kept track of him and found out that he has a job. So his check has been garnisheed to pay off his bill. How much is he paying? "Well, my take-home is $140 a week," he told me, "and the hospital takes $40. That sure don't leave much, does it? So I guess I ain't seeing any of these doctors anymore." I asked him if he didn't think it's interesting that the same hospital that didn't seem to care enough for him to find an appropriate place for him to convalesce could still track him down when it came to getting him to pay their bill. He just smiled.

Providers' Barriers to Health Care for Homeless People

The case history presented above points out two kinds of barriers to health care for homeless people on the part of the providers. The first kind comes about because of problems in the health care system; the second results from the attitudes of health care professionals.

LACK OF TRANSPORTATION. To begin with, Art did not have transportation to get to a hospital. Phoenix, like many cities, simply does not provide transportation for those who are not perceived to be in a crisis situation. This, in the case of the homeless, often results in being unable to obtain any kind of medical care.

LACK OF INSURANCE. The majority of homeless people are, like Art, uninsured (3–6). In Phoenix, 89 percent of homeless interviewees did not have any form of health insurance, while 60 percent did not even know that there was a state health insurance program for the indigent, AHCCCS (6). In a similar study carried out in Los Angeles, 81 percent of the respondents had no health insurance coverage whatsoever (4). Few homeless people have the documentation needed to apply for any form of health insurance. In fact, lack of documentation is often used as a form of "admission diversion" to keep people off the medical insurance rolls (3). Another problem is that without a fixed residence or address, homeless people are unable to apply for medical insurance. The end result is that the vast majority of homeless people have neither applied for nor received any form of health insurance coverage.

LACK OF FINANCIAL RESOURCES. Art was fortunate that he had a friend (myself) who could pay $25 so that he could enter the emergency room. Otherwise he might have been turned away. In Phoenix, as well as in many other parts of the country (3), it is generally impossible to enter an emergency room without some sort of payment "up front." For homeless people, for whom emergency rooms are often the only source for any kind of medical attention, such fees are out of the question, and thus health care is frequently unattainable.

LACK OF ADEQUATE DISCHARGE PLANNING. One of the biggest problems that hospitals have in caring for homeless patients is finding placements for them upon discharge (7,8). This is particularly true when a homeless patient needs bed rest after an inpatient stay. If Art had not been homeless, he probably would have returned home and spent the following weeks "taking it easy"—resting a good deal of the time and eating nutritious foods. As it was, he was simply given a ride to a shelter that was open only at night, meaning that he had to spend his days on the streets, and he was relegated to eating one starchy meal a day. His nutrition, like that of homeless people elsewhere, was probably of little help to the healing process (9,10,11). One might argue that even without the availability of convalescent facilities, the hospital, in Art's case, could at least have found out what services were available at the shelter and could perhaps have located a more appropriate environment for his convalescence. In fact, in the best of worlds, hospital personnel might have thought of providing some sort of case management in order to keep track of Art's progress (8). This was certainly not the case.

BILLING. There is no "free ride" in medicine today. This is certainly true for homeless people (4). After being released from the hospital, Art was billed for $1,800 plus another $600 for the anesthesia he received during surgery. His bills are in the hands of a collection agency, which has garnisheed his wages. As a result, he is paying $40 weekly out of a $140 paycheck. At this rate, it will take him a little over a year (60 weeks) to pay off his bills. In the meantime, he will be lucky to be able to support himself on the $100 per week that remains from his paycheck. Should the cost of his housing be raised by even a few dollars, or should he miss any time at work, his fragile economic situation may cause him to become homeless again. No wonder he is reluctant to submit himself to any more medical bills by seeking follow-up care.

Besides these barriers that stem from the delivery system, there are also problems that arise from the attitudes of health professionals who deal with homeless people.

THE EMERGENCY ROOM OPTION. My first suggestion upon meeting Art in the park was that he should seek help in an emergency room. It was obvious to me, and probably to Art as well, that a visit to a doctor's office would be impossible. Poor people, even those who have insurance, are rarely welcome in physicians' waiting rooms. Their shabby appearance often provides too great a contrast between themselves and middle-class patients (4,10,12–14). Beyond this, there is often a great reluctance on the part of physicians, in Phoenix as in other parts of the country, to treat those who seem to have no way to pay for their services. Thus the only option available for many homeless people, if indeed they can manage to be admitted, is the emergency room of a local hospital (8). They will go there, as Art did, only after having experienced medical crises. As a result, the care they receive is generally fragmented and often of little long-term value (3).

LACK OF RESPECT. One of the most common problems experienced by homeless people is the lack of respect they are afforded by health care professionals. In Art's case, this was most apparent in the treatment he received from the admitting clerk in the emergency room. It is doubtful that such an individual would have talked in a loud voice in front of a patient who was not homeless about his or her perceived inability to pay. Nor would the clerk probably have tried to make unilateral decisions, without any input from the patient or the physician, as to where the patient would receive future health care. In Art's case, it was fortunate that he had an attending physician who was willing to place the health needs of his patient before the economic considerations of the hospital.

The opposite side of the coin was the attention that Art received once he was admitted as an inpatient. Cleaned up, dressed in a hospital gown, he was no different from any other patient in the eyes of the floor staff, who cared for him with respect and compassion. What was also revealing was the way his own attitude and self-image improved as a result of the sympathetic care he was given.

In general, the treatment of homeless people by the health profession is based on a rather rigid set of middle-class standards. It is expected that the patient will have access to transportation as well as insurance or the means to pay for his or her medical bills. It is also assumed that the patient will have a place to recuperate after being discharged from a hospital. If such a situation does not exist, health professionals' solution to the problem has been to ignore it or deny that it exists. Patients without transportation often do not get medical care unless their situation is serious enough to warrant being transported in an emergency vehicle. Patients who are shabby and without apparent means of support are often made to feel unwelcome or are turned away from doctors' offices. At times, they may simply be turned out onto the streets. If individuals cannot fit into the health care system, they are often simply left out of it. Thus they must fend for themselves, hoping never to get sick enough to have to attempt to penetrate a system that is resistant to their presence.

Homeless People's Barriers to Their Own Health Care

Although a certain amount has been published recently about barriers created by providers, there has been little written about those created by homeless people themselves. Writers who have referred to this problem have usually made reference to the facts that (a) homeless people are often reticent about seeking health care until they are very sick, and (b) they often have trouble following up on health care offered to them. Both problems are often blamed on a life-style that is described as "disorganized" (9:116) or "unstructured" (3) and that values food and shelter above health care. Actually, this description is only partly true. Although homeless people do place an emphasis on securing food and shelter, their life-styles are by no means disorganized. To be able to survive on the street requires a great amount of self-discipline and organization (15). For example, in order to get a bed in a shelter, a homeless person must be in line by a certain time; in order to eat, he or she must arrive punctually at the hour during which a congregate meal is served. A homeless person must also be aware of the schedules of food and clothing banks, public buildings in which free rest rooms are located, walk-in clinics, and so on. Whereas a domiciled person can eat whenever and wherever he or she desires, go to bed at any time, and buy food or clothing whenever convenient, all such necessities are available only on a very limited and tight schedule for a homeless person. Organization, or at least some short-term planning, is very important in order to live successfully on the street. Therefore, if we rule out a "disorganized" life-style as a major barrier to medical care on the part of homeless people, we must look elsewhere for factors that separate homeless people from the health care they need.

DENIAL OF HEALTH PROBLEMS.   Art's first response to his illness was to deny it. This was, in a way, a typical attitude on the part of a homeless person. In a study carried out in Phoenix in 1983, 60 percent of homeless respondents stated that they had been in good health during the previous six months (16). Yet in another study undertaken less than a year later, 65 percent of those who were interviewed had experienced some sort of serious health problem during the previous six months. The reason for the difference between the two figures may be that homeless people do not like to acknowledge bad health or medical problems. As stated in the second study: "It is interesting to note that the surfacing of this information [about health problems during the previous six months] really took some probing on the part of our interviewers. Many individuals at first said no [they hadn't had any health problems]; however, as the interviews progressed, they would mention some incident, usually concerning health. The interviewers would ask, 'Well, didn't that cause you . . . (such and such) . . . health problem?' To which, most would say yes!" (6:1).

There is a kind of macho bravado that is adopted by homeless people, the idea being that to survive on the street one has to be tough and resilient. This would rule out admitting any weakness, especially a medical problem. This is exemplified by an interview with Henry, a homeless man in his mid-sixties. Henry was asked whether he had experienced any medical problems during the previous six months. In another part of the interview, he was asked whether he had been assaulted or had experienced any kind of crime perpetuated against him during that period. Henry answered no to both questions. It was then that the interviewer noticed a deep gash in Henry's head. When she asked him about it, he explained that he had recently been stabbed by a man who had tried to steal his sleeping bag. When asked if he didn't regard a stab wound as a medical problem, of the attempted robbery as a crime, he responded that he didn't. After all, the stab wound was healing all right without any medical attention, and he had kept the would-be thief from getting away with his sleeping bag. Henry is a survivor, and part of being one entails not admitting that one has any kind of problems, whether they be medical, or due to assault. Like Henry, homeless people in general tend to deny that they have medical problems, and are therefore apt not to search for medical attention when the need arises. This generalization is supported by a Los Angeles study in which 47 percent of a group of homeless individuals with chronic health problems stated that they had not consulted a doctor during the previous 12 months; 30 percent said they had not done so because the problem was not serious enough (4). A similar denial of health problems as a coping mechanism has also been pointed out in residents of single-room occupancy hotels in Saint Louis (17) and San Francisco (chapter 9).

LACK OF KNOWLEDGE OF MEDICAL FACILITIES. Homeless people, like Art, often do not know where they can receive medical attention. They are often unaware of the fact that there may be free clinics, publicly funded primary care centers, or emergency rooms at public hospitals that will help them (5). In Phoenix, 14 percent of homeless individuals interviewed did not know where to go to receive medical attention (6). In a similar study with data from Los Angeles, 8 percent of those interviewed did not know how or where to find a doctor (4).

A lack of knowledge of health care facilities should probably not be seen as indicating a total lack of interest in health. Many homeless people have very limited knowledge of the communities of which they are a part. A study carried out in Phoenix points out that homeless people tend to maintain daily schedules limited primarily to securing the "basics" for their survival (shelter, food, clothing, work, etc.). It also found that such individuals carry out their activities in relatively circumscribed geographic areas (18). Part of this may be because the basic necessities of their lives are often located in a particular area of a city, but part of this geographical circumscription may also be because of a need to have a feeling of control—to be totally familiar with the ins and outs of one's environment. This may entail limiting one's daily activities to a specific location, and not expanding into unknown territory where one might feel potentially vulnerable. Thus, it is not unusual to find homeless people who stay in a circumscribed area of a city, rarely wandering outside its limits and thus knowing little of the institutions, including medical facilities, that are not within its perimeter.

PERSONAL HYGIENE. Although it is often mentioned that medical practitioners are frequently disturbed by the presence of shabbily dressed homeless people in their offices, the belief appears to be that it is only the middle-class individual who has this feeling and that the homeless person is unconscious of his or her often dirty and odoriferous state. This is generally not the case. With the exception, perhaps, of some chronically mentally ill people, homeless individuals are generally as self-conscious as anyone about their personal appearance. Art is only one example of a person who was mortified about his bodily appearance when asked to disrobe. The middle-class adage that recommends "wearing clean underwear because you never know when you might be in an accident or find yourself in a hospital" is subscribed to as much by homeless people as by any others. It is also, in candid moments, a reason that is given for not seeking medical care. As one homeless man stated when questioned as to why he didn't try to find medical attention for an ulcerated leg: "I haven't showered in three weeks. My clothes are filthy and my body stinks. Do you really expect me to go see a doctor like this?"

FEAR OF LOSS OF CONTROL. One of the main goals of most homeless people is to maintain some sort of control over their daily lives, especially in a world where so much is outside their command. As noted earlier, the smallest and most habitual events of a homeless person's life are controlled by others—where to sleep, at what time to sleep, where to eat, what to eat, and so forth. When this is acknowledged, one can perhaps more easily understand the importance of maintaining control over what is left. In some instances, this may include a few possessions. Art did not want to leave his shopping cart, which contained all of his earthly belongings. Had he had a home, he would simply have locked the door, leaving his possessions safely inside. On the street, one does not have that kind of luxury.

Perhaps more important to homeless people, as the primary possessions over which they still exert some control, are their physical selves—their bodies. In response to the suggestion that a homeless individual seek care, one often hears the answer: "No. I'm not going to the hospital. I don't want them cutting on me." There is also the deep-seated belief that poor people are often used by hospitals as guinea pigs (12). However, we must not overlook the fact that when homeless people do feel that they have control over a situation, they are willing to use their bodies in ways that may seem distasteful to others—in particular, their weekly sale of plasma for a small amount of cash. We must remember that this is a voluntary process, with the individual in full control of his or her actions.

The other side of the fear of loss of control is an aversion to authority. Many homeless (and domiciled) people believe that once they enter a hospital, they are subject to the whims of authorities who often have little or no concern for their feelings. Such was the case with Art when he was privy to the argument as to whether or not he should be moved to another hospital. At no time were his own desires taken into account.

LACK OF FINANCIAL RESOURCES. Unlike the stereotypes often perpetuated about poor people, homeless individuals are not generally abusers of either medical or social services. Most studies show that homeless people have generally had very little access to entitlements that might be available to them, including health insurance (chapter 11). Lack of insurance or of the financial wherewithal to pay for medical services has meant that many homeless individuals simply do not seek the medical attention they need. In a Los Angeles study, 81 percent of those interviewed reported having no health insurance, while 24 percent stated that a lack of insurance or the cost of treatment was their reason for not having a regular source of medical care. Of those suffering from acute illnesses or injuries, 23 percent reported that they did not seek help from a doctor because they could not afford it (4). There is often a feeling among homeless people that medical services must be paid for and that one will not receive treatment, even for an acute illness, if one cannot pay for it.

LACK OF FOLLOW-UP. A problem that has often been noted by those who work with homeless people is the difficulty that arises in persuading them to participate in follow-up care. For instance, in a study carried out in San Francisco only 28.6 percent of homeless patients with infected lacerations returned for follow-up care after their initial treatment (19). Art did not return to see his doctor because he did not have the resources to pay for additional care. This, indeed, is an important aspect of homeless people's reluctance to continue with follow-up care. There may also be an aversion to coming back into an environment perceived as hostile and authoritarian, over which one has little control (20). Beyond this, homeless individuals often feel that it is difficult to include such appointments in a daily schedule. A person who has been homeless for a while often falls into a cyclical kind of time frame. In order to accomplish certain survival goals every day, he or she must adapt to the daily schedules of organizations (e.g., shelters, food programs, clothing banks, and spot labor pools) that supply the necessities of life (21). As a result, the homeless person may find it difficult to integrate a new one-time activity into the repetitive cycle of which he or she is a part. Often one hears: "If I go to an appointment at 1:00 PM, I won't be able to make it back to the dining room for lunch." The meal always has precedence, not only because it is seen as important for survival but also because it is part of the patterning of the day, a pattern that many homeless people find very hard to break.

Discussion

As we have seen, the strategies that are used by homeless people to cope with a potentially very dangerous and unmanageable environment are often those that, ironically, serve as barriers to the provision of care for what are often very serious health needs.

The barriers to health care which have been erected by homeless people are in direct contrast to those raised by medical professionals. The latter are part of a health care system geared to middle-class clients who have transportation; a well-kept appearance; the ability to pay, or insurance that will cover medical expenses; and a place to recuperate.

Starting in 1985, some of the barriers to health care for homeless people began to be removed through a number of innovative programs funded by the Robert Wood Johnson Foundation and the Pew Trust, and subsequently, beginning in 1988, by the federal government's McKinney Act (PL 100-97). By removing the barriers that have long kept homeless people from health care, the grantees of these programs have managed to make health care available to this sector of society. Health programs have been located in shelters, so that such factors as lack of transportation or ignorance of clinic locations are no longer problems. The costs of medical care are underwritten by the grants or by

Medicaid, so that homeless individuals need not fear that they cannot pay for the services they receive, or that they will be denied treatment because of their economic situation. Individuals working in the clinics are selected and trained to treat their clients in a nonjudgmental way, and with respect and understanding. And a few programs have instituted respite beds in neighboring shelters where an individual can recuperate from an illness with continued care and tranquillity. As a result, homeless people are starting to drop some of their reserve as they have begun to realize that they can still exert some control over their lives while receiving the medical attention they need. The walls that have separated them from the medical profession are beginning to be lowered. It should be noted, however, that the programs funded by the Robert Wood Johnson Foundation and the Pew Trust were located in only 22 cities, and the federal Health Care for the Homeless program of the McKinney Act consists of 109 projects in 42 states, the District of Columbia, and Puerto Rico (22). This still leaves large numbers of homeless people with limited access or no access to health care.

Phoenix was fortunate enough to have received both Johnson-Pew and McKinney funding. The local health care for the homeless program that has been developed has many of the components necessary for breaking down barriers to the delivery of health care to homeless people. Not only does the program offer a health care clinic next door to the city's largest shelter but it also includes a mobile outreach team, free transportation, and public health services. The program also contracts for case management, advocacy for entitlements, and substance abuse services. However, in interviews carried out in 1989 with 8,848 single homeless men, only 903 (10%) had health insurance through AHCCCS, the local Medicaid program (23). Yet as the Institute of Medicine's Committee on Health Care for Homeless People states, "Homeless people have many obstacles in obtaining access to health care, but the single greatest problem is . . . [that] they are unable to pay for health care, and therefore do not receive it" (24:4).

The mortality rate among the homeless population of Phoenix, even with improved health care, is still much higher than that associated with domiciled people. In 1987 121 adult men and women out of a local homeless population estimated at 25,000 were known to have died while homeless (25). This would amount to 484 deaths per 100,000 population, a death rate more than twice (484/238) that of white males aged 35–44 in the general population.

From the perspective of Phoenix, a city that has had access to the funding necessary to develop specialized health programs for its homeless citizens, the problem of the poor health of homeless people has not been solved. This is in part because the health problems of homeless people are caused by their lack of a home. Homelessness causes some illnesses, while it exacerbates other health problems by thwarting the efforts needed to cure them (24). While many health programs have succeeded in breaking down the barriers to providing medical services to homeless people, the health problems of such individuals will not be solved until the ills of a nation that has denied millions of its citizens a right to decent and affordable housing are cured.

References

1. Kirkman-Liff BL. *Refusal of Care: Evidence from Arizona*. Tempe, Ariz.: Arizona State University, Center for Health Services Administration, 1984.

2. Brickner PW, et al. (eds.). *Health Care for Homeless People*. New York: Springer, 1985.

3. Elvy A. Access to care. In Brickner et al. (eds.), *Health Care for Homeless People*, pp. 223–231. See ref. 2.

4. Robertson MJ, Cousineau MR. *Health Status and Access to Health Services among the Urban Homeless*. Los Angeles: University of California–Los Angeles, School of Public Health, 1985.

5. Lumsden GH II. *Issues Associated with the Health Care for the Homeless Project in the City of Dallas*. Dallas, Tex.: Dallas Department of Health and Human Services, 1984.

6. Brown C. *The Health Needs of Homeless People*. Phoenix, Ariz.: Phoenix South Community Mental Health Center, 1984.

7. Bond GL, Wilkinson K, Mang M. A public hospital in a community network of services for the homeless. In Brickner et al. (eds.), *Health Care for Homeless People*, pp. 259–277. See ref. 2.

8. Bargmann E. Washington, D.C.: The Zacchaeus Clinic—A model of health care for homeless people. In Brickner et al. (eds.), *Health Care for Homeless People*, pp. 323–332. See ref. 2.

9. Kellogg FR, et al. Hypertension: A screening and treatment program for the homeless. In Brickner et al. (eds.), *Health Care for Homeless People*, pp. 109–119. See ref. 2.

10. Winick M. Nutritional and vitamin deficiency states. In Brickner et al. (eds.), *Health Care for Homeless People*, pp. 103–108. See ref. 2.

11. Crane J. Springfield, Massachusetts: The Sisters of Providence Health Care for the Homeless program. In Brickner et al. (eds.), *Health Care for Homeless People*, pp. 311–321. See ref. 2.

12. Breakey W, Fischer P. Can they go home again? *Johns Hopkins Magazine 36(3)*: 16–24, 1985.

13. Erkel E. The implications of cultural conflict for health care. *Health Values 4:*51–57, 1980.

14. Weir S. Contact before crisis point for those who need care most. *Health and Social Services Journal 25:*332–333, 1977.

15. Stark L. Strangers in a strange land: The chronically mentally ill homeless. *International Journal of Mental Health 14:*95–111, 1986.

16. Brown C, et al. *The Homeless of Phoenix: Who Are They? And What Should Be Done?* Phoenix, Ariz.: Phoenix South Community Mental Health Center, 1983.

17. Ehrlich P. *St. Louis "Invisible Elderly": Needs and Characteristics of Aged "Single-Room-Occupancy" Downtown Hotel Residents*. St. Louis, Mo.: St. Louis University, Institute of Applied Gerontology, 1976.

18. Stark L, McDonald-Evoy KE, Sage AJ. *A Day in June: A Sample of the Daily Activities of the Homeless in Phoenix*. Phoenix: Arizona Ecumenical Council, 1983.

19. Kelly JT. Trauma: With the example of San Francisco's shelter programs. In Brickner et al. (eds.), *Health Care for Homeless People*, pp. 77–91. See ref. 2.

20. Baxter E, Hopper K. The new mendicancy: Homeless in New York City. *American Journal of Orthopsychiatry 52:*393–408, 1982.

21. Murray H. Time on the streets. *Human Organization 43:*154–161, 1984.

22. Mitchem F, Weiss S. *Homeless Health Care Projects.* Washington, D.C.: National Association of Community Health Centers, 1990.

23. Maricopa County. *Homeless Characteristic Report.* Phoenix, Ariz., October 12, 1990.

24. Altman D, et al. Health care for the homeless. *Society 26(4):*4–5, 1989.

25. Stark L. *Mortality Rates for the Homeless of Maricopa County.* Phoenix, Ariz.: Community Housing Partnership, 1987.

PART II

Interventions Directed at Homeless People

CHAPTER 11

Services for Homeless People:
An Overview

René I. Jahiel, M.D., Ph.D.

Interventions with homeless people have several objectives: to minimize damage to the person and improve his or her functional status (tertiary prevention), to return the person to a home (secondary prevention), and to prevent the recurrence of homelessness (primary prevention). The impact on the individual is limited to preventing further suffering and damage, strengthening the person, and making him or her better able to compete in the lower socioeconomic strata of our society. However, for a person who is homeless, this intervention and this impact are all important.

The growth of services for homeless people has been accompanied by the emergence of a "homelessness industry" to provide services and goods to homeless people; of state and local administrative entities that grew as shelters and other tertiary prevention services became the focal point of governmental action in the early 1980s (1); of an ambiguous reaction of the community at large (2); and of further growth of advocacy services (chapter 19).

This chapter is organized according to services: sheltering, food, general health, mental health, substance abuse, employment, education, social service, and transitional housing. In each instance, a brief description of the services is followed by recent studies, cost estimates, and a summary of federal intervention.

Sheltering

The term *sheltering* refers to the provision of lodgings that are not homes. It includes shelters as well as hotels or motels where a room for a family or individual is paid for by an agency. There are diverse sheltering arrangements. In some shelters, homeless people stay only for the night and have to find shelter anew each night. In others, a person can stay only for a given period, for

RENÉ I. JAHIEL

instance, two weeks. In still others, individuals or families can stay for several months or longer. Some shelters give only a cot for the night; others provide meals and allow people to stay in during the day; still others offer social work and other services (3).

The quality of shelters varies. The best ones provide not only resting places but also sites where the strengthening and social rehabilitation of homeless people can begin. Others do not provide as much but are not deleterious to the individual.

Some shelters or hotels are terrible. A lawsuit on behalf of homeless families with children lodged in welfare hotels in New York City cited lack of heat, hot water, refrigeration or cooking facilities; inadequate beds so that infants fell on the floor; infestation by rats, mice, cockroaches, lice, bedbugs and other vermin; plaster and paint chips falling from the walls; door locks that did not work; missing window guards on high floors; widespread robberies and burglaries; prostitution; drug traffic; attacks and beatings (4:219–225). In mass shelters, men, women, infants and children slept in tightly packed rows of cots, without separation by partitions; the most basic furnitures were lacking; children were unable to do their homework; communal bathrooms lacked security and were sites for molestation; sanitary facilities were grossly inadequate for the size of the shelter population, filthy, and frequently inoperative; the risk of airborne infection was magnified by the tight packing which left only one or two feet between beds (4:225–227).

STUDIES ON SHELTERS

SHELTER CAPACITY IN THE UNITED STATES. There have been two recent studies—a survey of shelters in cities of more than 100,000 population, conducted by the Urban Institute in 1987 (5) and a nationwide survey by the U.S. Department of Housing and Urban Development (HUD) in 1988 (6). The Urban Institute researchers found 1,700 shelters with a total of 120,000 beds in cities over 100,000 population (which together constitute 25% of the U.S. population), and HUD found 275,000 beds nationwide. Thus, cities over 100,000 would have 44 percent of the beds. There are no independent ways to check the accuracy of these figures. The shelters were identified by compiling an initial list of shelters from information given by local public and voluntary agencies, using shelters on that list to identify other shelters, and so on. This method—snowballing—has been criticized, since it leaves out shelters outside the main networks.

The relation of the demand for shelter to the number of beds available has been studies by the United States Conference of Mayors every year since 1984 in large U.S. cities. While the shelter capacity steadily increased, the demand kept ahead of it, and every year applicants had to be turned down for lack of space. In 1989 an average of 22 percent of requests for shelter had to go unmet (7).

SURVEYS OF SHELTERS IN LOCAL AREAS. Very few studies have been done which survey the shelters within local areas. The studies of Alice K. Johnson in Saint Louis stand out. Her survey shows the great diversity of that city's shelters, particularly with regard to size (i.e., number of beds); extent and type of services; and number and kind of personnel, including the relative participation of volunteers in the total work force (8). A similar diversity was noted in Chicago (9).

THE COST OF SHELTERS

There have been surprisingly few reports on the cost of shelters or welfare hotels. Not unexpectedly, in view of the diversity of shelters, the cost varies markedly across shelters. In Chicago in 1986–87 the yearly budget was found to range from $121,000 for a 75-bed shelter to $1.2 million for a 120-bed shelter. Typically, the budget cost per bed per year was $3,300 (range, $1,183–10,000), corresponding in 1986–87 to $275 per month (range, $135–810), or $9 per day (range, $4.50–27.00) (9).

In Saint Louis in 1987 the mean cost per bed was found to be $2,555 per year (i.e., $213 monthly, or $7 daily) for shelters providing only bed and board, and $8,395 per year (i.e., $700 monthly, or $23 daily) for those with casework (8).

HUD's 1988 national survey of shelters revealed a total shelter operating cost of $1.564 billion (of which $560 million came from private sources and $1.004 billion from governmental ones). Based on 275,000 shelter beds nationwide, the mean cost per bed would be $5,687 per year, $474 per month, or $15.60 per day (6).

These are low estimates, because the cost of sheltering has increased in the years since the surveys and because not all forms of sheltering were included, particularly welfare hotels. There is little information about the latter. However, in New York City in 1987 a hotel room for a family cost the city $1,612 per month (chapter 20). Furthermore, if the shelter option for lodging homeless people is fully implemented, additional sheltering capacity would be needed for homeless people whose applications for shelter are turned down (22% in 1989) (7) and for many street-bound or doubled-up homeless people who did not apply because they thought that sheltering was unavailable or that it was of poor quality. Additionally, the budgets reported above are primarily for operating expenses. Capital expenses (e.g., new construction, rehabilitation, and new equipment) and interest on capital constitute an additional major category of expenses. Finally, there is considerable pressure to improve the terrible environmental conditions of many of the present shelters, at considerable additional expense. Taking all these factors into account would markedly increase the cost of sheltering, even without an increase in the homeless population. There is an acute need to include these various factors in estimated projections of the national cost of sheltering homeless people, and also to break down operating costs into room, board, and casework costs, so that the shelter option may be meaningfully compared to other options such as transitional or permanent housing.

GOVERNMENTAL INTERVENTION

Local and state governments have markedly increased their role in the provision of shelter since 1980. *Callahan v. Carey* in New York and other court actions elsewhere (chapter 2) have been instrumental in this respect. At the state level, the National Association of Housing and Redevelopment Officials (NAHRO) has recently reviewed the states' programs for assisting the homeless, which include, among other services, shelters (10).

At the federal level, the Stuart B. McKinney Homeless Assistance Act (PL 100-77, July 22, 1987) and its 1988 amendments (PL 100-628, November 7, 1988) authorized appropriations in the range of $100 million (fiscal year [FY] 1987) to $125 million (FY 1990), with matching requirements, for the operation, renovation, or rehabilitation of emergency shelters. This is in addition to other federal funds for shelters, such as those of the McKinney's Act's Title III, which are administered by the Federal Emergency Management Agency (FEMA), and supplemental funds for sheltering families (Title IV-C, see below). As noted earlier, the total governmental funds spent on shelters in 1988 were slightly over $1 billion, one-fourth of which came from federal funds and the rest from state and local governments (5).

Food Programs and Services

Food programs that serve homeless people may be classified into four groups: food stamp programs, which enable recipients to buy food in supermarkets or other collaborating stores; food pantries, which provide groceries, usually gratis, to homeless people; soup kitchens (meal services), which provide prepared meals to homeless people; and those shelters or day programs where meals are served.

In addition, there is a complex system of back-up services to provide food to pantries, soup kitchens, and shelters (3). It includes (a) food banks (warehouses that collect or buy, and store, large quantities of surplus food to distribute or sell at nominal prices to the various food services); (b) clearinghouses and distributors (which together comprise the first link in the programs' food chain, collecting surplus food—fresh produce and canned or stored food—from various sources and distributing it to food banks, pantries, or other services); (c) private sources of food (e.g., individuals who make small donations; and farmers or businesses who sell or donate surplus food, or foodstuffs that have damaged packaging or are too old to sell at market rates); (d) public sources of food (e.g., the U.S. Department of Agriculture [USDA], FEMA, and the Department of Defense [DOD]); and (e) regulatory programs (e.g., state or local health departments' licensing and regulation of food services, regulations imposed by the source of funds or foods [e.g., USDA], and the requirements of state and federal taxation offices for tax-exempt food services).

STUDIES OF FOOD PROGRAMS FOR HOMELESS PEOPLE

THE SELECT COMMITTEE ON HUNGER. Following a hearing on hunger and the homeless on March 6, 1986 (11); the House Select Committee on Hunger sent a mailed questionnaire to shelter providers on March 20, 1986. The sample, which was not intended to be representative of the U.S. shelters, was selected by three umbrella agencies serving the homeless (the Emergency Food and Shelter National Board Programs; the Salvation Army; and the National Coalition for the Homeless). Responses from 140 shelters in 24 states showed that at full capacity, these shelters served 7,663 homeless people daily, including 1,416 children. Half of the shelters provided less than two meals a day, and 27 percent provided no meals.

Among the clients identified as being eligible for food stamps (roughly half of the study population), 45 percent were reported not to be receiving them. In family shelters, 49 percent of clients were not receiving food stamps. Five main causes of failure to receive benefits were identified: (a) incorrect denial of eligibility by state or local offices, based on the lack of a permanent address, the absence of cooking facilities, or the interpretation that residence in a shelter was residence in an institution (the Food Stamp Program allows none of these as grounds to deny eligibility); (b) inadequate documentation on the part of homeless people who lacked both the necessary documents and the financial means to acquire them; (c) inadequate program information and outreach; (d) a definition of *household* for purposes of food stamp eligibility which eliminated otherwise eligible individuals who doubled-up with noneligible households; and (e) complex application forms, requirements for repeated visits, lack of funds for transportation, and high client caseload per food stamp eligibility worker (12).

THE URBAN INSTITUTE STUDY. In March 1987, Urban Institute researchers conducted in-person interviews of 1,704 homeless adults selected with a probability-based, three-stage (cities, provider facilities, and homeless adults) random sample of homeless adults who use shelters or soup kitchens in U.S.

cities of 100,000 or greater population. The provider population was 47 percent shelters with meals, 42 percent soup kitchens, and 12 percent shelters without meals (5).

Interviews with shelter and soup kitchen staff, coupled with direct observation of the food served, showed that the variety and nutritional content per meal in proteins, vitamins, and calories was generally adequate. The mean number of calories per meal was 1,023, that is, 38 percent of the recommended daily level for men and 51 percent of that for women. However, while the nutritional content per meal was rather good, many homeless people did not eat three meals a day. A total of 321,000 meals per day were served to 229,000 homeless people who used the shelters or soup kitchens (i.e., 1.4 meals per day per person). Interviews with homeless people showed that 75 percent ate no more than two meals per day, and 36 percent went a day or longer per week without any food. Homeless people who did not use these services might be expected to have still fewer meal resources.

THE UNITED STATES CONFERENCE OF MAYORS SURVEYS. Yearly surveys of large U.S. cities by the United States Conference of Mayors included surveys of the demand for emergency food assistance since 1984. The data were summarized in the 1989 report (7). The average demand increased every year by 18–28 percent and 15–23 percent of requests went unmet. In 1989, there was a 19-percent increase in demand, and 17 percent of requests went unmet. The reasons given for the unmet need in 1989 were increased demand, reduction in USDA surplus food and FEMA funding, and decreased food donations from companies.

THE QUALITY OF FOOD SERVICES. Many homeless people have special nutritional needs. Among them are adults and children who experienced malnutrition in the past and who are still undernourished; elderly people; people with anemia, diabetes, hypertension, or other chronic illness requiring special diets; people with a history of alcohol abuse; pregnant women; and infants. Food pantries and soup kitchens are often unable to meet the nutritional needs of people in these categories (13). Assessment of the distribution of special nutritional needs among homeless people based on the knowledge we already have of the features of the homeless population (chapter 4) can pave the way for a strategy to meet these needs.

For most people, meals are not merely an intake of nutrients but also an opportunity to rest, relax, and socialize. Meal providers should give homeless people due respect. National surveys to assess these features of meal services are needed.

THE COST OF MEALS

The average cost of food served per meal ranged across providers from $0.36 to $0.58, according to the Urban Institute study (5). Thus, the total cost of food served in cities with more than 100,000 population would be about $150,000 per day, or $55 million per year. Paid staff time devoted to meal services was estimated at $5 million per year. This relatively low staff cost is explained in part by the extensive use of volunteers, whose work would have amounted to another $5 million at the minimum wage. The study did not estimate other expenses, including transportation, public relations, dissemination of information, administration of meal services, and budgeting for food bank and clearinghouse personnel, nor did it estimate the cost of meals obtained at food pantries or with food stamps. It did not include food expenses for homeless people in cities of less than 100,000 or in rural areas. Thus, even when the value of donated food is not included, food-related expenses for homeless people are far greater than the figures given above.

GOVERNMENTAL INTERVENTION

Funding for emergency food assistance comes from locally generated revenues, state grants, Community Development Block Grants, and Community Services Block Grants (7). The McKinney Act authorizes the Emergency Food and Shelter Grants (Title III-B) and the Temporary Emergency Food Assistance Program (Title VIII-B). That eligibility for food stamps does not require a permanent address was reaffirmed by federal legislation in 1986 (the Omnibus Budget Reconciliation Act of 1986 [OBRA 1986; PL 99-509] and the Homeless Eligibility Clarification Act [PL 99-570]). Title VIII-A of the McKinney Act revised the definition of *household* to maintain a household's eligibility when it is doubled up with another household, and provided a method for giving expedited food stamp service within five days of application. These various governmental interventions can greatly improve food services for homeless people. However, continuing vigilance is needed to ensure that they are appropriately funded and implemented.

General Health Care

Health services are categorized into primary, secondary, and tertiary care. Primary care includes ambulatory care within the expertise of primary care physicians, nurses, or physicians' assistants; first-contact medical care, triage, and referral to appropriate specialized care; outreach, disease prevention, and health education; social services liaison; and in some instances, certification of disability. Secondary and tertiary care involve more specialized services, including surgical services, specialized clinics, inpatient hospital care, and re-habilitation services.

THE DEVELOPMENT OF GENERAL HEALTH SERVICES
FOR HOMELESS PEOPLE

Homeless people have more health problems and a higher mortality rate than do comparison groups of the general U.S. population (chapter 4), yet they had virtually no health services adapted to their needs till the 1970s. During that decade, a model of health care for homeless people was developed by Philip Brickner and his staff at Saint Vincent's Hospital, in New York City (14). It is based on primary care delivered by a team (physician, nurse, and social worker) in clinics or at the sites where homeless people live; back-up secondary and tertiary care facilities are available if needed. Important features of the model are a humane and respectful attitude toward homeless people, adaptation of services to their circumstances, and a comprehensive approach to care which includes rehabilitation and social services.

The model was implemented on a larger, though still limited, scale in the Health Care for the Homeless program of the Robert Wood Johnson Foundation and the Pew Trust (JP/HCH), which was directed by Brickner (15). The 19 programs that were funded in the same number of cities with a total of $25 million for 1985–89 had to be community-based; supported by local coalitions of service organizations for homeless people; and integrated with services such as job finding, housing assistance, and assistance with entitlements. The basic team unit was the same as in the original model. Otherwise, there was considerable flexibility and diversity across programs in such matters as local program structure; service delivery sites; referral arrangements; mental, alcohol, dental, or podiatry services; respite services for parents; and additional funding (16). All programs had a uniform reporting requirement, and there was centralized clinical information storage and analysis at the University of Massachusetts in Amherst.

The Johnson-Pew program paved the way for a similar Health Care for the Homeless program, funded by the federal government under a new section 340 of the Public Health Service Act mandated by Title VI-A of the McKinney Act (the legislation was passed in 1987 and implemented in 1988). Some 104 health care delivery projects were funded in 41 states (17). These projects are required to

- Provide primary health care in locations accessible to homeless people;
- Provide care for mental health or substance abuse problems, or referrals for such care;
- Provide access to emergency health services;

- Provide referrals to necessary hospital services;
- Conduct outreach services; and
- Assist homeless people in establishing eligibility for assistance and in obtaining services and benefits under entitlement programs (18).

The projects supported by the McKinney Act gave health services to about 230,816 persons in 1988, the first full year of operation (18). This is a relatively large number, yet it represents only a fraction of the homeless population, since I estimate that at least 2 million people during the course of each year were expected to be literally homeless (i.e., living in the streets, shelters, or similar sites) by the end of the 1980s (chapter 22).

THE FUNDING OF HEALTH SERVICES PROVIDED
BY THE MCKINNEY PROJECTS

The funds allocated to the McKinney projects in FY 1990 amounted to about $33 million, that is, $140 per person if one assumes the same number of people served as in 1988, or $100 per person if one assumes that the number of users increased to 330,000 in FY 1990. The optimal average personal health care costs per homeless person are not known. Elderly people, who consume a disproportionate amount of health services, are underrepresented among the homeless population. On the other hand, homeless people have a much higher frequency of injuries and diseases than is found in samples of the national U.S. population (chapter 4). A personal health services budget of $100 to $150 per individual is thought to represent no more than one-tenth of the cost of the general health services needed by homeless people. This highlights the importance of other sources of funds besides the ones provided directly by the McKinney Act.

The funds available from those other sources are also very limited. The 1988 report on the McKinney Act's Health Care for the Homeless program shows that 76 percent of the clients had no health benefits, 21 percent had Medicaid, and 3 percent had Medicare, veterans' benefits, or private insurance (18). Similar findings prevailed in studies of the homeless population served by the Johnson-Pew projects (19). Since more than 21 percent of the McKinney study population consists of children under 19, and in addition there is in that population a large number of pregnant women, single parents, and mentally ill or otherwise disabled people eligible for SSI (i.e., people who are eligible for Medicaid in most states), it follows that there must have been in the McKinney projects' 1988 population a significant number of people who were eligible for Medicaid but were not covered by it.

The two main governmental programs that provide funds for personal health services of homeless people—Title VI-A of the McKinney Act, and Title XIX of the Social Security Act (Medicaid)—have already been discussed. Something must be said about the implementation of these programs. There are 9 states, as well as several large cities in the other 41 states, that have no McKinney projects (18). As for Medicaid, the Homelessness Eligibility Clarification Act, passed in 1986, mandated state Medicaid plans to provide a method of making Medicaid eligibility cards available to eligible homeless individuals (20). By 1990, nearly all states had incorporated that provision into their state Medicaid laws and plans. However, the actual implementation of that provision by measures such as outreach programs or coordination with the states' Comprehensive Homeless Assistance Plans (CHAPs) had not occurred by spring 1990 in most states, and the matter appeared to have low priority for state Medicaid officials according to a telephone survey of these officials (21).

Mental Health Services

TYPES OF MENTAL HEALTH SERVICES

Services may be classified according to structure of content. Classification according to structure may be based on the environment in which the services are delivered, mental hospitals, mental health clinics, community mental health centers (CMHCs), or streets and shelters—the two last-named served by outreach or crisis intervention teams.

Classification according to content breaks down mental health care into counseling and other forms of psychotherapy, chemotherapy, case management, and treatment of alcoholism or drug abuse. Therapeutic approaches have been discussed in the American Psychiatric Association's book *The Homeless Mentally Ill* (22) and subsequent publications (23).

The objectives of mental health services include the care of homeless individuals with overt mental illness; accurate diagnosis, and reassessment of medication; management of the demoralization of homelessness; and emergency mental health services for people (with or without antecedent mental disorder) who are in a state of crisis following some of the very traumatic events that occur not infrequently in the homeless environment (e.g., having been raped; having seen one's friend killed; having been robbed of one's last possessions or documents; having been separated from one's children who were placed elsewhere).

The federal government, through the National Institute of Mental Health (NIMH) responded to the increased number of chronically mentally ill people in the community in the 1970s (24) by introducing in 1977 the Community Support Systems (CSS) program to aid localities in providing comprehensive management (25). As the problem of meeting the needs of homeless mentally disordered people grew, the NIMH undertook studies of service needs. Among the problems identified were the inadequate service system for people with chronic mental illness and substance abuse (26–28); the stress on psychotherapy rather than emergency needs or housing assistance by the CMHCs (9), inadequate monitoring of mentally disabled people at risk of homelessness because of eviction notices (28); inadequate access to specialized treatment services (9,26); and inadequate discharge procedures for inpatients (9,27).

The ability of the mental health care system to adapt to the homeless situation has also come under scrutiny. Breakey (29) discusses three types of deleterious attitudes of providers: some have a bias against homeless people; others, in their zeal to avoid "blaming the victim," underemphasize the significance of personal as opposed to social factors; and still others underestimate the difficulties encountered by homeless people. Program features may be deterrent to needed care when they pose or are perceived to pose a threat to homeless people's hard-won adjustment to homeless life and when the hierarchy of needs of homeless people are not appreciated. Late in the 1970s, a psychiatrist, Rodger Farr, moved mental health services into Skid Row and started to adapt them to the local situation. Eventually, this approach was developed into the program discussed in chapter 12. Another approach to adaptation of services is presented in chapter 13.

GOVERNMENTAL INTERVENTION

Title VI-B of the McKinney Act provides Community Mental Health Block Grants to the states ($27.7 million in FY 1990) and Community Mental Health Services Demonstration Project Grants ($6.0 million in FY 1990). Using the working estimate that about 200,000–450,000 homeless people of all ages might need mental health services during the year,[1] many of them on a chronic basis, this funding would correspond to about $75–169 per person per year. By itself, this is grossly insufficient. Therefore, if this program is to meet the population's needs, it must be enlarged or supplemented.

Programs for Alcohol Abuse

Alcohol abusers are a very heterogeneous population, who can be grouped into several etiologic subtypes (30). Many have symptoms and biological markers

---

177

of an underlying depressive state. The alcohol dependence syndrome (31,32) and the severity of alcohol abuse are other important variables. The latter is measured not only by the amount of alcoholic beverage ingested and the duration of alcohol abuse but also by the biomedical effects of alcohol abuse on the individual and the severity of associated problems with work, marriage, and other interpersonal and financial situations. At least in its severe form, alcohol abuse is connected to the affected individual's entire outlook on his or her life and to his or her ability to give it a meaning (33).

Traditional homeless alcoholics were alcohol abusers before becoming homeless. However, there are "nontraditional" homeless alcoholics who acquired their habit after becoming homeless (34). These "environmental alcohol abusers" made great progress, in one study, after they were helped to relocate in another part of the city (35).

TYPES OF ALCOHOL ABUSE PROGRAMS

Alcohol abuse treatment includes detoxification and treatment of withdrawal symptoms; counseling and psychotherapy; provision of alcohol-free environments; treatment with peer support groups such as Alcoholics Anonymous (AA); social support and rehabilitation, including provision of jobs and housing; and treatment of underlying conditions such as depression, or associated conditions such as drug abuse, as well as of medical problems.

The facilities that provide alcohol abuse programs include medical or social detoxification centers; residential alcohol treatment centers; alcohol treatment clinics in hospitals or other settings; and transitional, alcohol-free housing with social support. Some facilities provide outreach services in the streets or shelters. Homeless people may self-refer themselves, be referred by their providers, or be assigned to the facilities by the authorities because of public inebriation or other alcohol-related offenses.

RECENT STUDIES

There have been several reviews of traditional and innovative services for homeless alcohol abusers (36–38). In general, the methods used are similar to those used for low-income or indigent domiciled alcohol abusers. There is a trend toward nonmedical (i.e., social) detoxification. However, the indications for the two types of detoxification need to be more firmly defined (39). Outreach programs based on the principle of symbolic interaction have given encouraging results in helping homeless substance abusers who are wary of services (40). Chronic public drunkenness offenders treated with behavior modification techniques have shown decreased recidivism and increased job retention (41). Alcohol-free living environments for homeless alcohol abusers have given encouraging results (42–44). In an older study of Skid Row inebriates, the ability to form enduring relationships affected significantly the chance for recovery (45). In a more recent study, employment and income, family contact, and development of new friendships were associated with the recovery process (46).

Premature withdrawal from treatment and relapses after successful short-term treatment are two common problems. In a cross-sectional study (including a four-year follow-up) of alcoholics who varied widely in duration of absti-nence, it was suggested that "the key to full recovery in alcoholics are [sic] abstinence and time, which are necessary for recovery from a protracted with-drawal syndrome and brain dysfunction, for the repair of social relationships, for vocational rehabilitation, and for abstinence itself to become stable" (47:693). This would indicate that most alcohol treatment programs in current use are too short to assure long-term success. Various facilitative strategies for retaining alcohol-dependent clients in outpatient departments have been de-scribed (48). Cultural bias factors that greatly limit the effectiveness of therapy have also been described. The implication is not that counselors should neces-sarily be from the same culture as the patient but rather that they should be knowledgeable about and sensitive to cultural differences (49).

Most evaluation studies of programs for homeless substance abusers are naturalistic (i.e., without strict comparison with other programs). A new re-search program has been initiated by the National Institute on Alcohol Abuse and Alcoholism (NIAAA) to perform case-comparison studies of innovative and traditional programs. Comparability across programs will be enhanced by the use of common instruments to measure alcohol or drug use, general func-tioning, and work and housing stability (50–53); and by a standardized study design (54).

Most studies of intervention have focused on alcoholism rather than abuse of other drugs, possibly because the reported frequency of the former is greater than that of the latter (55). Studies of drug abuse services for homeless people are likely to increase in the future.

GOVERNMENTAL INTERVENTION

Federal intervention has been minimal throughout the 1980s. The main con-tribution of the McKinney Act was treatment demonstration programs, funded at a level of $16.3 million in FY 1990.

Employment Services

Providing a homeless person with a well-paying, stable job is a major way of breaking the cycle of homelessness. This requires actions directed at the job market and at homeless people. The former actions expand the job market to make more openings available, and increase employers' receptivity to hiring homeless people. The latter actions provide homeless people with skills that meet market needs and facilitate job hunting. Securing a job may involve four or more parties: homeless people, employers, the public, and employment services. Homeless people in general want jobs (chapter 4), but the jobs have to be relatively well-paying, otherwise they may remain homeless or run a high risk that homelessness will recur. Employers need employees when there is a shortfall of labor, but they must be reassured that the homeless employees will function adequately. Further, homeless applicants may be attractive to them because of the possibility of hiring them at lower wages than other workers, an attitude that may open the door to exploitation. The public may be reluctant to have homeless workers in the community because of prejudice. Once that barrier is overcome, the beneficial effects that homeless workers may have in the community, either as workers or as consumers, may be appreciated. On the other hand, if homeless workers are perceived as competing for jobs with unemployed community residents, the barriers may become formidable. Providers of employment services (employment agencies, shelters, etc.) may advocate for homeless people, but in general their primary interest is in their own jobs, which entail obligations to their own bosses and the employers to whom they bring potential employees.

The types of jobs that homeless people get depend on these factors as well as on the local job market and the ability of the homeless individuals to develop vocational and social skills. One may classify the jobs at five levels: (a) work for room and board, in a shelter or shelter-owned business; (b) sheltered work that pays well below the minimum wage; (c) jobs at or slightly above the minimum wage that do not provide enough income for a family or even an individual to break out of homelessness (in my opinion, in 1991 such jobs are those with an hourly wage below $5 for a single individual or $6–9 for somebody who has a family to support in an area with an average cost of living); (d) jobs that pay well enough for an individual or family to break out of homelessness; and (e) self-employment, that is, setting up a business. Only jobs at the latter two levels would help to break the cycle of homelessness for a household. This must be kept in mind in assessing employment services for homeless people. These services include training and placement programs and job development programs.

TRAINING AND PLACEMENT PROGRAMS

A survey of 33 ongoing programs supported by the Department of Labor under the McKinney Act shows that the majority use a case-management approach that includes outreach and initial assessment of the homeless client's work capabilities and potential; counseling; development of an individual vocational plan, with vocational training and remedial education as needed; training in job-seeking skills; placement; and postplacement follow-up and support. Vocational training usually lasts from 8 to 26 weeks. The program descriptions show a high expected attrition rate; for instance, 30–50 percent of those who start vocational training get jobs that they keep for 90 days, according to the stated expectations of many of the programs. A disturbing feature of many programs is that the jobs homeless clients are trained for are expected to pay $4–5 per hour, which may not be enough to bring the clients out of homelessness (56).

Job Programs

Several current job programs have been described. The more interesting ones are programs that involve job development following a study of the local job market. Restart, a temporary shelter in Kansas City, has a small-scale loan program that has helped two homeless people to start their own businesses—a pest control business and a towing service. In Los Angeles, the Skid Row Development Corporation leases two industrial buildings to companies that are required to hire local Skid Row residents, many of whom are homeless. In Denver, Osage Initiatives, a cooperative effort of private industry, government, and community agencies, spearheaded by U.S. West, developed several new business ventures employing homeless or economically disadvantaged people. The businesses include an asbestos-abatement service, a parking lot mainte-nance and repair service, a landscape maintenance service, painting services, and a manufacturer of plastic containers. While such expansion of the labor market is attractive because it minimizes competition between homeless and domiciled workers, it must be assessed very critically to ensure that the home-less workers are not exploited financially, exposed to dangerous environments, or used as pawns in conflicts between management and unions (57).

Binding Together, a new copy, collating, and binding shop organized by Small and Associates in New York City (58), combines an expanded vocational training program with a job program. The workers are former homeless sub-stance abusers. It was created as follows: (a) market research was done, which showed that the copying industry had a demand for technically trained labor in New York City; (b) young, motivated homeless substance abusers were given a battery of needed services—counseling, substance abuse treatment, work preparation, remedial education, and housing in a treatment center—while they learned the trade on the job and were paid competitive wages from the beginning; and (c) part of their pay was held in escrow till they finished the training program and, now having savings and stable jobs, were ready to move into their own apartments.

RENÉ I. JAHIEL

THE COST OF TRAINING PROGRAMS

The cost of training programs varies from $3,000 to $12,000 per trainee (57,58), depending upon the duration of training and the nature of the program (the latter figure is that of the Small and Associates program (58); however, close to half of this sum was later reimbursed out of work-incurred profits). These costs do not include room and board.

GOVERNMENTAL INTERVENTION

The federal government has intervened in the job market to provide work for unemployed poor people since the early 1960s. According to Thomas Bailey, the issue about such intervention is "whether unemployment results primarily from the absence of jobs (that is insufficient demand) or from lack of skills among the unemployed (that is unprepared labor supply)" (59:164).

The Manpower Development and Training Act of 1962 and other 1960s programs were labor-supply programs, meant to train various special categories of workers. They were consolidated in 1973 with the Comprehensive Employment and Training Act (CETA), administered by local governments. CETA made public-service jobs available to poor people, that is, it was a demand-side program that created job openings. In 1978, CETA's funding was $9.5 billion. Because the program was seen as providing "subsidized work," it was cut markedly during the Carter and Reagan administrations. It was replaced in 1983 by the Job Training Partnership Act (JTPA). The public-service (demand) program was discontinued. Instead, a training (labor-supply) program was installed, with a major role for local Private Industry Councils (PICs) and private employers. Funding fell to $2.6 billion in 1985. This decline from $9.5 billion to $2.5 billion is highly likely to have caused unemployment in the population served by CETA and to have been a contributing factor to homelessness in the 1980s.

The McKinney Act made the following funds available in FY 1990: $7.4 million for adult remedial education, through the Department of Education (Title VII-A); and $9.4 million for grants to public and private agencies and business for job training administered by the Department of Labor (Title VII-C). At a cost of $4,000 per person (a conservative estimate for training programs), the Title VII-A and VII-C programs, which together are funded at about $16 million, would be able to train only 4,000 homeless people, a negligible number given the size of the homeless population. Furthermore, the McKinney act does not even begin to address the needs of the homeless people who have work skills and are eager to use them. In a study of 793 homeless men, First and Toomey found that almost one-half were displaced from the work force but capable of working, one-third needed a moderate range of

182

services to become capable of working, and about one-quarter were so severely disabled that they would not be able to work in the foreseeable future (60). The first group is estimated to include 440,000–1 million literally homeless people annually.[2] While the much larger pool of JTPA funds might be used for them, they would have to compete in that pool with a much larger group of millions or even tens of millions of unemployed or underemployed domiciled workers. The surest way to help the large group of homeless people with work skills would be a demand-side approach that would open up to them jobs that would provide wages high enough to pay for low-income housing. In large cities, the rent and utilities for low-income housing of a single person amount at least to $350 a month. Using the standard 35-percent ratio of housing costs to income, this corresponds to an income of about $1,000 per month, that is, an hourly wage of about $6.60, in 1989. This is well above the minimum wage, even after the increases planned for the 1990s.

The Education of Homeless Children

Recent estimates of the number of homeless school-age children in the U.S. range from 220,000 (61) to 750,000 (62). Many of them do not attend school— 30 percent according to a 1989 report of the U.S. Department of Education (61); 57 percent according to the National Coalition for the Homeless (62); and 43 percent according to a 1988 Child Welfare League of America study (63). The New York State Department of Education reports erratic attendance (four or more days absent per week) for 55 percent of homeless high-school students and 28 percent of homeless elementary-school students (64).

Furthermore, homeless children experience a very high rate of transfers among schools. Yvonne Rafferty and Norma Rollins, working for Advocates for Children of New York, interviewed 277 families in 10 New York City shelters and welfare hotels in 1988–89. There were 427 children between the ages of 6 and 19. There were frequent moves from one shelter to another, which were associated with frequent transfers of children among schools—more than 20 percent of the children had transferred twice since they became homeless, and 10 percent had transferred three to six times. Rafferty and Rollins' analysis of a New York City Board of Education data base on 8,070 homeless children in regular education showed that the percentage below grade level in reading and mathematics was well above the citywide rate, and the holdover rate (i.e., the percentage of those repeating a grade) appeared to be significantly higher. Students requiring special education programs have especially severe problems when they are homeless (chapter 7). In the Rafferty-Rollins study, only 30–60 percent of students who had been in special programs when they had homes attended them after becoming homeless (65).

Costs

To my knowledge, there are no accurate currently available estimates of the cost of educating homeless children, including the costs of remedial education and related health, mental health, or transportation services. Such data are urgently needed for adequate planning. Furthermore, at the policy-making stage, such costs should be compared with the projected future lifespan costs of services and subsidies that would be incurred as the children grew up with suboptimal education and neglect of their stresses and needs.

Governmental Intervention

Education is the responsibility of local authorities at the primary and secondary school levels. With the McKinney Act, the federal government has intervened in the following ways: (a) It stated the policy of Congress that homeless children and youths should have access to free, appropriate public education, and that states have to revise any residency requirements for such education to make it accessible to homeless children (section 721). (b) It made grants to states ($5 million in FY 1990) to carry out the policies of section 721; to establish an office of Coordinator of Education of Homeless Children and Youth, who will gather data on the number and location of homeless children and youths and on problems of access to and placement in appropriate schools, as well as develop and carry out a state plan; and to prepare and carry out the state plan to ensure that local educational agencies continue to educate children or youths in the school district of origin or of current residence (whichever is in their best interests, and whether they are living with homeless parents or not) and maintain records so that they are promptly available when a child or youth enters another school district (section 722). (c) Exemplary grants, funded at $2.5 million per year for the nation, will be used to develop programs that specifically meet the needs of homeless children (section 723). Sections 722 and 723 are important not so much for the funds they provide (which are very small), but as catalysts to induce states and localities to spend more and modify their programs to the benefit of homeless children.

However, no matter how good such programs might be, they cannot overcome the harmful effects of life in shelters or hotels on the children's educational, emotional, and social development. The first priority for the children's education, as well as their other needs, is to move the families out of shelters and hotels and into their own housing. Thus the recent introduction in the McKinney Act of the Transitional Housing Demonstration Program of Aid to Families with Dependent Children (see below) is on target. However, its funding level, $20 million in FY 1990, is suitable only because it is a demonstration project. The funding would have to be increased severalfold to have any impact.

Social Services, Case Management, and Networking

THE FUNCTIONS OF SOCIAL SERVICES

Social workers are at the junction between the homeless person's world and the society at large. One of their functions is to engage homeless people in interactions with the system of services. This is hard when the latter are demoralized or psychotic, or have had bad experiences with the system. Strategies to facilitate this process (40,66) are described in chapters 12 and 13.

Another of their functions is to help clients obtain benefits they are entitled to under programs including general assistance, provided locally; federal programs such as the Food Stamps Program, Social Security Old Age and Survivors Insurance (OASI), Aid to Families with Dependent Children (AFDC), Social Security Disability Insurance (SSDI, for disabled people with work histories), Supplemental Security Income (SSI, for disabled people), veterans' pensions and benefits, and Medicare (health insurance for aged people eligible for Social Security); and the federal-state program Medicaid (health benefits for certain groups of poor people, with benefits and eligibility that vary within certain limits among the states). There are several barriers to such benefits. Homeless people may not know that they are eligible or how to apply; they may not have the documents needed to qualify; the application forms are often complex; decisions by mid- or low-level administrators sometimes make it more difficult to obtain the benefits (67,68); and changes in laws or regulations or state-to-state variation in eligibility may create barriers. Comparison across JP/HCH projects in different states using multiple regression analysis showed that differences among states in eligibility were the most influential factor in explaining differences across JP/HCH centers (19).

CASE MANAGEMENT AND NETWORKING

Most homeless people have to deal with a multitude of problems. Getting food and housing; applying for jobs or benefits; taking care of children; managing physical, mental, or substance abuse disorders, or problems with the law; and getting standard education, remedial education, or retraining are some of the external problems. Demoralization; difficulty in managing one's money; difficulty in keeping control of one's actions; and management of damaged identity or of injured self-respect (chapter 9) are some of the internal problems. Intervention with a single problem may not be effective in many instances because of interactions between problems or the need to solve several problems simultaneously or in sequence. For instance, getting a job may require not only seeking and applying for the job but also getting remedial education or special training, improving one's appearance, finding resources to care for children while one is at work, controlling substance abuse, and dealing with demoralization or identity problems. Two methods—case management and networking—have been devised to coordinate action on multiple problems.

In case management, one professional coordinates the various services or interventions needed. The clinical and administrative functions of case management include outreach, assessment, service planning, advocacy, benefit acquisition, service linkage, and service monitoring (69). Case management has been used extensively with people who are chronically mentally ill (70) or substance abusers (71). The tasks of the case manager, according to a list that was initially developed for the treatment of alcohol abusers but is applicable to other homeless clients as well, include (a) providing individual support to the client and his or her family; (b) helping the client to solve immediate problems; (c) helping to secure the support of the client's family or relevant others; (d) acting as a readily accessible link between the client and the treatment system; (e) facilitating access to resources and entitlements; and (f) remaining alert to the client's changing needs (71).

Networking is a more complex undertaking, involving the formation of linkages among professionals, laypeople, clients, facilities, and agencies to provide in appropriate sequence the system of services needed by homeless clients. This is described in chapter 14.

Housing

The McKinney Act provides housing programs for different constituencies within the homeless population. Some homeless families with children and homeless individuals with mental disabilities have access to supportive transitional housing for up to 24 months (or longer if so determined by the secretary of housing and urban development). This demonstration program is funded with $111 million for FY 1990, under Title IV-C, section 422(12)(A). Its object is to determine the capital and operating costs of supportive housing and the outcomes of this approach. The funding for capital acquisition or substantial rehabilitation is very limited, and the emphasis is on moderate rehabilitation and operating expenses (housing proper, and support services). Although the total funding is substantial, it should be seen in the context of the estimate that about 135,000–305,000 households fall into the target categories.[3] For instance, if the average funding is $10,000 per household, only 11,000 households will be served.

Other federal housing programs, as well as the provision of permanent housing by city, county, or state authorities, represent interventions in the social context of homelessness. These are discussed in chapters 17 and 18.

Empowerment

Empowerment of people refers to their acquiring the ability to participate in and influence their social environment (72,73). The empowerment of homeless people may take place at several levels. At one level, it means giving them technical and social skills and linkages with organizations, so that they are better able to compete for jobs, entitlements, or housing. At this level, social workers and clients collaborate as peers in problem solving (74). The degree of agreement between social worker and client on service needs has major impact (75). At the next level, homeless people form groups to participate together in activities and, together, influence their microenvironment. A client's self-determination is essential in engaging the client in the group. An example is tenants' meetings in transitional housing (76). At the third level, homeless people and/or their advocates organize to change the social conditions that have led to homelessness or to improve the quality of homeless people's lives. At this level, homeless people and their advocates act as a pressure group that competes with other pressure groups. An example is the legal actions that affirmed homeless people's right to vote (77). Another example is the organization of homeless people in the Union of the Homeless (78:243–247).

Notes

1. A working estimate that about 130,000–300,000 homeless adults might need mental health services during the year was derived as follows. Three estimates of the point prevalence of literal homelessness were used: Burt and Cohen's, 679,000 (5); my low estimate, 1,157,000; and my high estimate, 1,535,000 (chapter 22). I estimate that 64 percent of homeless people are homeless as single individuals (chapter 22), that 30 percent of them have mental disorder, on the basis of hospitalization history, test instruments, or psychiatric diagnosis; and that 50 percent of those so categorized actually need mental health services. Applying these factors to the estimates of point prevalence yields, respectively, 65,184; 111,072; and 147,360 single, literally homeless adults who need mental health services. To extrapolate to the annual need, the ratio of annual prevalence to point prevalence was assumed to be 2.0:1.0 (chapter 22), yielding, respectively, 130,368; 222,144; and 294,720 adults who are homeless as single individuals and need mental health services.

For children, the same estimated numbers of all literally homeless people were multiplied by 0.25 (on the assumption that children comprise 25% of the literally homeless population) and then by 0.2 (on the assumption that 20% of homeless children need specialized mental health services [chapter 5]) to yield, respectively, 33,950; 57,850; and 76,750 literally homeless children who need special mental health services on any given day. These figures were then multiplied by 2.0 to obtain the corresponding annual numbers of literally homeless children who need special mental health services: 67,900; 115,700; and 153,500.

Adding the two sets of figures (for adults and for children) yields 198,268; 279,994; and 448,220 literally homeless people who need mental health services.

It should be emphasized that these estimates are based on very soft data. As pointed out in chapters 5 and 24, the prevalence of mental disorder among homeless adults cannot be estimated accurately with the data that are now available. The estimates for children are based on very scant data (chapter 5). They may be understated, in view of the considerations raised in chapter 7 and the studies of homeless youths discussed in chapter 5. Additionally, the ratio of annual prevalence to point prevalence of literal homelessness is based on very soft data; further, it is not known whether it is the same for homeless people with mental disorders as for the total literally homeless population.

2. The working estimate that, during a year, about 440,000–1 million literally homeless adults would be able to work without significant work rehabilitation other than retraining was obtained as follows. I used the same three estimates of point prevalence given in note 1: 679,000; 1,157,000; and 1,535,000. I assumed that 75 percent of homeless people are adults (chapters 4 and 22), that 36 percent of literally homeless people are in family groups, and that there are on average 3.5 individuals per family group (chapter 22). I assumed that one adult in each family group is unavailable for work other than taking care of the household, so that 10.3 percent of literally homeless people are excluded from work. Of the remaining adults, I assumed that 50 percent (i.e., 220,000; 375,000; and 516,000; respectively, on any given day) are able to work without work rehabilitation other than job retraining (60). Finally, I assumed that the ratio of annual prevalence to point prevalence of literally homeless people is 2.0:1.0. With these assumptions, the number of literally homeless adults capable of working without rehabilitation other than job retraining is, respectively, 440,000; 750,000; and 1,032,000 during the year.

Again, these estimates are based on soft data. The estimate that 50 percent of literally homeless people are capable of working without rehabilitation other than job retraining is based on only one study of homeless men (60). Furthermore, the ratio of annual prevalence to point prevalence of literal homelessness is based on very soft data, and it is not known whether it is the same for homeless people who can work without work rehabilitation other than job retraining as it is for the total literally homeless population.

3. The estimate that, on any given day, about 70,000–158,000 housing units with support services are needed for literally homeless families was arrived at as follows. I used the same estimates for the point prevalence of literal homelessness (679,000; 1,157,000; and 1,535,000) as in note 1, and the same estimates for the number of people who are homeless in family groups (36%) and the average size of the family group (3.5 persons) as in note 2, to arrive at an estimate of 69,844; 119,000; and 157,890 housing units needed on a given day for literally homeless family groups.

With regard to housing units needed for literally homeless people with mental disorder who need services, I assumed that nearly all of them were homeless as single individuals, and I used the same numbers as in note 1, i.e., 65,184; 111,072; and 147,360, respectively.

Therefore, the total number of housing units with support services needed for these two groups is, respectively, 135,024; 230,078; and 305,250.

References

1. Stern MJ. The emergence of the homeless as a public problem. *Social Service Review* 58:291–301, 1984.
2. HomeBase. *Neighbors, after All: Community Acceptance for Siting, Housing, and Serving Homeless People*. San Francisco: HomeBase, 1990.
3. U.S. Department of Health and Human Services. *Helping the Homeless: A Resource Guide*. Washington, D.C.: Government Printing Office, 1984.

4. *Yvonne McCain et al. v. Edward I. Koch*, Court of Appeals, State of New York, no. 41023/83, November 14, 1986. Reprinted in Hayes RM (ed.), *The Rights of the Homeless*. New York: Practising Law Institute, 1987, pp. 205–302.

5. Burt MR, Cohen BE. *America's Homeless: Numbers, Characteristics, and Programs That Serve Them*. Washington, D.C.: Urban Institute, 1989.

6. U.S. Department of Housing and Urban Development. *A Report on the 1988 National Survey of Shelters for the Homeless*. Washington, D.C.: HUD, Office of Policy Development and Research, 1989.

7. Reyes LM, Waxman LD. *A Status Report on Hunger and Homelessness in America's Cities, 1989*. Washington, D.C.: United States Conference of Mayors, 1989.

8. Johnson AK. *A Survey of the St. Louis Area Emergency Shelters for the Homeless*. St. Louis, Mo.: Homeless Services Network Board, 1988.

9. Sosin MR, Colson P, Grossman S. *Homelessness in Chicago: Poverty and Pathology, Institutions and Social Change*. Chicago: Chicago Community Fund, 1988.

10. Nenno MK (ed.). *Assistance for Homeless Persons: A NAHRO Resource Book for Housing and Community Development Agencies*. Washington, D.C.: National Association of Housing and Redevelopment Officials, 1988.

11. House Select Committee on Hunger. *Hunger among the Homeless*. Hearing before the Committee, 99th Cong., 2d sess., March 6, 1986.

12. House Select Committee on Hunger. *Hunger among the Homeless: A Survey of 140 Shelters, Food Stamps Participation, and Recommendations*. Committee Print, 100th Cong., 1st sess., March 1987.

13. Winick M. Nutritional and vitamin deficiency states. In Brickner PW, et al. (eds.), *Health Care of Homeless People*. New York: Springer, 1985, pp. 103–108.

14. Brickner et al. (eds.). *Health Care of Homeless People*. See ref. 13.

15. Wright JD. The National Health Care for the Homeless program. In Bingham RD, Green RE, White SB (eds.), *The Homeless in Contemporary Society*. Newbury Park, Calif.: Sage Publications, 1987, pp. 150–169.

16. Institute of Medicine. *Homelessness, Health, and Human Needs*. Washington, D.C.: National Academy Press, 1988.

17. National Association of Community Health Centers. *A National Directory of Homeless Health Care Projects Funded through the Stewart B. McKinney Homeless Assistance Act of 1987*. Washington, D.C.: NACHC, 1989.

18. Lewin ICF. *The Health Needs of the Homeless: A Report on Persons Served by the McKinney Act's Health Care for the Homeless Program*. Washington, D.C.: National Association of Community Health Centers, 1989.

19. Wright JD, Weber E. *Homelessness and Health*. New York: McGraw-Hill, 1987.

20. *Medicare and Medicaid Guide: New Developments, September 1986–December 1987*. Chicago, Ill.: Commerce Clearing House, 1986–87, pp. 13231–13232.

21. Meyer J, Jahiel RI. Medicaid and homeless people. Paper presented at the meeting of the Foundation for Health Services Research, Washington, D.C., June 17, 1990.

22. Lamb HR (ed.). *The Homeless Mentally Ill*. Washington, D.C.: American Psychiatric Association, 1984.

23. Bassuk EL (ed.). *The Mental Health Needs of Homeless Persons*. New Directions in Mental Health Services, no. 30. San Francisco: Jossey-Bass, 1986.

24. Goldman HH, Morrissey JP. The alchemy of mental health policy: Homelessness and the fourth cycle of reform. *American Journal of Public Health 75*:727–731, 1985.

25. Levine IS, Lezak AD, Goldman HH. Community support systems for the homeless mentally ill. In Bassuk (ed.), *Mental Health Needs of Homeless Persons*. See ref. 23.

26. Morse G, et al. *Homeless People in St. Louis: A Mental Health Program Evaluation*,

Field Study, and Follow-up Investigation. Jefferson City: Missouri Department of Mental Health, 1985.

27. Mulkern V, et al. *Homelessness Needs Assessment Study: Findings and Recommendations for the Massachusetts Department of Mental Health.* Boston: Human Service Research Institute, 1985.

28. Vernez G, et al. *Review of California's Program for the Homeless Mentally Disabled.* Santa Monica: Rand Corporation, 1988.

29. Breakey WR. Treating the homeless. *Alcohol, Health, and Research World 11(3):*42–47, 1987.

30. Chaudron CD, Wilkinson DA (eds.). *Theories on Alcoholism.* Toronto: Addiction Research Foundation, 1988.

31. Pattison EM, Sobell MB, Sobell LE. *Emerging Concepts of Alcohol Dependence.* New York: Springer, 1977.

32. Edwards G. The alcohol dependence syndrome: A concept as stimulus to inquiry. *British Journal of Addiction 81:*177–183, 1986.

33. Flores PJ. Alcoholics Anonymous: A phenomenological and existential perspective. *Alcohol Treatment Quarterly 5:*73–94, 1988.

34. Koegel P, Burnam MA. Traditional and nontraditional homeless alcoholics. *Alcohol, Health, and Research World 11(3):*28–34, 1987.

35. Shandler IW, Shipley TE. New focus for an old problem. *Alcohol, Health, and Research World 11(3):*54–57, 1987.

36. National Association of State Alcohol and Drug Abuse Directors. *Innovative State Activities Relating to Alcohol and Drug Treatment Services for the Homeless Population.* Rockville, Md.: National Institute on Alcohol Abuse and Alcoholism, 1987.

37. Wittman FD, Madden PA. *Alcohol Recovery Programs for Homeless People: A Survey of Current Programs in the U.S.* Rockville, Md.: National Institute on Alcohol Abuse and Alcoholism, 1988.

38. National Institute on Alcohol Abuse and Alcoholism. *Synopses of Community Demonstration Grant Projects for Alcohol and Drug Abuse Treatment of Homeless Individuals.* Rockville, Md.: Alcohol, Drug Abuse, and Mental Health Administration, 1988.

39. Sadd S, Young DW. Nonmedical treatment of indigent alcoholics: A review of recent research findings. *Alcohol, Health, and Research World 11(3):*48–49, 53, 1987.

40. Blankertz LE, Cnaan RA. Symbolic interaction: A framework for outreach. Paper presented at the 8th meeting of the Homelessness Study Group, at the annual meeting of the American Public Health Association, Chicago, Ill., October 21, 1989.

41. Miller PM. A behavioral intervention program for chronic public drunkenness offenders. *Archives of General Psychiatry 32:*915–918, 1975.

42. Korenbaum S, Burney G. *Alcohol-free Living Environments for Homeless Individuals.* Rockville, Md.: Alcohol, Drug Abuse, and Mental Health Administration, 1986.

43. Korenbaum S, Burney G. Program planning for alcohol-free living centers. *Alcohol, Health, and Research World 11(3):*68–73, 1987.

44. Koreloff NM, Anderson SC. Alcohol-free living centers: Hope for homeless alcoholics. *Social Work 34:*497–504, 1989.

45. Turner S. Community residential treatment for skid row alcoholics. *Health and Social Work 4:*163–180, 1979.

46. Fagan RW, Mauss AL. Social margin and social reentry: An evaluation of a rehabilitation program for Skid Row alcoholics. *Journal of Studies on Alcohol 47:*413–425, 1986.

47. De Soto CB, O'Donnell WE, De Soto JL. Long term recovery in alcoholics. *Alcoholism: Clinical and Experimental Research 13:*693–697, 1989.

48. Zweben A, et al. Facilitative strategies for retaining the alcohol-dependent client in

outpatient treatment. *Alcoholism Treatment Quarterly 5:*3, 1988.

49. Chapman RJ. Cultural bias in alcoholism counseling. *Alcoholism Treatment Quarterly 5:*105–113, 1988.

50. McLellan AT, et al. An improved diagnostic instrument for substance abuse patients: The addiction severity index. *Journal of Nervous and Mental Disease 168:*26–33, 1980.

51. Horn JL, et al. *Alcohol Dependence Scale (ADS).* Toronto: Addiction Research Foundation, 1984.

52. Endicott J, et al. The Global Assessment Scale: A procedure for measuring overall severity of psychiatric disturbance. *Archives of General Psychiatry 33:*766–771, 1976.

53. Barrow SM, et al. *The Personal History Form, and the Personal History Follow-up.* New York: New York State Psychiatric Institute, Epidemiology of Mental Disorders Research Department, 1985.

54. National Institute on Alcohol Abuse and Alcoholism, and National Institute on Drug Abuse. *Request for Applications AA-90-01: Cooperative Agreements for Research Demonstration Projects on Alcohol and Other Drug Abuse Treatment for Homeless Persons.* Rockville, Md.: Alcohol, Drug Abuse, and Mental Health Administration, January 1990.

55. Milburn NG. Drug abuse among homeless people. In Momeni J (ed.), *Homelessness in the United States: Data and Issues.* New York: Praeger, 1990, pp. 61–79.

56. U.S. Department of Labor. *Synopsis of Homeless Job Training Demonstration Projects.* Washington, D.C.: The Department, 1989.

57. Kincaid NM, Farber M, Unger M. *Evaluation of Opportunities for Revenue-generating Programs Employing the Homeless.* Eugene: University of Oregon, Department of Planning, Public Policy, and Management, 1989.

58. Murnion KW. Incorporating innovation. *Worklife 2(1):*10–11, 1989.

59. Bailey T. Employment and training programs. In Brecher C, Horton RD (eds.), *Setting Municipal Priorities, 1988.* New York: New York University Press, 1987, pp. 163–196.

60. First RF, Toomey BG. Homeless men and the work ethic. *Social Service Review 63:*113–126, March 1989.

61. U.S. Department of Education. *Report to the Congress on State Interim Reports on the Education of Homeless Children.* Washington, D.C.: The Department, February 15, 1989.

62. National Coalition for the Homeless. *Broken Lives: Denial of Education for Homeless Children.* Washington, D.C.: The Coalition, 1987.

63. Maza PL, Hall JA. *Homeless Children and Their Families: A Preliminary Study.* Washington, D.C.: Child Welfare League of America, 1988.

64. New York State Department of Education. *Report on the Homeless in New York State.* Albany: The Department, 1988.

65. Rafferty Y, Rollins N. *Learning in Limbo: The Educational Deprivation of Homeless Children.* Long Island City, N.Y.: Advocates for Children of New York, 1989.

66. Cohen MB. Social work practice with homeless mentally ill people: Engaging the client. *Social Work 34:*505–509, 1989.

67. Burt MR, Pittman KJ. *Testing the Social Safety Net.* Washington, D.C.: Urban Institute, 1985.

68. Schmidt L. *Management of Alcohol and Homelessness Services in a California County Welfare System.* Paper presented at the National Institute on Alcohol Abuse and Alcoholism conference entitled Homelessness, Alcohol, and Other Drugs, San Diego, Calif., February 2–4, 1989.

69. Row Sciences. *Services for Homeless People with Alcohol and Other Drug Problems: A Taxonomy for Reporting Data.* Rockville, Md.: National Institute on Alcohol Abuse and Alcoholism, 1989.

70. Schwartz SR, Goldman HH, Churgin S. Case management for the chronically men-

tally ill: Models and dimensions. *Hospital and Community Psychiatry 33:*1006–1009, 1982.

71. Timney CB, Graham K. A survey of case management practices in addiction programs. *Alcoholism Treatment Quarterly 6(3-4);*103–127, 1989.

72. Freire P. *Pedagogy of the Oppressed.* New York: Continuum, 1970.

73. Rose S, Black BL. *Advocacy and Empowerment.* Boston: Routledge and Kegan Paul, 1985.

74. Solomon B. How do we really empower families? New strategies for social work practitioners. *Family Resource Coalition 3:*2–3, 1985.

75. Plapinger J. *Program Service Goals: Service Needs, Service Feasibility, and Obstacles to Providing Services to the Mentally Ill Homeless.* New York: New York State Psychiatric Institute, 1988.

76. Cohen MB. Tenant organizing with the mentally ill homeless. *Catalyst 4(22):*33–37, 1988.

77. Buschman RM. Overview of the voting rights of homeless individuals. In Hayes (ed.), *Rights of the Homeless,* pp. 95–107. See ref. 4.

78. Hope M, Young J. *The Faces of Homelessness.* Lexington, Mass.: Lexington Books, 1986.

CHAPTER 12

Skid Row–based Services
for People Who Are Homeless
and Mentally Ill

Elaine Lomas, L.C.S.W.

Since 1963, federal legislation has allocated monies for an alternative community mental health system to support the deinstitutionalization effort.
Unfortunately, the dollars allocated over the years by federal, state, and local
levels of government to the community mental health system have not made up
for the reduction in services formerly provided by the state psychiatric hospitals, that is, basic life support, supervision, protection, evaluation and treatment by physicians, and social and recreational services, all under one administration and in one location (1).

Furthermore, substantial outpatient services were diverted to better-
functioning populations as a result of the emphasis on prevention and the
philosophy that community mental health services should be available to anyone in need of them (2). Since the mental health system is underfunded relative
to the need for services, community-based outpatient programs face a grave
disparity between the number of people they can serve and the demand. The
traditional organization of services limits the number served, because of the
usual practice of providing services to those who request and keep appointments on a first-call, first-served basis. When resources are scarce, waiting lists
delay initial appointments for weeks after the initial contact. When patients fail
to keep appointments or come in at unscheduled times, they may not be given
services, except in emergencies; rather, they are asked to return for other
scheduled appointments, which they may also not keep. Thus, the emphasis on
scheduled appointments and on one specified therapist who assumes full responsibility contributes to the loss of the more dysfunctional and reluctant
severely mentally ill people, who are the most in need but take the least
initiative to secure services. The need for flexibility and for a range of programs

that provide for individuals' dependency needs and yet allow considerable freedom of movement is now being addressed (3).

In general, it has become apparent that the community mental health system is serving better-functioning people, even among the chronically mentally ill patients. The structure and requirements of community mental health programs are factors contributing to this circumstance. Another factor may be therapists' inclination, when the demand for services exceeds the availability of clinicians, to select patients according to social characteristics rather than degree of disability. The literature supports the use of the social selection process (based on characteristics such as youth, competence, communication skills, and motivation) even in determining the form of social treatment (group v. individual) patients receive in the psychiatric hospital (4).

Homeless mentally ill people generally underutilize the traditional system of community-based mental health care. They may avoid psychiatric hospitalization, particularly if they remain in areas such as Skid Row, where their bizarre symptoms and dysfunctional behavior are either unnoticed or tolerated. In the past, the mental health system has viewed this population as unable or unwilling to use community-based mental health services (5).

This paper describes the development of a community mental health program designed to serve the homeless, severely and chronically mentally ill population. This program, the Skid Row Mental Health Service (SRMHS), is operated by the Los Angeles County Department of Mental Health. Due to the increasing number of homeless mentally ill people, and the increasing public awareness of this problem, the SRMHS began to experiment with new approaches to reach this population (6). Contrary to the commonly held belief that homeless mentally ill people will not use such services, this pioneering program shows that they will use appropriately designed community mental health services.

Most of SRMHS is funded by regular California Department of Mental Health Short-Doyle, MediCal, and county match dollars. A portion is also funded by State Categorical Bronzon Bill Homeless dollars. Money management is funded by a Federal Block Grant Demonstration.

The Target Population

The Los Angeles Skid Row is approximately two square miles, with a perimeter formed by three freeways and the Los Angeles River. About 7,000–15,000 homeless people reside in the area, depending on the time of year. The homeless population consists of many subpopulations, among whom are the chronic alcoholics; other substance abusers; people with personality disorders, including those with criminal histories; and people who are chronically mentally ill,

SKID ROW SERVICES FOR HOMELESS MENTALLY ILL

or chronically mentally ill with substance abuse. Research shows that the frequency of severe mental illness is many times as great in Skid Row as it is in adjacent areas. For example, schizophrenia occurs 38 times as frequently and manic-depressive illness 25 times as frequently as elsewhere in Los Angeles (7).

The SRMHS serves people who tend to have the following characteristics:

- Severe and chronic major mental illness (schizophrenia, major depression, manic-depressive illness, chronic brain syndrome);
- A pattern of moving in and out of living arrangements or living in situations that are not meeting their basic health and safety needs;
- A lack of or failure to use entitlements to meet basic life-support needs;
- A lack of support system or disrupted support systems;
- Poor hygiene relative to most homeless people;
- Underutilization of the community mental health system; and
- Current undertreatment for their mental illness, so that they may be grossly psychotic.

Program Development

From 1981 till the spring of 1984, the primary mental health service provided by the Los Angeles County Department of Mental Health (DMH) to the Skid Row area was outreach, along with consultation and minimal direct services to the Skid Row agencies that already had some contact with the target population, such as the local Department of Social Services and several missions and shelters. These agencies were only able to mange minimally and sporadically the large numbers of psychotic people in the area. This early clinical work and National Institute of Mental Health–sponsored research done by the DMH highlighted the need for innovative services and led to ideas for program development and advocacy for funds (8). Thus, in the spring of 1984, the DMH placed a multidisciplinary team consisting of a full-time psychiatrist, a clinical psychologist, a psychiatric social worker, a psychiatric registered nurse, and clerical support staff in Skid Row to provide continuing outreach and direct services, including assessments, medication, crisis intervention, and case management. In following years, SRMHS incrementally expanded program components and added new ones. Since there were no models for such a program, the first effort was to determine what would work.

STAFF COMPOSITION. Starting in the spring of 1984, SRMHS decided to develop a highly qualified, multidisciplinary mental health team, despite the popular view that many homeless people will not talk to professionals. This approach was undertaken because of the success of the initial professional outreach staff in eliciting a positive response from agencies and from many homeless people, and because the other Skid Row agencies had competent paraprofessionals and street people on staff who were eagerly seeking assistance from mental health professionals. In other words, the program decided to provide a service that was not yet in existence by maintaining professional identity and skills. The current staff consists of 30 people, including psychiatrists on site six days a week, clerical support, and a multidisciplinary staff of professionals and paraprofessionals.

From the spring of 1984 on, all staff members were recruited and selected for their commitment to working with the target population. Several of the first staff members had newly acquired degrees and little experience; the full-time psychiatrist had years of public service experience and wanted to spend his last few years before retirement making a special contribution. After the program became more visible, SRMHS easily recruited staff with clinical experience with the mentally ill population.

After a drop-in triage service had been operating for several months, SRMHS added two security guards to the program. They remain primarily in the triage area, because of the continuing threat of violence by some individuals who may carry weapons. The presence of the security guards is reassuring to staff and clients, and it did not lead to decreased utilization by the target population.

Despite the stressful nature of the work, staff turnover has been low. This may be due to staff members' strong commitment and to the fact that they are doing something worthwhile for people who are homeless and mentally ill; as well as to their identification with the development of a unique program; the frequent acknowledgment of their work by top county officials, the department head, and the media; competitive salaries; and their orientation to finding gratification in the accomplishment of even small goals for their homeless and mentally ill clients.

ACCESSIBILITY. Locating the program in Skid Row was the first step in making it accessible. However, location in Skid Row was not sufficient by itself. Massive outreach was initially necessary and continues to be necessary to reach the fearful, reluctant population of those who are homeless and chronically mentally ill.

Program design is as important as location and outreach in creating an accessible program for this target population. Program design to create accessibility for this population includes an emphasis on a non-appointment, drop-in system, a team response to allow a maximum "give them what they need when they are there" response, and a nondemanding approach, with minimum requirements for both performance and demonstration of motivation for change. Our chronically mentally ill population responded to such accessibility with a gradual increase in utilization of a range of mental health services.

An additional approach to managing scarce resources, managing workload, and maintaining accessible resources is to limit services to a designated target population. SRMHS limits formal mental health services to people who are homeless and severely, chronically mentally ill.

RELEVANCE. In order to be effective, programs must also be appropriate to the circumstances, mental state, and capabilities of the population. Over several years, SRMHS added program components by trial and error to meet the needs of this population. Ultimately it developed a balance between innovative, flexible program components and traditional treatment components.

Program Components

OUTREACH. Outreach is the backbone of accessible services for the homeless mentally ill population. Outreach to agencies consists of consultations for specific homeless individuals; consultation about the management of homeless individuals; seminars on the nature of mental illness, and on symptoms and behavior; information about the mental health system as well as our program; and assistance and support in making successful referrals to the program.

Outreach to homeless mentally ill people also takes place in the streets, where staff repeatedly approach people who appear to suffer from mental illness. At times, staff members have successfully completed Social Security evaluations in the street for people reluctant to come to the base program. They have eventually persuaded others to come in and use the range of services. Staff members provide involuntary hospitalizations from the street for those who refuse services and appear to be at great risk to themselves or others or are so gravely disabled that their lives are at risk due to deteriorating health. Since street outreach attempts to reach the most alienated individuals, the linkage of people to services usually comes slowly (9). Staff members also seek out those who have stopped coming to the base program.

DROP-IN TRIAGE. The drop-in triage component, open seven days a week from 8:00 AM to 6:00 PM, is the hub of activity for the base program. The staff members respond to all homeless people who come in regarding services. Activities consist of screening and referral; immediate assessment, including the evaluation of medication; case management; crisis intervention; and evaluations for commitment to an institution.

The crux of the drop-in program's accessibility is the non-appointment system. When staff at other agencies identify homeless mentally ill people in need of services, they can send them or walk with them to the program at that time. When homeless people decide to seek services and come in, they receive services at that time. The experience of SRMHS with the non-appointment system is that it is successful. Homeless mentally ill people may not keep appointments, but they do continue to come in, some sporadically and others frequently, to secure services when the agency is responsive at the time when they come.

The non-appointment system requires a team response to patients. Staff members, assigned by rotation to the triage area, see the people who come in without appointments. This system is more difficult for staff, because most professional people prefer their own clearly identified caseloads for which they feel fully responsible. Traditionally trained therapists experience a stressful loss of the sense of being "on top of the case." In this system, the assigned therapist–case manager may actually see the patient only a small fraction of the times the patient seeks services. The therapist–case manager does the initial assessment, develops a treatment plan and presents it to the disposition case conference, submits the Social Security evaluation, and performs administrative tasks for the patient, while other team members may also provide crisis intervention and case management services in the drop-in area.

RESTRICTION OF SERVICES TO A SPECIFIED POPULATION. SRMHS limits formal mental health services to the homeless, severely and chronically mentally ill target population and refers other homeless people—usually those who are more assertive in securing services—to other agencies. The restriction of services to a specific target population requires skilled differential diagnosis, a strong sense of mission, and determination to reach the most underserved population. Professional staff members require further training to refine their differential diagnostic skills, particularly in differentiating between primary substance abuse and major mental illness with substance abuse. Staff members also require training and substantial support to effectively work in the triage and referral process in the face of people who are homeless and may have multiple problems, including mental health ones.

MAIL AND CHECK PICK-UP. SRMHS allows members of the target population to pick up their checks and mail at the program site. This service allows homeless mentally ill people to stay connected with their checks, and it also increases contact with the mental health staff for those who initially avoid other services. The mail pick-up service facilitates the Social Security application process for those who require addresses and provides some oversight through the process.

SOCIAL SECURITY EVALUATION. The Social Security evaluation is crucial for the long-term care of chronically mentally ill people because the income Social Security provides allows for life-style alternatives and Medicaid (MediCal) benefits for medical and psychiatric care.

The Social Security program consists of supporting the patients through all the steps necessary to secure Social Security benefits. Those who do not have Social Security benefits are referred to the Social Security Administration (SSA) liaison who comes to SRMHS one day each week. The liaison reviews information in the SSA computer files, assists the patients in filling out application forms, and assists Supplemental Security Income (SSI) recipients with other business.

The SRMHS initial assessment form has the typical clinical assessment sections and the SSA evaluation requirements. Thus evaluation for both purposes can be done at the same time. SRMHS maintains a log to monitor the application process, including the timely submission of SSA evaluations.

CASE MANAGEMENT. SRMHS maintains a large case management program. All staff, whether professional or paraprofessional, regardless of discipline (except for psychiatrists), serve as therapists and case managers for patients. Homeless mentally ill patients come to the program whenever they feel they need assistance. The program's philosophy is to respond when they come in with a "catch as catch can" team case management. The therapist–case managers strive to meet the basic needs of the target population (e.g., food, shelter, showers, clothing, and income) as well as to provide support to help the clients accept mental health services and other support services. The staff members make efforts to contact clients' support systems, including those in other states. Since homeless mentally ill people tend to move in and out of facilities, have difficulty in maintaining benefits, and are suspicious of the traditional service system, informal and immediate response increases their use of services.

The most important aspect of the long-term case management program is the concerted effort to obtain SSI for the clients, many of whom have never obtained benefits or have lost them due to lack of follow-through. SRMHS places clients outside the dangerous Skid Row area, but not to the extent originally conceived, primarily because of the paucity of appropriate low-cost housing and because the entire system is just beginning to redesign programs so that they are more accessible to the target population. It is imperative that appropriate long-term living alternatives—such as hotels or boarding houses with mental health case management, on-site staff, and good linkages to flexible mental health services—be developed for the many homeless mentally ill people who will never tolerate more traditional residential care.

MONEY MANAGEMENT. Los Angeles County has recognized for many years the need for a representative payee program within the existing extensive case management system. Many mental health professionals were skeptical that the program could be instituted in a large bureaucracy, while others were concerned about management of patients who may be psychotic and aggressive regarding their money. Without a model, procedures, or know-how, they were apprehensive of taking this responsibility.

SRMHS was confronted daily with the need for a representative payee money management program. In collaboration with SSA and Mental Health Advocacy, SRMHS designed a money management–case management program for chronically mentally ill people who remain homeless in Skid Row despite their Social Security incomes. It consists of case managers located at SRMHS; accounting and check-writing services in the Administrator–Public Guardian Office, using its computers and accounting staff; and a local check-cashing service. The Department of Mental Health is the representative payee for those—the majority—who require payees.

Money management has successfully served as a means of maintaining regular contacts with mentally ill people who underutilize the mental health system. The case managers provide the typical services of intensive case management programs, including planning, advocacy, linkage to services, and support regarding daily living activities. Their primary responsibility is to resolve the social problems of the people they serve (10). Patients who have lost benefits due to lack of compliance with procedures have successfully maintained their entitlements. The frequent contact has usually led to the use of other mental health services, such as medication or socialization. In several instances, patients discharged from psychiatric hospitals returned immediately to the money management staff in a much more stable and cooperative mood, and they were persuaded to continue in the SRMHS medication service. This led to continued and increased stability for patients who had previously used the psychiatric hospital and refused appropriate follow-up programs in the community.

MEDICATION AND MEDICATION SELF-HELP. SRMHS provides physician coverage most hours the program is open, along with a self-help medication program that gives some oversight and assistance for patients who wish support with their medication program. While many homeless mentally ill patients are initially reluctant to take medication due to side effects or other complaints (11), others see medication as bringing relief from frightening psychotic symptoms. Patients may have difficulty in taking the medication regularly because of their homeless life-style and environment and their lack of social support systems. SRMHS stores the medication and maintains a record of medication intake for selected patients who come to the program almost daily for money management and socialization. A psychiatric registered nurse leads a weekly group for patients to discuss the role of medication in reducing unpleasant symptoms, and various concerns regarding medications and their side effects. The aim is to give the patients the opportunity to discuss the advantages and disadvantages of taking medication, and to encourage them to work with staff regarding their medication plans. The group is well attended and appears to lead to greater participation in the medication program.

SOCIALIZATION DAY CARE. Socialization day care provides a safe haven from the dangers of Skid Row street life and reduces social isolation in a low-expectation, nonthreatening environment. The primary emphasis is on providing an atmosphere of acceptance and friendliness in which the participants begin to develop basic life skills and have whatever degree of social interaction they can tolerate. This program component is structured to require less from the participants in the way of commitment to regular attendance, specific goals to work toward, and level of participation than the typical day care program does (12).

Socialization day care provides several program levels simultaneously and at different times of the day to accomodate several levels of functioning of the patients. Also, the same patients may participate in a highly structured program for part of the day and in a very slightly structured one, such as watching television with staff oversight, at other times.

Examples of objectives for clients include developing acceptable personal hygiene and grooming habits, increasing effective use of life management skills, enhancing social and leisure skills, and taking prevocational training programs. Examples of activities include breakfast, snack, and lunch; hygiene (including shower and laundry time); community meeting; paper recycling group (to earn some cash); crafts; community outings, parties, and holiday dinners; and sports at the local YMCA. The expectation for performance and attendance remains low, as the main function of the program is to provide a protective environment and reduce isolation.

SPECIALIZED SHELTER. The specialized shelter is a cooperative arrangement between selected Skid Row shelters and the SRMHS to provide time-limited life support services (food, showers, beds, change of clothes, and supervision) and case management for vulnerable homeless chronically mentally ill adults who have no resources and no alternatives but the streets or shelters. As one component in the continuum of care for homeless people, the specialized shelter increases clients' access to other services by providing stability, care, and access to the case management support staff.

SRMHS screens and makes all referrals to specialized shelters. Outreach and case management staff provide support to the shelters; transportation of clients to the shelters; and incomplete case management to develop plans, establish linkages, and secure benefits. The SRMHS six-day socialization program and seven-day walk-in response provide back-up and support to the specialized shelter. The specialized shelter also serves as an alternative temporary placement for patients who have temporary difficulties during treatment and require additional support and oversight.

Although the specialized shelter provides a lower level of care than do any of the residential models, it is more acceptable to many homeless mentally ill people because it is less structured and less demanding of clients, particularly in terms of pressure to accomplish objectives beyond the most basic. Ironically, severely dysfunctional mentally ill people (who are not violent or suicidal) may respond best to this form of life-support care.

SPECIALIZED HOTEL. The Single Room Occupancy Corporation dedicated in 1988 a newly renovated hotel, the Golden West, for chronically mentally ill people screened and approved by SRMHS. The corporation provides additional hotel staff and case managers through a HUD grant. SRMHS provides on-site case management and a socialization program, as well as assessment, money management, and medication at the main clinic two blocks away. The corporation also funds recreational activities and field trips and one hot meal a day. Residents pay a low rent, easily affordable within their Social Security incomes. The hotel has 45 furnished rooms, with 30 available for the target population, and a large lobby for recreational purposes. The hotel maintains staff on duty 24 hours a day, including a security guard at night. The SRMHS and corporation staffs work together to accept new residents, plan and provide programs, develop policies and procedures, and resolve problems.

The specialized hotel is an alternative for those homeless mentally ill people who are somewhat stable after intervention by SRMHS, reject the traditional residential programs outside of Skid Row, and prefer the relative freedom of the hotel life-style yet cannot manage well on their own. It provides a balance of independence and support acceptable to them.

PSYCHIATRIC HOSPITAL. Many homeless chronically mentally ill people who avoid community-based care continue to use the hospital sporadically, usually involuntarily. The psychiatric hospital continues to be an important resource for the SRMHS target population. Because of easy access to SRMHS, patients continue to come to the program as they deteriorate, refuse to take medication, and increase their threats of violence, finally resulting in involuntary hospitalization. Upon discharge, those who ordinarily refuse all community services may return to SRMHS in a much more stable, lucid, and cooperative mood.

Although the overall use of the hospital by SRMHS's caseload is substantially reduced because SRMHS is maintaining clients who would otherwise be high hospital users in the community, some who would avoid appropriate hospitalization are hospitalized.

Changes in Patients' Service Utilization

The treatment histories of patients for two years before admission to SRMHS and for one year after admission to SRMHS, including any services received in the state-funded mental health system, were obtained from the Management Information System of the Los Angeles County Department of Mental Health. The total sample consisted of 291 patients. Table 12.1 presents service utilization data by type of program. The results show a marked decrease in hospitalization and an increase in nonhospital service utilization after admission to SRMHS.

TABLE 12.1   PATIENTS' USE OF SERVICES BEFORE AND AFTER ADMISSION
TO THE SKID ROW MENTAL HEALTH SERVICE PROGRAM

Type of Service	Units of Service[a] in the Two Years before Admission		Units of Service[a] in the One Year after Admission	
	No. of Units	%	No. of Units	%
24-hour care	2,256	67.83	512	4.78
Day treatment (socialization)	114	3.43	2,197	20.52
Case management and/or outpatient services	956	28.74	7,998	74.70
Total	3,326	100.00	10,707	100.00

Source: Ron Honnard and Roger Rice, Program Review and Evaluation Division, Los Angeles County Department of Mental Health.

[a]Units of service: For hospitals, units of service represent 24-hour days; for day treatment, full or part days; for case management, hours; for outpatient service, sessions.

Case Examples

Mr. C., a black male in his late forties, was first contacted in July 1986 by street outreach staff. He was psychotic and fearful, and very poorly groomed, with long hair and scruffy beard. After many street outreach contacts, he finally came to the drop-in area in April 1987 because he wanted to secure an income. Staff called the Social Security Administration (SSA) and secured his SSA number, drove him to the local Department of Social Services office, and with the assistance of the Protective Services staff, secured General Relief benefits. Mr. C. accepted a full assessment, and staff processed an SSI application. He accepted medication, had decreased delusions and hallucinations and improved sleep, and is now living in a hotel.

Mrs. P., a Caucasian female in her late sixties who had been homeless for 18 years, was referred by SSA. She reluctantly signed a voluntary consent for the Department of Mental Health to be her representative payee and for money management. She was delusional, angry, and verbally abusive toward staff. She had no regular place to stay, was poorly groomed, took poor care of her basic needs despite her income, and was isolated. She gradually accepted guidance from the case managers who had daily contact with her. She accepted placement in a hotel in the same building as the SRMHS program, and she kept her room clean with the oversight of case managers. She began to take Prolixin shots. Overt signs of her psychosis abated. She accepted dental care. She began to take increasingly better care of her appearance and to attend socialization work. She contacted her youngest daughter, and this led to a reunion with her two daughters and grandchildren. Mrs. P. moved into permanent housing and continued contact with the money management staff. Her level of functioning has remained stable.

Discussion

The Skid Row Mental Health Service was initiated to provide mental health services to people who are homeless and severely chronically mentally ill. Because traditional mental health approaches have proved of little value to this population, it was essential to deliver the type of mental health care they can accept, with a balance between innovative and traditional features. An informal, nontraditional approach that includes coordination of mental health programs with existing and accepted homeless shelter programs has proven successful in increasing service utilization where traditional approaches have failed.

Outreach, particularly the collaboration with Skid Row agencies, succeeded beyond expectations in connecting the homeless population to mental health staff and services. Over the past few years, outreach programs have been developed in cities throughout the United States. Congress has allocated funding for them through the National Institute of Mental Health, and there is growing interest at all levels of government in developing programs for the homeless mentally ill population (13,14). To have significant impact, outreach must be connected to services that are accessible and acceptable to this population. The solution, in Skid Row, was to create a new program with a relevant range of mental health services for this population rather than to continue to try to increase the accessibility of existing community programs based outside the immediate area. The various components of the SRMHS program—outreach, drop-in triage, mail and check pick-up, Social Security evaluation, medication and medication self-help, socialization day care, and specialized shelter and hotel—were each designed especially for the homeless chronically mentally ill population. Clients participate according to their tolerance for structure and involvement. Thus the mental health program, which also included food, shelter, warm clothing, medical care, and a safe environment as part of mental health treatment services, was able to provide meaningful assistance to the chronically mentally ill homeless population.

References

1. Lamb R. Deinstitutionalization and the homeless mentally ill. *Hospital and Community Psychiatry 35:*899–907, 1984.
2. Lamb R. What did we really expect from deinstitutionalization? *Hospital and Community Psychiatry 32:*105–109, 1981.
3. Recommendations of APA's Task Force on the Homeless Mentally Ill. *Hospital and Community Psychiatry 35:*908–909, 1984.
4. Link B, Milcarek B. Selection factors in the dispensation of therapy: The Matthew effect in the allocation of mental health resources. *Journal of Health and Social Behavior 21:*279–290, 1980.
5. Farr R. Clinical insights. In *Treating the Homeless: Urban Psychiatry's Challenge.* Monograph Series of the American Psychiatric Association. Washington, D.C.: American Psychiatric Press, 1986, pp. 66–90.
6. Farr R. The Los Angeles Skid Row Mental Health Project. *Psychosocial Rehabilitation Journal 8:*64–76, 1984.
7. Farr R, Koegel P, Burnam R. *A Study of Homelessness and Mental Health in the Skid Row Area of Los Angeles.* Los Angeles: Los Angeles County, Department of Mental Health, 1986.
8. Gold Award: A network of services for the homeless chronically mentally ill. *Hospital and Community Psychiatry 37:*1148–1151, 1986.
9. Cohen N, Putnam J, Sullivan A. The mentally ill homeless: Isolation and adaptation. *Hospital and Community Psychiatry 35:*922–924, 1984.
10. Rapp C, Chamberlain R. Case management services for the chronically mentally ill. *Social Work 30:*417–422, 1985.
11. Diamond R. Drugs and the quality of life: The patient's point of view. *Journal of Clinical Psychiatry 46:*29–35, 1985.
12. Harris M, Bergman H, Bachrach L. Individualized network planning for chronic psychiatric patients. *Psychiatric Quarterly 58:*51–56, 1986.
13. Lezak A. *Synopsis of NIMH Community Support Program Service Demonstration Grants for Homeless Mentally Ill Persons.* Rockville, Md.: Alcohol, Drug Abuse, and Mental Health Administration, 1985.

14. Axelroad S, Toff G. *Outreach Services for Homeless Mentally Ill People.* Proceedings of the First of Four Knowledge Development Meetings on Issues Affecting Homeless Mentally Ill People. Washington, D.C.: George Washington University, Intergovernmental Health Policy Project, 1987.

CHAPTER 13

Working with People
Who Are Mentally Ill and Homeless:
The Role of a Psychiatrist

Ezra Susser, M.D., M.P.H.

I t is now widely recognized that a psychiatrist can acquire specialized skills to work with chronically mentally ill people and to work in the public sector (1,2). Fellowships in public psychiatry and some residency training programs teach these skills. Less well recognized is the extent to which skills need to be creatively modified in some settings where chronically mentally ill people who are homeless might be treated, such as bus terminals, parks, and shelters. One enters an institutional and social milieu that is entirely different from that of the hospital or clinic. This chapter illustrates possible roles for a psychiatrist in clinical work with people who are homeless and mentally ill, and the adaptations required of the psychiatrist in filling them.

People who are homeless and mentally ill sometimes view mental health services with mistrust and give them a low priority (3–5). Mental health providers, for their part, often view homeless people as a potential liability, a subgroup with multiple and intractable problems and no financial resources. In spite of reluctance to work together, there is frequent contact, often on terms that are satisfactory to neither side, as when a homeless person requests a hospital admission as a form of shelter.

The prevailing relationship between people who are homeless and mentally ill and the mental health system is advantageous to none. The homeless people are denied the long-term rehabilitative services that they so desperately need. Instead, they are forced to "reinterpret" existing services to meet self-perceived needs, using shelters as day programs, and tertiary medical centers as sources of food and clothing. Providers then expend scarce resources inefficiently. When emergency rooms are used to get food, shelter, or routine medical care, the process seems needlessly expensive.

In an effort to improve the relationships, some cities have created special mental health programs to reach out to homeless mentally ill people (6,7). These programs have had some success in engaging people who are disconnected from the mental health system. Generally, they use a gradual and non-threatening approach. Food, safe shelter, a respectful listener, and other services are emphasized, in addition to mental health treatment per se. For instance, one outreach team initiates relationships with suspicious or paranoid street people by leaving a peanut butter sandwich (and a flier) next to the spot where the person stays. Within such programs, a more trusting relationship between homeless people and mental health providers often emerges.

Requirements that apply to other parts of the mental health system often have to be waived to permit these programs to operate effectively. Traditional mental health programs cannot reach out in the same way, even if they wish to do so, because they are encumbered by more restrictive regulations. For example, an outreach worker may need many brief contacts before a woman who sleeps in the park is willing to enter into a conversation. The program has to be reimbursed even for early contacts without having to provide a diagnosis at the onset.

Outreach programs are only a transitional stage. They depend on referrals to other providers for more comprehensive and long-term care. In the long run, their clients will interact predominantly with other mental health institutions. Clients may again meet with indifference or rejection from these agencies, or they may feel that the services offered do not correspond to their needs. Therefore the achievements of a transitional program may be only modestly reflected in lasting change (8).

Some strategies have now been developed to carry gains beyond the limited context of special programs. One approach is to provide incentives for broad institutional changes to better accommodate people who are mentally ill and homeless. A complementary approach is to work directly with homeless people in order to achieve long-term changes in the manner in which they interact with institutions. For example, "advocacy-empowerment" programs train people to extract resources from institutions (8). Clients are armed with a knowledge of their rights, and they become more effective in securing entitlements, food, housing, health care, and vocational training. These programs also encourage homeless people to develop a common identity as belonging to a community deserving of support. The shared social problems of homeless people are framed in terms of a social system that has failed them. For mentally ill people, the analogy is sometimes drawn between veterans of war and veterans of mental hospitals (8). Insofar as possible, people work together in groups to form a shared perspective. They take common action to improve their lot and increase their control over the circumstances in which they live.

The advocacy-empowerment strategy was derived from the work of Paolo Freire, who sought to organize poor communities in Brazil (9). Although Freire's philosophy has only recently been articulated as a theme for community mental health care in the United States (10), it has long been influential in other fields, such as health education. A health education project for elderly single-room occupancy hotel (SRO) tenants in San Francisco is a well-known example of its application in this country (11). "Facilitators" attempted to build support networks among tenants and to organize them to address threats of health such as high crime rates. They found it difficult to do so in a community where there was little sense of common identity. They concluded that Freire's methods are best suited to communities that are already socially cohesive but need to mobilize to gain resources. This experience in health education illustrates the central challenges in applying Freire's work to a group such as the homeless mentally ill. That is, one has to adapt methods and expectations that are relevant to a fragmented community. One can work only gradually toward group identity and cohesion.

Relatively few psychiatrists have played an important role in this process of experimentation at the level of direct services. Social workers and clergy, for example, have been far more prominent. There is, in fact, controversy over whether psychiatrists should be involved in special programs for homeless people. Concerns are voiced that psychiatrists will attempt to reintroduce the traditional hierarchy of mental health institutions, in which the psychiatrist is the director; that they will be unable to adapt their modes of care to match the problems of people who are homeless as well as mentally ill; and that in the eyes of the clients, the presence of a psychiatrist will identify the program with traditional mental health services. In spite of these concerns, most teams in the field would be happy to include a psychiatrist in some capacity because of the severity of the psychiatric and medical problems encountered and the difficulties inherent in the referral process. Yet there is no agreement as to the appropriate role of the psychiatrist in the team's work.

The programs that have claimed success are diverse in their philosophies, staffing patterns, institutional linkages, and settings. Some retain the goals and services of traditional mental health services but modify the services to make them more accessible and attractive. Other radically redefine goals. Most, though not all, include paraprofessionals as case managers, but the extent and type of professional staffing—for example by social workers, clergy, or nurses—varies a great deal. Programs may be hospital-based or affiliated with schools of social work, or they may be instituted as independent not-for-profit corporations. They may operate in the streets, small church shelters, large municipal shelters, or SROs. The characteristics (e.g., age or cultural background) of the homeless people reached by otherwise similar programs also differ considerably.

A psychiatrist working with people who are homeless and mentally ill has to adapt to the program and to its setting. In contrast to hospital wards or clinics, where a psychiatrist is likely to be in authority, the team may be led by a nurse, a social worker, a priest, or perhaps a paraprofessional. In addition, since the task is to "reach the unreached," the clients are often in a position of setting the terms of service. Thus, the success of a psychiatrist depends on the capacity to modify psychiatric practice to make it meaningful within diverse and unusual programs and communities.

Psychiatrists working in this fashion rarely publish their experiences, and as a result, there is no basis to compare the methods applied in these hetero-geneous circumstances. Those of us who are involved in developing programs cannot draw on the experience of others. In this chapter I present a personal case history, to help build a literature that will permit us to do so. It describes my experience in a transitional residence for homeless women. I detail the adapta-tions required to integrate my work with that of the mental health team and the community, and suggest that psychiatrists can play a direct and meaningful role in the continuing effort to reach out to people who are homeless and mentally ill.

The Setting

The transitional residence was an SRO in midtown Manhattan that housed 36 women. It was rented from the landlord by a community service agency that hired a devoted and competent staff to run it. The paraprofessionals who "man-aged" the desk at the entrance 24 hours per day were always available for chatting or counseling in an "open-office" arrangement. Although the hotel had originally been designated a transitional residence, few of its residents had been able to find alternative housing, and for the majority, it was a de facto home. Thus, barriers to entry were minimal, and women who could not comply with the stricter demands of a licensed community mental health residence could get a room.

The hotel community included women who had a profound mistrust of mental health professionals, especially psychiatrists, and yet were in great need of their services. Some examples illustrate this point. One highly educated and intelligent tenant had episodes so disabling that she could not cope even with basic hygiene. However, between episodes she called on a legal consultant to draw up papers requesting that involuntary hospitalization or medication be forbidden, should she become ill again. A second example was an elderly tenant who held a high status in the community and was widely recognized as a leader. Although she clearly had multiple delusions and pressing medical prob-lems, she could not be induced to visit either a psychiatrist or an internist. This tenant had publicly denied for years that she had any need for doctors, and the perception that she might lose face if she changed her stand added another level to her hesitancy. A third example was a tenant with a delightful sense of humor and a large repertoire of jokes who was also paranoid and delusional. She maintained a high degree of interaction with hotel staff, but in a confrontational style that mingled wit and hostility. For example, she often accused staff of giving or taking bribes. In spite of her evident symptoms and dependence on contact with staff, she not only asserted that she had no mental problems but was highly critical of those who, in her view, did. Thus, her involvement in a mental health program would have been something worse than joining a political party that one adamantly opposes.

The Community Support System Program

A community program affiliated with a school of social work contracted to provide mental health and related services in the hotel, with Community Support System (CSS) funding. The on-site team was led by a social worker with an M.S.W. degree who supervised a second social worker, a paraprofessional case manager, and two social work students (12). The CSS team was not directly linked to any medical institution or department.

The CSS team blended emerging modes of care for the chronically mentally ill, such as assertive case management and rehabilitation, with the above-described advocacy-empowerment approach. The team helped tenants to develop a knowledge of their rights and to take advantage of opportunities to exercise choices effectively or to make demands. In a traditional approach, the emphasis is more likely to be on the tenants' individual or shared deficits and on their adaptation to existing services. The advocacy-empowerment philosophy does not imply a naive denial of individual deficits or of the need for mental health treatment. Instead, it proposes the basis of an alliance between the tenants and the CSS workers.

In this hotel, advocacy was communicated on a case-by-case basis as tenants sought health services, supportive work programs, legal services, and entitlements. Empowerment, that is, the formation of social networks and the identification of shared goals, was facilitated mainly by group meetings. Change was slow. Only over years was there a progression from getting together to make community meals to the formation of a tenants' association. Thus, the approach had to be translated into a form and pace that was meaningful in hotel life.

The advocacy-empowerment strategy in mental health was developed in counterpoint to psychiatrically defined services, although this CSS team attempted to integrate the two. The more radical proponents of advocacy-empowerment specifically exclude psychiatrists, whom they perceive as representatives of the "medical model," from their program staffs. My inclusion in the CSS team, as a consultant working one day per week, was seen as an experiment.

Group Work

My first task was to devise, with the CSS team, a strategy to integrate a psychiatrist into the life of the hotel. The hotel was a small, tight-knit community with strong group norms. It was also perceived as home. Many of the women were former state mental hospital patients who were wary of an intrusion by a psychiatrist into their home. Also, some stigma was attached to mental illness within this community. When I was first introduced at a tenants' meeting, it was with some apprehension as to what the response would be.

We knew that a successful approach had to respect a central feature of hotel life: that the women were tenants, not residents of a facility for the mentally ill, a feature essential to acceptability to many of the women. If my appearance appeared to violate that understanding, it would fuel mistrust. Therefore, my entry had to be nonintrusive. Nevertheless, my presence had to be made known to a large number of the women and had to be positive and influential enough to alter their perceptions about psychiatrists. Some of the women most in need of an on-site psychiatrist were also likely to be the most suspicious. It was imperative to establish some distinction between my work at the hotel and their prior experience with psychiatrists.

The solution was simple, though it required what might be considered an extreme adaptation for a psychiatrist. I began with a job that, while valued in this community, was totally incongruous with the women's perceptions of a psychiatrist—namely, running the weekly bingo game. Bingo was the most culturally accepted, best-attended, and least-threatening group activity in the hotel. For some, this presented an unusual opportunity, in meeting with a doctor, to put their best foot forward, as one does for a guest at home. For instance, a tenant might offer me a better seat or a refreshment, or ask whether I had had to travel far. Thus, instead of exposing weakness and seeking help, the tenants could assume a position of strength on the first encounter. Sheer curiosity tempted some of them to approach me, to find out what a psychiatrist was doing running the hotel bingo game. Many women who were intensely suspicious of psychiatrists were quite comfortable meeting me on these terms. By the end of six weeks, almost everyone knew who I was, and I had informal contacts with many of the women in the hotel. I quickly became an accepted feature of the community.

My next task was to orient the group work in a direction that would be useful to both clinical treatment and advocacy-empowerment. In this endeavor, we hoped to benefit from the mystique associated with doctors, having minimized the negative connotations. I began a group entitled "Talking to the Doctor." The theme, at first, was the experience of the consumer of medical care. Every tenant would have some experience to contribute, and she could choose one that was not emotionally laden if she wished. Even tenants who were withdrawn, or easily agitated, could participate in the discussion group, since it was acceptable just to chat if one so wished, or to sit at a distance, or to wander in and out. The theme naturally led to discussions of issues in clinical treatment. In addition, it lent itself to transition to the advocacy-empowerment strategy. For instance, the discussion often focused on how to get better medical care, or how to get information about the medication the tenants were taking. The process could not be rushed, however, for the primary purpose of the first several months was to foster group cohesion.

From these modest beginnings, the group underwent a number of transitions. The theme of "sharing experiences with doctors" was followed by a phase of "health education." There was considerable discussion about differing practices for coping with health problems (e.g., thresholds for seeking medical care, and the use of social networks). Guest speakers were invited to answer questions about health problems and access to services. The health education theme diminished after its strongest supporter among the tenants, an elderly woman, suffered a debilitating stroke. The group then became an open forum for the discussion of a diverse range of life problems. It was also used on an ad hoc basis by women who had suffered severe stresses in the preceding week (e.g., the death of a relative, or a major fight with a friend) and were in need of a setting where they could count on group support. Sometimes the group meeting became a stage for community endorsement of necessary but painful decisions, for example, to place the tenant who had suffered a stroke in a nursing home, or to involuntarily hospitalize a tenant.

Some of the uses of the group were unpredicted and were determined more by the participants than by myself. An example illustrates how the employment of a psychiatrist to run such a group partly fashions its nature. When the elderly tenant mentioned above suffered a severe stroke, the women asked me to visit her in the hospital and to bring back an assessment of her condition. The decision as to whether she could return to her room rested with the hotel staff and the hospital doctor, but the tenants were reluctant to accept an eviction decision that was not endorsed as a necessity by a doctor they trusted. At a large group meeting, we discussed the problem and reached a consensus that the only real option was to get her the best alternative placement, and to keep visiting once she was in the nursing home. Her unrivaled leadership and fighting spirit were recalled. People such as a doctor or a priest, if available, are likely to be called on in such circumstances.

Some of the themes I proposed for the group were flatly rejected. On several occasions, I suggested that, since most participants had been on psychotropic medications, at least episodically, they could use the opportunity to learn about their medications and so assume more control in their own treatment. The topic was of little or no interest. Life experiences with friends, lovers, family, housing, or work were always more absorbing. For instance, the pain of placing a child in foster care or of losing contact with him or her, an experience shared by several women, was of more immediacy and could not be disregarded in favor of a seemingly dry alternative topic such as medication.

More than a year passed before the group began to approximate the process we had originally envisioned. Fluctuating membership and variable attendance, a feature of every group activity in the hotel, delayed the attainment of group cohesion and the emergence of leaders. Sometimes there were as few as 2 in the group, and sometimes as many as 15. Eventually, the focus indeed shifted to demands for tenant participation in hotel management. The group also became a training program for tenants to learn how to run a group of their own. This was consistent with our prior intentions. However, the earlier themes recurred intermittently and were important to the participants. Even after several years, these themes were more crucial to group cohesion than was the discussion of tenants' rights and group action.

Group work paid off in a number of ways. The group process itself was therapeutic, as the group evolved into a more cohesive entity and broadened its focus. In addition, the group permitted the psychiatrist to maintain a place in the social life of the hotel. Thus I could check the pulse of the community, maintain contact with women who did not see a psychiatrist formally, and gather enough firsthand knowledge to be useful in consultations with the CSS team and the hotel staff.

Clinical skills help in leading such a group. However, this alone might not justify the use of a psychiatrist in the role of group leader. While the group is valuable in itself, the group also brings to its leader the knowledge and the contact with the tenants which are a precondition for other work in the hotel, described below.

Individual Work

Since the intent of the program was to train tenants to make effective use of community services, regular on-site psychiatric care was not offered to most tenants. An exception was made for a few who had a pressing need but had repeatedly aborted prior referrals. I saw two of them on a weekly basis. The accessibility and flexibility of on-site psychiatry was an inducement to continue treatment, but other factors were also important, such as the degree of control the patient was given over her treatment and over the psychiatrist's knowledge about her life circumstances. A convenient medication prescription, unaccompanied by a therapeutic relationship as a basis for compliance, would not have sufficed in those cases. Both women made dramatic progress. One was the tenant referred to above who had drawn up legal papers to preclude further treatments by psychiatrists. Whereas in the past she had spent months in an incoherent state, covered with lice, she now emerged as a leader and caretaker among the tenants.

Acute crises—fights, suicide attempts, or psychotic decompensation— arose frequently. In these cases, an on-site psychiatrist was of help even when the tenant had an outside psychiatrist. More information was available to an on-site psychiatrist in an assessment. Also, effective planning of intervention required a knowledge of community norms as well as of individuals, especially in a hotel where almost any workable plan had to be acceptable to the tenant herself.

An unpredicted form of individual work was created by the tenants. They used me as a consultant on mental health issues on an ad hoc basis. One tenant who had been in a fight asked to see me a few times to "sort things out." A recently bereaved tenant sought advice on how to cope with the feelings of distress associated with the burial of her ex-husband. A third asked for help in securing treatment for a psychotic sister. Although an average of two tenants a week requested a session, inappropriate or excessive consultation was rare. Tenants approached me directly in the afternoon to ask for an evening consultation. They often did not discuss the reason with their case manager first, but saw it as a private matter. An understanding was developed with the CSS team and with the tenants to allow both for the sharing of information with case managers and for sufficient privacy in consultation, which seemed to be valued by the clients. The intrinsic benefit of these ad hoc consultations was complemented by the network of relationships I formed in this way with tenants, which equipped me, in turn, to be helpful when crises arose.

Individual work in the hotel demanded flexibility. Those most in need were often discouraged by minor barriers. I saw a tenant in my office, in her room, or in the corner of a community lounge, depending on her preferences. The timing of a session was adjusted according to the tenant's ability to wait for an appointment, and the length according to her tolerance. Prior knowledge of the community and informal contact with the individual were indispensable to making these arrangements.

Teamwork

Few would argue that a psychiatrist has no special skills to contribute to a team planning services for chronically mentally ill people. However, a psychiatrist can be a hindrance as well as a help. To be helpful to the CSS team required direct knowledge of hotel life. This applied both to my role as a consultant at weekly team meetings and to my role in staff education. Some of the modes of response learned in hospitals or outpatient clinics would have had no relevance to the team's work or would have been counterproductive. To apply clinical skills in a novel context, one first has to experience and understand the context.

The capacity to share leadership was also critical to effective work with this team. A social worker ran the program and, as a rule, made the final decisions if there was no consensus. However, there were a few exceptions, as when a tenant was suicidal and a decision had to be made about hospitalization. We never had a major dispute over who had the final authority. This may be attributed to the common philosophy of care and to a good working relationship between myself and the team leader. Still, while it can be a strength for authority to be divided, the potential difficulties of shared leadership cannot be disregarded.

This synopsis of an experience in a single setting is meant to be immediately useful for people who are involved in planning services for homeless mentally ill people, and to repair, a little, the deficiency of material on the role of psychiatrists. Few psychiatrists are interested in working with these people, whom they often perceive as unreachable and endlessly frustrating. Those of us whose experience is otherwise need to document that working with homeless mentally ill people can be creative and can lead to results.

Conclusion

Discussion of the role of the psychiatrist in the care of chronically mentally ill people has generally focused on hospitals and outpatient clinics, the settings where most patient care still takes place. To a lesser extent, the potential role of psychiatrists in assertive case management teams, clinic-based outreach programs, and rehabilitation programs has also received some attention. The psychiatrist is a relatively new entrant to the mental health programs for the homeless that have proliferated in the 1980s. The role of the few psychiatrists who have been employed by these programs has rarely been discussed explicitly.

Psychiatrists who work with homeless mentally ill people often know of no precedent, either for the type of clinical practice that seems to be required to adapt to the setting, or for the type of career that seems to arise from their work. The institutions that employ them likewise often know of no precedent to follow. They seek to employ and retain young psychiatrists in this field, but they do not know how to fashion their jobs. I have sought to illustrate that it is possible for psychiatrist and employer to experiment together to devise creative roles in which the psychiatrist can apply a broad training to best advantage.

References

1. Factor RM, Stein LI, Diamond RJ. A model community psychiatry curriculum for psychiatric residents. *Community Mental Health Journal 24*:310–327, 1988.

2. Faulkner LR, et al. A basic residency curriculum concerning the chronically mentally ill. *American Journal of Psychiatry 146:*1323–1327, 1989.

3. Ball FLJ, Havassy BE. A survey of the problems and needs of homeless consumers of acute psychiatric services. *Hospital and Community Psychiatry 35:*917–921, 1984.

4. Struening E. *A Study of Residents of the New York City Shelter System.* Report to the New York City Department of Mental Health, Mental Retardation, and Alcoholism Services. New York: New York State Psychiatric Institute, Epidemiology of Mental Disorders Research Department, 1986.

5. Gounis K, Susser E. Shelterization and its implications for mental health services. In Cohen N (ed.), *Psychiatry Takes to the Streets.* New York: Guilford, in press.

6. Barrow S, Lovell A. *Serving the Mentally Ill Homeless: Client and Program Characteristics.* New York: New York State Psychiatric Institute, Community Support System Evaluation Unit, 1985.

7. Cohen NL, Putnam JF, Sullivan AM. The mentally ill homeless: Isolation and adaptation. *Hospital and Community Psychiatry 35:*922–924, 1984.

8. Susser E, Goldfinger S, White A. Some aspects of clinical work with the homeless mentally ill. *Community Mental Health Journal 26:*459–476, 1990.

9. Freire P. *Pedagogy of the Oppressed.* New York: Herder and Herder, 1972.

10. Rose SM, Black BL. *Advocacy and Empowerment: Mental Health Care in the Community.* Boston: Routledge and Kegan Paul, 1985.

11. Pilisuk M, Minkler M. Supportive networks: Life ties for the elderly. *Journal of Social Issues 36:*95–116, 1980.

12. Cohen M. Mutual interaction in a program for the homeless mentally ill. Ph.D. diss., Brandeis University, 1988.

CHAPTER 14

Social Networking with
Homeless Families

William J. Hutchison, Ph.D., John J. Stretch, Ph.D.
Priscilla Smith, M.S.W., Larry Kreuger, Ph.D., M.S.W.

A mong social workers, the networking of services is neither an entirely new concept nor a new strategy for assisting people in need. However, in recent years the concept has been refined by a number of authors, and the range of strategies for networking has grown more sophisticated. Networking has been used with a variety of populations (e.g., elderly people, divorced people, and stepfamilies) and problems (e.g., day care and child development, mental health, health care, and health promotion) (1–5).

While there have been numerous descriptions of programs providing multiple services to homeless people (6–9), a paradigm for the integration of these services and their adaptation to the evolving needs of homeless individuals and families has not yet emerged. The problem is twofold—to integrate the services, and to provide the needed mix of services at the appropriate time. This chapter presents an approach that combines multilevel networking with staging of the needs of homeless families. It has been implemented since 1983 in an innovative program developed at the Salvation Army Family Haven in Saint Louis, in collaboration with the Saint Louis Community Development Agency.

We shall first describe four types of networking and then, using a five-stage model of the evolution of the needs of homeless families (starting at the time when they become homeless, and ending with their postshelter placement), show how the various types of networking may be used at different stages.

Four Types of Networking

NATURAL SUPPORT SYSTEMS.   A professional intervenes to assist a family or an individual by facilitating the linkage of clients to their "natural" support system, composed of family members, friends, or colleagues. For example, a social worker at the Haven assists a single parent to develop stronger ties with a sister who would provide shelter and baby sitting, so that the client can seek employment and have emotional support while she flees from an abusive situation with her spouse or boyfriend.

CLIENT-AGENCY LINKAGE. A professional intervenes to assist a family or an individual by facilitating the linkage of the client to other professional services or to agencies in the community. For example, a social worker at the Haven refers a mother and her developmentally disabled seven-year-old child to the Saint Louis Special School District and assists the client in enrolling her child in a special class. What is common to the first and second types of networking is that the professional intervenes with a client to link the client to a person or group providing some type of support or assistance. Both are forms of case management.

INTERPROFESSIONAL LINKAGES. Professionals network among themselves to link the goals of their respective agencies. For example, the housing specialist at the Haven collaborates with a program director at the Saint Louis Housing Authority to arrange to provide clients leaving the Haven with housing subsidized by Section 8 of the Housing and Community Development Act of 1974.

HUMAN-SERVICE ORGANIZATION NETWORKING. Coalitions are developed among agencies and administrative ties are established among them. For example, the executive director of the Haven facilitates a task force of 12 other agencies to develop a new model of providing health care for homeless people and to submit the plan to a foundation for funding.

In the next section, the five-stage model developed by the authors (Table 14.1) will be used to further illustrate networking in the primary and secondary prevention of homelessness (10).

The Five-Stage Model

PRIMARY PREVENTION

A review of the data kept by the Salvation Army Family Haven showed that the Haven received an average of 300 calls per month from people who felt that, without assistance, they would become homeless. To prevent this homelessness, the Haven developed a rental and mortgage assistance program. By networking with individual church organizations, it was able to set aside a pool of funds to assist temporarily unemployed people to remain in their own homes for a few months rather than being evicted and having to search for new housing. Another form of intervention was tenant-landlord mediation. The

TABLE 14.1 FIVE-STAGE MODEL: NETWORKING SERVICES FOR HOMELESS PEOPLE

PREVENTION STAGE
Assistance with rent, mortgage, or utilities
Counseling
Tenant-landlord mediation

CRISIS INTERVENTION STAGE
Hospitality House: Families-in-Crisis Center; Reception Center; Household Goods Network; Services for Displacement by City Condemnation
Emergency Lodge: Casework plan

STABILIZATION STAGE
Emergency Lodge Program
    Training sessions (budgeting; parenting; nutrition; home maintenance; tenant responsibilities; general educational and development classes)
    Child care (preschool and school programs)
    Individual and group counseling (women's groups; assertiveness training; short- and long-term life-goal setting; employment services)
    Housing search and assistance with landlord relationships

RELOCATION STAGE
Transitional Housing Program
Assistance in locating permanent housing
    Counseling, education and training, supportive programs

COMMUNITY REINTEGRATION AND FOLLOW-UP STAGE
Housing in permanent housing units (e.g., private and market-rate units; Section 8 housing; Ecumenical Housing Production Corporation units)
Participation in neighborhood groups and church activities
Involvement with training and employment goals
Achievement of self-sufficiency
Follow-up evaluation

Haven drew upon the resources of the local university's law school to establish a unit that assists clients with landlord-tenant relations.

CRISIS INTERVENTION

Since the Haven can admit only 20–25 of the 300 families who are eligible each month, the Haven intake worker has to screen applicants closely and accept those clients who are judged most likely to benefit from its intensive, family-focused case management approach. People who cannot be admitted are given information and referred to other agencies by the receptionist and the intake worker. At this stage, the families who are admitted are in a state of crisis, which has to be dealt with first.

Upon intake, a caseworker is immediately assigned to the family, and together they develop a casework plan. Children are included in the initial development of the plan, not only to familiarize them with their caseworker but also to make them realize that they are an integral part of the total plan and to let them know that they have an important role to play in carrying out the plan. The caseworker provides guidance and support to the family as they strive to identify the causes of their crisis situation and work on alternatives to prevent homelessness in the future.

A casework plan for a family consists of in-house and networked elements of two major kinds—for the parent, training in family finances, parenting skills, homemaking, and home maintenance skills; and for the child, emotional and educational testing, child care services, and school placement. The children are assured of continuity in their current school. The plan is a family-centered plan, case-managed by a trained Haven social worker. Medical screening and health care are provided by a citywide health care for the homeless program.

STABILIZATION

In this stage, the caseworker helps the family to develop new supportive networks and to improve their relationships in existing networks. Nearly all of the sampled families admitted to the Haven have nonsupportive networks or virtually no networks at all from which resources could be obtained. They have neither enough money to secure basic essentials nor family or friends who could temporarily provide them with supports. In addition, the parents usually lack the education or training needed to secure jobs. Often lacking, also, are social skills that are often necessary to make them acceptable to prospective landlords. Thus, in this stage, the caseworker develops networks among families, other agencies, and other Haven staff in the following areas: food, housing, counseling, clothing, medical care, utility assistance, jobs, and job training.

CASEWORK SUPPORT. Continued comprehensive support and services are provided. Individual and family sessions are conducted dealing with family relationships and with successes and failures in following through on the casework plan, always trying to create a supportive atmosphere.

TRAINING SESSIONS. As a condition for remaining in the Haven, residents must attend two training sessions each week. These provide adult education in budget control, family management, employment skills, housing, landlord-tenant rights and responsibilities, minor home repairs, nutrition, and parenting skills. Through this program, residents are prepared for permanent housing by providing them with the basic survival techniques needed to keep them from recycling through the emergency shelter system.

EMPLOYMENT PROGRAM. The majority of the parents served by the Haven have no employment. Their most common source of income is AFDC, which is extremely inadequate for the provision of a satisfactory life-style. An employ-

221

ment program has been established to provide a weekly employment support group. Providing clothing, transportation, telephone service, and counseling for parents who seek employment is part of that effort.

CHILD CARE.   One of the most important components of the Haven is its fully equipped child care center, which offers well-balanced educational, social, and recreational opportunities for the children. While the children are being taken care of, the parents can seek employment and housing.

Personal and social skills are enhanced through creative play and group activities that require social interaction. Fine motor skills are developed by participating in such activities as doing puzzles, playing with blocks, stringing beads, or doing art work. Language development and cognitive skills are addressed in educational activities with the alphabet, numbers, music, word games, and the like. Gross motor skills are developed through play on riding toys, and through exercise and active group games such as kickball and dodge ball. It is this dimension of the program which often reveals developmental delays. Many children progress during the two months they reside in the Haven. Others are just too far behind, need individual instruction, and are often referred to other resources.

SCHOOL PROGRAM.   The formal education of school-age children residing in the Haven does not need to be interrupted. For those currently enrolled in school, transportation is arranged through the board of education so that they may continue in their own school districts. This allows for some consistency in their lives, which is a vital component of the stabilization process.

The Haven has the option of enrolling children who are not currently enrolled in school in the neighborhood's elementary school. A unique professional relationship exists between the Salvation Army and the Cole School, which is located eight blocks from the Haven. At any time during the school year, the Haven can register children as necessary, whether it is for a few days or two months of continuous education. School officials keep in touch with casework staff if problems arise which would require intervention by the Haven. Upon discharge of the family from the Haven, Cole School is notified immediately, and it processes all transfer arrangements to the new school district.

RELOCATION

In this stage, the caseworker and the family work closely with the housing specialist and, in some cases, the transitional housing specialist. Mandatory housing sessions are provided by the housing specialist, wherein families are trained in the process of seeking housing and presenting themselves to prospective landlords. The housing specialist meets with each family and accompanies its members to prospective housing sites in the community. Families are encouraged to use their networks of family, friends, and other Haven residents, as well as newspapers, to develop leads on possible housing. The housing specialist secures several housing leads from residents and other Haven staff. This staff person also uses personal and professional contacts to obtain information about housing.

The Haven has placed many of its residents in Section 8 units (chapter 17). Most of them were secured by the housing specialist. As a result of their efforts to secure Section 8 housing, housing specialists have found that the key is in working with small developers of Section 8 housing. They have found that simply looking for existing Section 8 housing is not as productive as finding ways to help small developers create new Section 8 housing.

The housing specialist cooperates with the caseworkers by emphasizing to residents that those families that have secured jobs or job training while at the Haven have a better chance of obtaining housing. Program aides continue to provide support to residents, as well as helping to discover housing leads. Residents continue to attend training sessions and residents' meetings.

The Transitional Housing Program of the Salvation Army Family Haven was initiated in 1983 in an effort to provide a temporary bridge between residents at the Haven and independent community placement. Families who receive services from the Haven for up to 60 days but who are not deemed ready for permanent community placement are transferred to the Transitional Housing Program. Its staff provides counseling, education, vocational guidance, job readiness training, and supportive programs to ensure the successful reintegration of families in the community. Although the families served in the transitional housing are relatively few, they stay in the program for a considerably longer time than do other families. The average duration in residence in transitional housing has increased from three months in 1983 to over nine months in 1987. A three-month follow-up period is provided for families moving into permanent housing.

COMMUNITY REINTEGRATION AND FOLLOW-UP

In the community reintegration stage, families receive continued assistance directly or through networking. The following conditions have to be met for follow-up:

- The family must have stayed at the Haven for at least 14 days;
- The address of the family has to be known;
- The family has to reside in the metropolitan area of Saint Louis at the time of the 30-day follow-up contact; and
- The family has to reside outside of another shelter, transitional housing, or institution at the end of the Haven shelter stay.

These community-reintegrated families are followed up by caseworkers at 1-, 2-, 3-, and 12-month intervals after termination from the Haven. In the follow-up sessions, a community reintegration instrument is administered by the worker to aid in assessing the degree of stability of the families. This instrument, along with formal interviews, aids the caseworker in determining the need for any further referral, services, or networking to enhance community reintegration. When possible, the caseworker makes a visit to the family's residence. If a home visit is not possible, the caseworker contacts the family by phone, conducts the follow-up interview at the Haven, or gathers information from family, friends, or agency staff.

Although the family has secured permanent housing at this stage, they may be seeking to improve their housing conditions by upgrading their current residence or moving to another one. With the family's permission and cooperation, the caseworker may act as liaison between the family and the landlord of the current residence. In other instances, the caseworker may counsel, coach, and support the family in dealing with the landlord directly.

The caseworkers' services during the follow-up stage include supportive counseling and the issuance of vouchers. The family may need further support in pursuing job training, obtaining employment, or improving relations with family, friends, employees, or landlords. Several families receive assistance with food, transportation, clothing, medical care, and furnishings.

Case Example

Mr. and Mrs. B. and their two children entered the Haven in the early summer. The family had a transient history, with crisscrossing travels from New York to Kansas. Both parents were unemployed. They applied for AFDC while at the Haven. Then, near the final days of their two-month stay, Mr. B. abandoned his family, presumably to live with another woman.

Patty B. was selected for the Transitional Housing Program, and she moved into an Elmwood Park apartment in early fall. Patty, a 30-year-old, did not have a significant employment history and continued receiving an AFDC income of $261 monthly.

Neither of the children, Shawna, age 6, and Eddy, age 4, had previously attended school. The daughter was immediately enrolled in kindergarten, but the younger boy remained on the waiting list for a HeadStart preschool. Shawna soon began exhibiting learning deficiencies, and as months progressed, many tests indicated a learning disability caused, at least in part, by a hearing impairment. It was also obvious that there were speech problems. Further testing and numerous conferences with school officials followed, and Shawna received intensive teaching in a self-contained classroom. Medical treatment of the hearing condition continued. This worrisome development was compounded because Patty vividly recalled her early years in an archaic "special" school. Young Eddy was tested by Childcheck (a child-centered evaluation instrument) as a preventive measure before he entered school.

Patty found her niche in Elmwood Park. The housing project was plagued by unattended children in the streets, and vandalism and violence were consequently prevalent. She assumed the role of a block mother for the latchkey children. She fastens buttons and combs hair in the morning. Later, she opens her doors and prepares snacks at evening time. The city housing authority accepted Patty as a permanent tenant the next spring, primarily because of her positive impact in the neighborhood.

A Survey of the Program, 1983–1987

The findings of an ongoing survey and follow-up study of the program have been presented in detail elsewhere (11). Only the briefest summary is given here. The program reported on in this study is based on a joint project undertaken by the Saint Louis Community Development Agency and the Salvation Army to operate a 54-bed emergency housing shelter. By the program's eighth year, about half of the operating expenses of the shelter were paid by a Community Development Block Grant (chapter 17). Families of all sizes (from one person to more than five) who had become homeless for a variety of reasons were admitted to the shelter for a stay of up to two months. The trend in family sizes and the causes of homelessness changed during the five-year period because of changes in intake policy, the use of primary preventive interventions, and the increased availability of other facilities. Thus, by 1987, most of the families admitted had two to four members, as those with five or more tended to be served by other sectors of the Saint Louis Homeless Service Network. Loss of income had shown a relative decrease as a cause of homelessness, and the stranded and transient category had also decreased, while family friction had shown a relative increase. About one-third of the families had no source of income, and almost one-half had only AFDC or public assistance. The job skill level was "unskilled" in over 55 percent of the group, and about 45 percent had no high-school diploma. The estimated monthly income was none in 36 percent and less than $400 per month in another 49 percent.

The housing disposition (i.e., the type of housing the family went to upon leaving the shelter) over the entire study period was as follows: permanent housing, 51 percent (more than half of which was accounted for by Section 8); temporary housing, 19 percent; another shelter, 9 percent; and other, 21 percent (four-fifths of which was "left without specification"). The study's total population was 875. Forty-four families were admitted to the transitional housing program during the study period. Short-term follow-up (30, 60, and 90 days combined) allowed tracking of 76 percent of the families. Of those tracked, 88 percent were in permanent housing, 60 percent in Section 8 housing. A disturbing finding was that the average monthly income was low ($344 if those with no income were included, and $357 if they were excluded). Furthermore, the average income had decreased (i.e., it was lower in those followed up in 1987 than in those followed up in 1983).

In summary, the results show that the approach is feasible and is associated with good short-term (90-day) housing stability in these families, which were to some extent selected. The question of long-term stability requires further studies with long-term follow-up. That of the role of the program in assuring housing stability should be approached with case-comparison follow-up studies of homeless people exposed to the networking system and of a comparison group managed differently.

Discussion: Policies That Affect Networking

The networking system described in this chapter does not operate in a policy vacuum. Its effectiveness depends to a great extent upon policies that affect the various causes of homelessness. Needed are policies that reduce unemployment or prolong the period for which unemployment insurance is paid; increased Section 8–subsidized housing for families who have passed through the stabilization stage; local ordinances prohibiting housing discrimination against families with children; the support of emergency housing with the help of Community Development Block Grants or, perhaps, of a tax on room rates of hotels; an increase in welfare-adjusted payment to make families capable of affording low-cost housing; and programs and funds to help dischargees from mental hospitals to find and remain in adequate housing. No matter how well organized the service and social networks are, they cannot achieve full effectiveness unless these broad policy needs are addressed at every level of political jurisdiction. Neither one level, nor one approach, whether public or private, can do the job alone.

References

1. Gottlieb B (ed.). *Social Networks and Social Supports.* Beverly Hills, Calif.: Sage Publications, 1981.
2. Froland C. *Helping Networks and Human Services.* Beverly Hills, Calif.: Sage Publications, 1982.
3. Maguire L. *Understanding Social Networks.* Beverly Hills, Calif.: Sage Publications, 1983.
4. Whittaker JK, Garbarino J. *Social Support Networks: Informal Helping in Human Services.* New York: Aldine, 1983.
5. Sauer WJ, Coward RT (eds.). *Social Support Networks and Care of the Elderly.* New York: Springer, 1985.
6. U.S. Department of Health and Human Services. *Helping the Homeless.* Washington, D.C.: Government Printing Office, 1984.
7. Wittman FD, Madden PA. *Alcohol Recovery Programs for Homeless People: A Survey of Current Programs in the U.S.* Rockville, Md.: National Institute on Alcohol Abuse and Alcoholism, 1988.

8. Vernez G, et al. *Review of California's Program for the Homeless Mentally Disabled.* Santa Monica, Calif.: Rand Corporation, 1988.

9. *This Line Is No Place to Be: Improving the Delivery of Support Services to Homeless People.* San Francisco, Calif.: HomeBase, 1990.

10. Hutchison WJ, Searight PR, Stretch JJ. Multidimensional networking: A response to the needs of homeless families. *Social Work 31:*427–430, 1986.

11. Stretch JJ, et al. *The Homeless Continuum Model: Serving Homeless Families.* St. Louis, Mo.: Salvation Army, Midland Division, and St. Louis Community Development Agency, December 1988.

PART III

The Social Context
of Homelessness

CHAPTER 15

The Changing Context
of Subsistence

Jill Hamberg, Ph.D. Cand., and Kim Hopper, Ph.D.

This chapter will sketch the trend lines for a number of developments in the 1970s and early 1980s that conspired to produce widespread homelessness in our time (1). The relevant developments occurred in five areas: (a) household income and the sources of that income; (b) household composition; (c) characteristics of the housing stock; (d) regional population shifts; and (e) specific governmental policies affecting income, housing, and the situation of people with disabilities. It is this cluster of factors, their changes over time, and their reciprocal interaction at any one time that provide the essential background against which crises of dislocation have been played out. Thus, depending on the constellation of factors at a given time and place, the forces of displacement may be more or less severe, and the effect of losing one's home may be more or less transient.

Developments in the 1970s

INCOME. In the 1970s, real wages declined on average 7.4 percent. Nonetheless, median household income kept pace with inflation, but only because more households had more than one wage earner (2). The stability of the median obscures a more pertinent fact—the growing polarization of income, which reversed what had been the post–World War II trend toward greater income equality. The shrinking of the middle-income range, in turn, had its roots in four developments: (a) structural changes in the U.S. economy, specifically the declining importance of the manufacturing sector and the concomitant loss of middle-income unionized jobs, and the parallel rise of low-paid retail and service-sector work (3); (b) the accelerated formation of single-parent households (by 1982, half of all black and one-sixth of all white children lived in such families, the majority of whom subsisted below the poverty line) (4); (c) recurrent high levels of unemployment and underemployment; and (d) the erosion of benefit levels in means-tested assistance programs (the real value of AFDC payments fell by 28 percent in the 1970s, while the comparable figure for general assistance was 32 percent) (2).

HOUSEHOLD COMPOSITION. Average household size declined steadily between 1950 and 1970, from 3.37 to 3.14. It then fell another 13 percent in the following decade to reach 2.73 (2). By 1980, nearly two-thirds of all renter households were made up of one or two persons (5). In the same decade, the divorce rate doubled, further explaining the trend toward disaggregated households of smaller size (6).

HOUSING. Three developments were significant. The first was a decline in the percentage of families who could afford to purchase homes—only a quarter of all families in 1976 (7). The second was a steady rise in the proportion of income paid for rent. From 1970 to 1980, the median ratio of rent to income increased from 20 percent to 27 percent (8). Again, this obscures developments at the margins. For the very poor, the 2.7 million households with annual incomes of less than $3,000, the decade was disastrous. Half of such households spent at least 72 percent of their total income on rent, compared with 34 percent in 1970. Overall, 7 million households were spending at least 50 percent of their income to cover shelter costs in 1980. Nearly three-quarters of those were renter households with median annual income of $4,000–5,000 (9). The third significant development was the loss of low-income single-room occupancy units. Nearly half of all such units were removed from the nation's housing stock in the 1970s. In certain rapidly gentrifying areas, single-room occupancy hotels (SROs) faced extinction. For instance, New York City lost 87 percent of its low-rent SRO units in 1970–82 through inflation, conversion, demolition, and abandonment (10).

POPULATION SHIFTS. With the demise of a number of smokestack industries, part of a more general trend toward "deindustrialization" (11) in the northeast and north central United States, more and more laid-off workers and their families sought employment elsewhere. Some found jobs (at much lower wages) in the growing service sector, but many chose to leave their regional economies altogether. Between April 1980 and July 1982, the north central states lost nearly a million people to migration (12). All too often, the new arrivals found that the fabled job-rich areas of the Sunbelt were experiencing their own local employment difficulties and that their attitude toward additional competitors was less than hospitable.

DEINSTITUTIONALIZATION OF MENTALLY ILL PEOPLE. Deinstitutionalization had begun in the 1950s. The second phase of the movement—restrictive admission policies—took on greater importance as the 1970s progressed. The story is a familiar one. What needs to be stressed is the lag between the intensive early phase of depopulation of state hospitals and the later appearance on the streets of both ex-patients and those who had never been hospitalized. Clearly, intermediate factors were at work, chief among them the loss of affordable housing (13,14).

The general consequence of the developments discussed above was the slow march of more and more households toward the brink of destitution. Official poverty rates, which had been declining steadily since 1960 (except for a brief elevation at the time of the 1973–75 recession), began to climb upward in 1978. These trends continued in the 1980s. Some, in fact, worsened. All were exacerbated by the combined effect of the twin recessions of 1979–82 and the Reagan budget cuts (15).

Developments in the Early 1980s

The restructuring of the economy that began in the 1970s continued in the early 1980s, accelerated by policies of the Reagan Administration.

INCOME.   The earlier trend toward a bipolar distribution of income intensified. The average weekly wage fell 12 percent during the four recession years (16). In the first four years of the decade, the average disposable income of the poorest fifth of the population fell by nearly 8 percent, from $6,913 to $6,319 (17). The number of people officially living in poverty grew by 40 percent between 1978 and 1983, and their proportion of the population increased from 11.4 percent to 15.2 percent (18).

Unemployment took on markedly harsh overtones. Those who lost jobs were less likely to regain them once the recession ended. Over half of the new jobless in 1981–82 were permanently separated from their old jobs, compared with just over a third in the three recessions of the 1970s (19). Many unemployed people were also likely to stay jobless for extended periods. In January 1984, when unofficial unemployment rates had fallen to their prerecession levels of 8 percent, there were 2 million people who had been out of work for six months or more (20). At the same time, surviving while jobless became more difficult, since unemployment benefits were reduced by legislative changes. Less than half of those who lost their jobs in 1982 received unemployment benefits, as compared with 78 percent in the previous (1973–75) recession (21). By June 1984, the percentage of the officially unemployed collecting benefits fell to a record low of 29.2 percent. With "discouraged" workers (who do not appear in official tallies of the jobless) included, the figure was 25.4 percent (22).

Despite the upward climb of the number of Americans living in poverty, benefit programs were cut, further contributing to this surge. Means-tested assistance programs were reduced 16.4 percent between 1980 and 1984 (23). The real value of AFDC benefits fell a further 7 percent between 1981 and 1983 (24). New eligibility rules meant that 50 percent of the working poor collecting AFDC were dropped from the rolls. Another 40 percent of such families had their benefits reduced (25).

Recipients of disability benefits were treated especially harshly. Nearly half a million (one-sixth of the total) were expunged from the rolls (26), often with no more notice than a barely comprehensible letter informing the individual that under new review standards he or she was now considered able to work (27). For the most part, safeguards against arbitrary judgments were nonexistent except in instances where those affected appealed the ruling, usually successfully. One federal judge was moved to condemn the Department of Health and Human Services as a "heartless and indifferent bureaucratic monster" (28).

Elsewhere, applicants for general assistance, and even those suspected of being "not truly homeless," were subjected to new rules designed to minimize potential demand. In Sacramento, California, the workhouse was reinstituted, as able-bodied applicants for general assistance were offered the sole choice of living in a county-operated shelter and performing labor in exchange for room and board (29). Pennsylvania restricted similarly situated individuals to three months of assistance for any calendar year; for the rest of the time, they were expected to shift for themselves (30).

Food stamp programs were reduced, forcing growing numbers of households to resort to soup kitchens and food pantries to supplement their meager budgets. Hunger resurfaced in a country where it had been all but eliminated (31).

HOUSING. With interest rates soaring, homeownership was put out of the reach of more and more households. An estimated 4 million households remained in the rental market who formerly would have purchased homes (32). The measured prevalence of doubling-up increased twofold between 1978 and 1983—from 1.3 million to 2.6 million families (33). Rents began to increase faster than inflation: in the 12 months ending in July 1983, the rent component of the Consumer Price Index rose at a rate of 5.4 percent, compared to 2.2 percent for prices generally (34). The federal government responded by gutting low-income housing programs across the board. Severe reductions were made in programs that directly add to the stock of low- and moderate-income housing, rent subsidies were cut drastically, and maintenance of public housing declined, with some units being removed from publicly owned stock altogether (35; and chapter 17).

Conclusion

There is little doubt that the crisis deepened throughout the 1980s (chapters 16 and 17) and shows no sign of abating in the 1990s. Granted, it can be difficult to discern the causal linkages between the Federal Reserve Bank's prime rate and a given instance of homelessness, and the argument given here makes no pretense of doing so. It merely suggests that individual failures to procure stable housing have their roots in larger, systemwide tendencies that have made the satisfaction of basic needs an increasingly uncertain affair for a growing segment of the population (chapter 20). The specific plight of such groups as mentally disabled homeless people must be placed in the context of intensified competition for an increasingly scarce and costly commodity. Shrinking incomes and a depleted stock of affordable housing create less than optimal circumstances for anyone seeking decent quarters. They are surely formidable obstacles for someone whose mental health may be precarious. So there is not much that should provoke wonder in the present spectacle of homelessness. That such people often fail to find or to hold onto housing—and that their failure often takes the form of an unseemly affront to this society's pretensions to civilization—may be disturbing eventualities, but they are not mysterious ones.

The intent of this exercise has been to suggest the dimensions and scope of what might be called the field of requisite complexity that must be covered in contemporary analyses of homelessness. Much of the current interest in evaluating the role of context in the production of individual instances of homelessness, it seems to us, has been taking place in unduly restrictive fashion. The term *context* is often limited to the notion of immediate environment and precipitating events. Our concern here has been with those broad, historical limits and pressures that exert their influences over time in slow, unobtrusive ways that often escape the notice of actor and observer alike.

References

1. Hopper K, Hamberg J. The making of America's homeless: From skid row to new poor, 1945–1984. In Bratt R, Hartman C, Meyerson A (eds.), *Critical Perspectives on Housing.* Philadelphia: Temple University Press, 1986, pp. 12–40.
2. Bureau of the Census. *Statistical Abstract of the United States, 1982–83.* Washington, D.C.: Government Printing Office, 1982.
3. Bluestone B, Harrison B. *Storm Cloud on the Horizon: Labor Market Crisis and Industrial Crisis.* Brookline, Mass.: Economic Education Project, 1984.
4. Bureau of the Census. *Current Population Reports,* ser. P-23, no. 130, *Population Profile of the United States, 1982.* Washington, D.C.: Government Printing Office, 1983.
5. Downs A. *Rental Housing in the 1980s.* Washington, D.C.: Brookings Institution, 1983.

6. Hacker E (ed.). *U/S: A Statistical Portrait of the American People*. New York: Viking, 1983.

7. Stone M. Housing and the economic crisis: An analysis and emergency program. In Hartman C (ed.), *America's Housing Crisis: What Is to Be Done?* Boston: Routledge and Kegan Paul, 1983, pp. 99–150.

8. Bureau of the Census. *Annual Housing Survey, 1980*, ser. H-150-80, pt. C, *Financial Characteristics of the Housing Industry, United States and Regions*. Washington, D.C.: Government Printing Office, 1981.

9. Dolbeare C. The low-income housing crisis. In Hartman (ed.), *America's Housing Crisis*, pp. 29–75. See ref. 7.

10. Green C. *Housing Single, Low Income Individuals*. New York: New York City Setting Municipal Priorities Project, 1982.

11. Bluestone B, Harrison B. *The Deindustrialization of America*. New York: Basic Books, 1982.

12. Herbers J. Industrial flight from the North. *New York Times*, April 12, 1983, pp. D1, D19.

13. Fischer P, Breakey W. Homelessness and mental health: An overview. *International Journal of Mental Health 14*:6–41, 1985–86.

14. Roth D, et al. *Homelessness in Ohio: A Study of People in Need*. Columbus: Ohio Department of Mental Health, 1985.

15. House Committee on Ways and Means, Subcommittee on Oversight and Subcommittee on Public Assistance. *Effects of the Omnibus Budget Reconciliation Act of 1981 (OBRA), Welfare Changes, and the Recession on Poverty*. Washington, D.C.: Government Printing Office, 1984.

16. U.S. Department of Labor, Bureau of Labor Statistics. *The Unemployment Situation, November 1984*. Bull. no. 84-502. Washington, D.C.: The Department, December 7, 1984.

17. Moon M, Sawhill IV. Family income: Gainers and losers. In Palmer JL, Sawhill IV (eds.), *The Reagan Revolution*. Cambridge, Mass.: Ballinger, 1984, pp. 317–346.

18. Bureau of the Census. *Current Population Reports*, ser. P-60, no. 145, *Money, Income, and Poverty Status of Families and Persons in the United States, 1983*. Washington, D.C.: Government Printing Office, 1984.

19. Bednarzik RW. Lay-offs and permanent job losses: Workers' traits and cyclical patterns. *Monthly Labor Review*, September 1983, pp. 3–11.

20. Center on Budget and Policy Priorities. *Long-term Unemployment*. Washington, D.C.: The Center, 1984.

21. Burtless G. Testimony before the House Committee on Ways and Means, October 18, 1983. Typescript.

22. Center on Budget and Policy Priorities. *Unemployment Issues in June 1984*. Washington, D.C.: The Center, 1984.

23. Ridgeway J. The administration's attack on the homeless: Building a fire under Reagan. *Village Voice*, February 14, 1984.

24. House Committee on Ways and Means, Subcommittee on Oversight and Subcommittee on Public Assistance. *Background Material on Poverty*. Washington, D.C.: Government Printing Office, 1983.

25. Congressional Budget Office. *Major Legislative Changes in Human Resource Programs since January 1981*. Washington, D.C.: Government Printing Office, 1983.

26. Social Security agency halts cutoffs of disability benefits. *New York Times*, December 10, 1983.

27. Cuomo MM. *Never Again*. A report to the National Governors' Association, Task Force on Homelessness. Albany: New York State Executive Chamber, 1983.

28. *Merli* v. *Heckler.* District Court for the District of New Jersey, Civil Action no. 83-189, 1984.

29. Segal S, Specht H. A poorhouse in California, 1983: Oddity or prelude? *Social Work* 25:358–363, 1983.

30. Robbins W. Welfare cutoff swelling Philadelphia's homeless. *New York Times,* September 18, 1983, sec. 1, p. 20.

31. Physicians' Task Force on Hunger. *America's Hunger Crisis.* Boston: Harvard University School of Public Health, 1985.

32. National Housing Conference. *Housing Costs in the United States.* Washington, D.C.: The Conference, 1984.

33. Stegman M. *Rental Housing in New York City.* New York: New York City Department of Housing Preservation and Development, 1984.

34. Schecter HB. Closing the gap between need and provision. *Society 21(March–April)*:40–47, 1984.

35. Hartman C. Housing policies under the Reagan administration. In Bratt R, Hartman C, Meyerson A (eds.), *Critical Perspectives on Housing.* Philadelphia: Temple University Press, 1986, pp. 362–376.

CHAPTER 16

The Income Side of Housing Affordability: Shifts in Household Income and Income Support Programs during the 1970s and 1980s

Martha R. Burt, Ph.D.

The decreasing availability of affordable housing in the 1980s is the factor most often cited as a cause of homelessness. Housing costs are one side of the equation of housing affordability. Chapters 17 and 18 examine recent changes in the cost of housing that may have contributed to homelessness. The other side of the equation of affordable housing is income—how much money households have available for purchasing housing and other necessities. If income increases faster than housing costs rise, affordability increases even if housing costs also increase. Conversely, if incomes fall faster than housing costs drop, affordability decreases even when the cost of housing goes down. If affordability drops enough, some people may not be able to afford housing and risk becoming homeless.

Homeless people are extremely poor. In a national interview study of homeless users of soup kitchens and shelters conducted in 1987, single men reported a mean income of $143 for the preceding 30 days; single women reported $183; and women with children reported $300. Typically, the latter households consisted of a mother and two children. If annualized, these mean income levels represent about $2,000, or about one-third of the federal poverty level for a one-person household, and only $3,600, or 40 percent of the poverty level for a family of three (1,2). Other studies of homeless people in specific cities have found comparably low incomes (chapter 4). (*Median* incomes of homeless people were even lower. Single homeless people reported a median monthly income of $64, which, if annualized, amounted to $768 per year.) In comparison, even very poor people with homes have substantially higher incomes.

Rossi reported a mean income for Chicago's homeless of $168 per month in 1985–86. This compares unfavorably to a 1985 mean monthly income of $580 for Chicago's single-room occupancy hotel (SRO) residents (3:107).

This chapter describes the shifts during the 1970s and 1980s in the levels of poverty, household income, and major governmental sources of income support. Circumstances may differ from state to state and from locality to locality, affecting homelessness differently in each place. But the general picture is important, and I focus on national shifts in this chapter. I first examine changes in the numbers of people in poverty and in poverty rates for all households and for selected household types. I then document changes in employment, unemployment, wage levels, and the minimum wage, and provide some information about unemployment compensation. The last part of the chapter describes changes in major "safety net" income benefit programs—Supplemental Security Income (SSI); Aid to Families with Dependent Children (AFDC); and the Food Stamp Program. As a cumulative result of many of these changes between 1970 and 1989, the resources available to many poor households decreased, leading to increasing difficulties in affording housing.

Changes in Poverty

Calculating how many people are poor is not a simple task, but researchers and policy makers have developed several alternative definitions over the years that give a good indication of who is poor and what helps them rise above the poverty line. The first data examined, in table 16.1, show the numbers in poverty and the poverty rates for all individuals, elderly individuals, and individuals living in female-headed families, from 1970 through 1987. "People in poverty" are all individuals still below the official poverty line when all cash income *plus* income from social insurance (e.g., unemployment compensation), Social Security, and means-tested benefits (e.g., AFDC, SSI, general assistance) is counted. The poverty rate is the percentage of individuals within a given category who are poor.

As Table 16.1 reveals, there were 3.9 million more poor people in 1980 than in 1970, an increase of 15 percent. The most precipitous increase in poverty shown in Table 16.1 occurred between 1980 and 1983, during which 6.0 million more people became poor—a 20-percent increase. Even in 1987, as the numbers in poverty shrank somewhat, there were still 3.3 million more poor people than there had been in 1980. The numbers of poor elderly people declined during the period, and the poverty rate of the elderly population dropped substantially in the early 1970s due to indexing and other changes in Social Security. It continued a slow decrease in later years. The pattern for individuals in female-headed families is not as sanguine. Many more individu-

TABLE 16.1   NUMBERS OF PEOPLE IN POVERTY AND POVERTY RATES, 1970–1987

	People in Poverty (in 1,000s)			Poverty rates (%)		
Year	All	Aged	Individuals in Female-headed Families	All	Aged	Individuals in Female-headed Families
1970	25,420	4,793	11,154	12.6	24.6	38.2
1971	25,559	4,273	11,409	12.5	21.6	38.0
1972	24,460	3,738	11,587	11.9	18.6	36.9
1973	22,973	3,354	11,357	11.1	16.3	34.9
1974	23,370	3,085	11,469	11.2	14.6	33.6
1975	25,877	3,317	12,268	12.3	15.3	34.6
1976	24,975	3,313	12,586	11.8	15.0	34.4
1977	24,720	3,177	12,624	11.6	14.1	32.8
1978	24,497	3,233	12,880	11.4	14.0	32.3
1979	26,072	3,682	13,503	11.7	15.2	32.0
1980	29,272	3,871	14,649	13.0	15.7	33.8
1981	31,822	3,853	15,738	14.0	15.3	35.2
1982	34,398	3,751	16,336	15.0	14.6	36.2
1983	35,303	3,625	16,713	15.2	13.8	35.6
1984	33,700	3,300	16,440	14.4	12.4	34.0
1985	33,064	3,456	16,365	14.0	12.6	33.5
1986	32,370	3,477	16,926	13.6	12.4	34.0
1987	32,546	3,491	16,912	13.5	12.2	33.6

Source: Data from House Committee on Ways and Means, *Background Material and Data on Programs within the Jurisdiction of the Committee on Ways and Means*. Washington, D.C.: Government Printing Office, 1989, pp. 944–945.

als in these families were poor in the 1980s than in the 1970s. Yet the rate of poverty in this group appears to fluctuate within a somewhat narrow range rather than showing a steady increase or decrease.

Because changes in Social Security during the 1970s raised many elderly people out of poverty, aged people dropped substantially as a proportion of the poor population. In 1970 they were 18.9 percent of the poor, in 1980 they were 13.2 percent, and by 1987 they were only 10.7 percent of the poor population. There was a drop of 30 percent between 1970 and 1980, and one of 19 percent between 1980 and 1987. On the other hand, people in female-headed families grew as a proportion of the poor, from 43.9 percent in 1970 to 50 percent in 1980 and 52 percent in 1987. The biggest jump for this group—14 percent— was in the 1970s.

Dramatic as is the increase in the numbers of poor people shown in Table 16.1, the jump would have been even more extreme if the definition of poverty had included the imputed value of noncash food and housing benefits and the effects of federal tax policy in moving people in and out of poverty. Under the definition of poverty used in Table 16.1, the number of people classified as poor increased 24.8 percent between 1979 and 1987, from 26.1 million to 32.6 million. Under a revised definition that includes noncash benefits and federal taxes, the number of people classified as poor increased almost twice as much during the same period, 41 percent, from 21.6 million to 30.4 million. Further, under the Table 16.1 definition the poverty rate increased only 15.4 percent, but under the extended definition it increased 37.4 percent (4). The results using the expanded definition are more extreme because noncash benefit programs served more people, noncash benefit programs were worth more, and tax policy was less punitive to low-income people in 1979 than in later years.

Table 16.2 starts with numbers in poverty and examines the sources of income that remove individuals from poverty. It also shows the changing effectiveness of these mechanisms from 1979 through 1987. The first row of Table 16.2 shows the number of individuals who would be considered poor if only cash income before transfers were counted. This cash income includes cash from earnings, pensions, savings, investments, self-employment income, and similar sources. The second and third sections of Table 16.2 show the numbers and percentages of people removed from poverty by various social programs. The final section shows the poverty rate that would result from different definitions of poverty. As the "cash income before transfers" line of this fourth section shows, between 19 percent and 23 percent of all Americans were poor during the years 1979–87 if one counts only cash income before transfers. For every year, this poverty rate is considerably higher than the official poverty rate after transfers and taxes given on the bottom line of the table.

The second section of Table 16.2 reveals that Social Security is the social program most effective at removing people from poverty. In every year from 1979 through 1987, Social Security lifted more than twice as many people out of poverty as did the means-tested cash, food, and housing benefits that form the core of public "welfare" spending. The third section reveals that in 1979 the means-tested benefits comprising the social safety net programs of cash transfers, food assistance, and housing subsidies removed from poverty 16.6 percent of those who would have been poor on the basis of cash income alone. This figure dropped to 14.6 percent in 1980, then fell even more dramatically during the first years of the Reagan administration to a low of 9.9 percent in 1983. The drop occurred as a consequence of provisions enacted in the Omnibus Budget Reconciliation Act of 1981 (PL 97-35), restricting eligibility for the major benefit programs.

A mechanism, such as the poverty line, that separates people into two groups, those who are poor and those who are not, is too simple in some important respects. One person is counted as poor with an income that is less than half of the poverty line, while another is counted as poor with an income only $1 below the poverty line. Yet the first person has only half the income of the second one. To capture the idea of the degree of poverty, the concept of the

TABLE 16.2 ANTIPOVERTY EFFECTIVENESS OF CASH AND NONCASH TRANSFERS (INCLUDING FEDERAL INCOME AND PAYROLL TAXES) FOR ALL INDIVIDUALS IN FAMILIES OR LIVING ALONE, 1979–1987

	1979	1980	1981	1982	1983	1984	1985	1986	1987
NUMBER OF INDIVIDUALS (IN THOUSANDS)									
Poor, by cash income before transfers	41,695	46,273	49,184	51,942	52,700	50,493	50,462	49,732	49,679
Removed from poverty due to									
—Soc. ins. other than Soc. Sec.[a]	1,860	2,257	2,210	2,953	3,232	2,253	2,254	2,236	1,948
—Soc. ins. incl. Soc. Sec.	13,849	14,635	15,275	15,738	15,772	15,241	15,291	15,168	15,299
—Means-tested cash, food, housing benefits	6,915	6,756	6,206	5,711	5,231	5,599	5,682	5,546	5,376
—Federal taxes	−675	−1,148	−2,280	−2,056	−2,226	−2,426	−2,351	−2,261	−1,396
PERCENTAGES									
Poor individuals removed from poverty due to									
—Soc. ins. (incl. Soc. Sec.)	33.2	31.6	31.1	30.3	29.9	29.9	30.3	30.5	30.8
—Means-tested cash transfers	6.3	5.5	4.8	3.9	3.6	3.9	4.1	4.4	3.7
—Means-tested cash, food, and housing benefits	16.6	14.6	12.6	11.0	9.9	11.0	11.3	11.2	10.8
—Means-tested cash, food, and housing benefits and federal taxes	15.0	12.1	8.0	7.0	5.7	6.2	6.6	6.6	8.0
Poverty rate on the basis of									
—Cash income before transfers	19.1	20.6	21.7	22.6	22.8	21.8	21.3	20.8	20.6
—Cash income before transfers plus social insurance (except Soc. Sec.)	18.3	19.6	20.7	21.4	21.4	20.8	20.4	19.9	19.8
—Cash income before transfers, plus soc. ins. (incl. Soc. Sec.)	12.8	14.1	14.9	15.8	15.9	15.3	14.9	14.5	14.3

—Cash income before transfers, plus soc. ins. (incl. Soc. Sec.), plus means-tested cash transfers	11.6	12.9	13.9	14.9	15.1	14.4	14.0	13.6	13.5
—Cash income incl. means-tested transfers; plus soc. ins. (incl. Soc. Sec.), plus food and housing benefits	9.6	11.1	12.2	13.3	13.7	12.9	12.5	12.2	12.0
—Cash income including means-tested transfers; plus soc. ins. (incl. Soc. Sec.) and food and housing benefits, less federal taxes	9.9	11.6	13.2	14.2	14.6	13.9	13.5	13.2	12.6

Source: Data from House Committee on Ways and Means; *Background Material and Data on Programs within the Jurisdiction of the Committee on Ways and Means*. Washington, D.C.: Government Printing Office, 1989, pp. 962–963.
[a]Soc. ins., social insurance; Soc. Sec., Social Security; incl., including.

"poverty gap" is used to measure the actual amount of money it would take to lift every poor person out of poverty. The poverty gap will be quite small if all poor people have incomes just under the poverty line, and it will be quite large if all poor people have incomes far below the poverty line.

In 1979 the poverty gap based on cash income before transfers was $100 billion (in constant 1987 dollars). It grew to $127 billion by 1983 and shrank only to $124 billion by 1987. By this measure, *poor Americans were 27 percent poorer in 1983 and 24 percent poorer in 1987 than they had been in 1979.* Social Security reduced the poverty gap by 48 percent in 1979 and 1980, by 46 percent in 1981, and by 44–45 percent in 1982–87. Means-tested cash transfers reduced the poverty gap by 16 percent in 1979 and by 13–15 percent in 1980–87. The imputed value of noncash means-tested benefits (food stamps, school meal programs, and housing) further reduced the poverty gap by 7–8 percent from 1979 through 1987 (4:962–963).

Thus, throughout the decade the antipoverty effects of Social Security were approximately three times as large as those of means-tested cash transfers and about twice as large as the combined effects of cash and noncash means-tested transfers. And of course the proportion of the poverty gap remaining after the effects of all income transfers are considered jumped from 29–30 percent in 1979–80 to 33–35 percent in 1981–87. This represents about a 20 percent increase in impoverishment and an equivalent reduction in the impact of government programs on the economic well-being of poor people (4:962–963).

The Committee on Ways and Means of the U.S. House of Representatives analyzed the factors contributing to the increase in poverty between 1979 and 1987 (4:974–983). It concluded that

changes in means-tested programs added 3.2 million people to the poverty population, changes in market income [i.e., what people earn from working] added 1.1 million, changes in federal tax policy added 0.5 million, and changes in the social insurance programs [including Social Security] added roughly 0.9 million. Population growth and all other changes added an additional 3.1 million. In percentage terms, the largest contributing factor was the reduced effectiveness of means-tested welfare programs (36 percent), followed by population growth (26 percent), changes in market income (13 percent), the reduced effectiveness of social insurance programs (11 percent), and the reduced effectiveness of federal tax policy (5 percent). . . . Population growth, changes in market incomes and other residual changes accounted for 50 percent of the increase in the aggregate poverty gap, followed by social insurance programs (26 percent), means-tested programs (21 percent) and changes in federal tax policy (2 percent). (4:974–976)

Individuals in single-parent families with children accounted for 46 percent of the total increase in the number of poor people, although they comprise but 12 percent of the population (4:974). These families were the hardest hit by changes in means-tested programs. All other household types comprised smaller percentages of the poor population than of the total population. Elderly households were most remarkable in this respect, experiencing an actual drop in their numbers in poverty despite considerable growth in their total numbers.

Changes in Employment and Unemployment

Both low earnings among workers and periods of unemployment affect the poverty of American households. In 1987 about one-third of all poor people over the age of 16 worked or looked for work for at least half of the year (5). About half of poor people work full time, but at minimum-wage jobs. Therefore, their wage level, rather than the amount of effort they put into supporting themselves, is implicated in their poverty. This circumstance highlights the importance of the federally mandated minimum wage for raising workers out of poverty.

From 1968 through 1973, the minimum wage was $1.60. Between 1974 and 1981 it rose in gradual increments to $3.35, almost keeping pace with inflation until 1979. It has stayed at $3.35 from 1981 to 1990. Legislation enacted late in 1989 raises the minimum wage to $4.25 by 1991, in two increments. Between 1970 and 1980, the minimum wage lost only 3 percent of its purchasing power; between 1980 and 1988, it lost about 23 percent of its purchasing power (5:12). Clearly, the federal government's failure to maintain the earning power of low-wage workers by increasing the minimum wage is responsible for some proportion of the increased poverty of the 1980s due to changes in market income.

Further, the loss of earning power in recent years is not confined to minimum-wage workers. Average annual earnings from employment, adjusted for inflation, have decreased for men in all but one age and education category since 1973. Only young college-educated men maintained their earning power. For all women, especially for those with college education, real average earnings from employment have risen substantially but are still only about 60 percent of men's earnings for people of the same age with equivalent educations. Men aged 25–34 with high-school educations lost the most purchasing power between 1973 and 1986—21 percent. College-educated women aged 35–44 gained the most—38 percent (6).

A shift in the distribution of American jobs from higher-skilled manufacturing jobs to lower-skilled manufacturing and service jobs is responsible for some of this drop in earning power. Between 1979 and 1987, the number of low-wage jobs—those in which a full-time year-round worker could not earn at least $11,611, the poverty level for a family of four—have "grown dramatically relative to middle and high wage jobs. Half of the 11.8 million payroll jobs created between 1979 and 1987 were low-wage jobs. Moreover, the share of low-wage jobs for many groups of workers and regions of the country has increased while the share of middle-wage jobs has dropped" (4:512). Younger men with fewer skills and less education experienced the largest of these shifts

(7), reducing their ability to support families, or perhaps even themselves. Note, also, that to make enough to exceed the low-wage cutoff of $11,611 per year, a wage earner working a 40-hour week, year round, would have to make at least $5.58 an hour. This figure is almost two-thirds more than the minimum wage in 1989. Looked at another way, it would take almost two full-time earners at the minimum wage to raise a family of four out of poverty.

Unemployment is another factor influencing poverty. In periods of high unemployment, which closely follow patterns of economic recession, unemployment is a strong contributor to poverty. Still, the persistence of poverty even with the substantial reduction in unemployment between the end of the 1981–82 recession and the end of the 1980s points to the greater long-run causal importance of low wages. Table 16.3 shows the annual fluctuations in the civilian unemployment rate from 1970 through 1988. The changes in this official rate reflect the major periods of downturn and upturn in the economy. Rates increased 73 percent between 1970 and 1975, decreased by almost one-third between 1975 and 1979, increased by two-thirds again through 1983, and then decreased through 1988 by 43 percent. Note, however, that the shifts in the numbers in poverty described in Table 16.1 are far less dramatic than these unemployment changes, suggesting that other factors contribute to poverty.

Table 16.3 also shows the proportion of unemployed workers covered by unemployment compensation. Coverage during the 1970s was generally higher than during the 1980s, helped by federal supplemental benefits during the recession and the high unemployment of the period May 1974–June 1977. Even with similar federal supplemental benefits for the period October 1982– June 1985, approximately 25 percent fewer unemployed workers received compensation by the end of the 1980s than at the beginning of the decade.

Income Support Programs

The homeless come from the ranks of the very poor (3,8,9). Often homeless people relate histories of having struggled to maintain an economic position that allowed them to afford housing, only to face a final crisis that precipitated an episode of homelessness. A number of federal social safety net programs were designed to help very poor people avoid complete destitution of this type. Chief among these are AFDC and SSI, which provide monthly cash benefits, and the Food Stamp Program, which provides coupons that can be exchanged for food in grocery stores. (Housing, another important area of federal assistance, is covered in chapter 17.)

The ability of these federal programs to meet the needs of all very poor people is severely limited by eligibility criteria. Only poor families with children may receive AFDC. SSI is only available to poor elderly people and to blind and disabled people. Food stamps are available to low-income groups

TABLE 16.3   UNEMPLOYMENT RATE AND PERCENTAGE INSURED,
1970–1988

Year	Yearly Average Unemployment Rate	Percentage of Unemployed Workers Insured
1970	4.9	48
1971	5.9	52
1972	5.6	45
1973	4.9	41
1974	5.6	50
1975	8.5	76
1976	7.7	67
1977	7.1	56
1978	6.1	43
1979	5.8	42
1980	7.1	50
1981	7.6	41
1982	9.7	45
1983	9.6	44
1984	7.5	34
1985	7.2	34
1986	7.0	33
1987	6.2	32
1988	5.5	32

Source: Data from House Committee on Ways and Means, *Background Material and Data on Programs within the Jurisdiction of the Committee on Ways and Means*. Washington, D.C.: Government Printing Office, 1989, pp. 442–70.

with gross household incomes up to 130 percent of the poverty level and net monthly incomes at poverty level or below. Poor childless able-bodied individuals—the most prominent category of homeless adults—are not eligible for any federal cash transfer program, although they are eligible for food stamps. Their only recourse is to locally administered general assistance programs (also called public assistance, home relief, or general relief), which provide relatively low monthly payments. Many communities have no general assistance programs; other communities exclude able-bodied individuals from eligibility. When general assistance programs accept able-bodied people, they usually require recipients to work or to look for work.

AID TO FAMILIES WITH DEPENDENT CHILDREN

AFDC was created by the Society Security Act of 1935 to provide "cash welfare payments for needy children who have been deprived of parental support or care because their father or mother is absent from home continuously (85.2% of the children in 1986), is incapacitated (3.2%), is deceased (1.9%), or is unemployed (7.4%)" (4:517). In 9 out of 10 AFDC families, no adult male is present and the mother is the only adult in the household. Receipt of AFDC categorically entitles a household to Medicaid (96% participate) and usually implies receipt of food stamps (82% participate) (4:1103).

AFDC is a combined state-federal program. Each state defines its need standard (the amount required to provide necessities), sets benefit levels (which may be less than the need standard), establishes income and resources limits within federal guidelines, and administers the program. Benefit levels vary widely. The maximum monthly AFDC grant for a three-person family in January 1989 ranged from $118 in Alabama and $120 in Mississippi to $809 in Alaska and $663 in California. The lowest benefits provided only 15 percent of poverty-level income for a three-person family, while the highest benefits provided 84 percent. The median AFDC state had a maximum AFDC grant for a family of this size of $360, which put the family at 46 percent of the federal poverty line (4:539–540).

AFDC benefits have been losing their purchasing power steadily for two decades. Table 16.4 shows this decline for selected years from 1970 through 1988. The first four rows give the average dollar benefit per family and per person, and the median and the maximum state benefit for a family of four for no income. The maximum state benefit is set by regulation in each state. The median state benefit is based on actual outlays.

The last two rows give the median and maximum state benefits in constant 1988 dollars. These figures permit calculation of the change in purchasing power between benefits available in one year and benefits available in another. These constant dollar figures reveal the shrinkage in the value of AFDC benefits, and also the shrinkage of the gap between the median and the maximum benefit amounts. Since most AFDC families do not receive maximum benefits, I focus the discussion on median benefit levels.

The median AFDC benefit lost 25.4 percent of its purchasing power between 1970 and 1980, and another 13.8 percent between 1980 and 1988, for a total reduction in value of 36 percent. Virtually all the change in the 1980s occurred between 1980 and 1984. Further, the median benefit level as a proportion of the maximum benefit fell to 50 percent after 1984, from a proportion that fluctuated between 1970 and 1984 but was as high as 62 percent in 1980. These reductions followed congressional action taken in the Omnibus Budget Reconciliation Act of 1981 (OBRA) and the Deficit Reduction Act of 1984 (PL 98-369). OBRA changes also resulted in the complete loss of AFDC eligibility for almost 500,000 families and the loss of a percentage of benefits for another 300,000 families, largely due to changed treatment of earned income. These families represented about 21 percent of 1981 AFDC families (4:617–618). The families that suffered most under OBRA were those with a working parent.

TABLE 16.4 HISTORICAL TRENDS IN AVERAGE AFDC PAYMENT PER RECIPIENT
AND PER FAMILY, AND MAXIMUM AND MEDIAN BENEfiTS FOR A FAMILY OF FOUR
FOR SELECTED YEARS FROM 1970 TO 1988

	1970	1975	1980	1984	1985	1986	1987	1988
Average monthly benefit								
—Per family	178	210	274	322	339	353	359	370
—Per individual	46	63	94	110	116	120	123	127
Median state benefit in July for family unit of four with no income	221	264	350	376	399	415	420	432
Maximum state benefit in July for family unit of four with no income	375	497	563	660	800	823	833	866
Median state benefit in July in constant 1988 dollars[a]	672	577	501	428	439	449	437	432
Maximum state benefit in July in constant 1988 dollars	1,140	1,086	806	751	880	890	867	866

Source: Data from House Committee on Ways and Means, *Background Material and Data on Programs within the Jurisdiction of the Committee on Ways and Means.* Washington, D.C.: Government Printing Office, 1989, pp. 547–548.
Note: Among 50 states and the District of Columbia.
[a]The constant-dollar numbers were calculated using the CPI-U monthly consumer price index series.

Poor children have also suffered under OBRA changes. From 1970 through 1981, on average, 72 percent of children in poverty got AFDC. From 1982, when the OBRA changes took effect, through 1987, on average only 54 percent of poor children got AFDC support (4:560). Thus, during the Reagan years, fully one out of four poor children who would have been covered by AFDC benefits under previous policies did not receive these benefits.

SUPPLEMENTAL SECURITY INCOME

The SSI program, begun late in 1974, supplements the incomes of poor people who are aged, blind, or disabled. It provides cash assistance (up to $368 per month for an individual and $553 per month for a couple in 1989) that, at its maximum, brings an individual and a couple to about 74–76 percent and 88–90 percent of the poverty line, respectively (4:889). SSI is indexed to the Consumer Price Index in the same way as are Social Security payments, so its purchasing power has not eroded in the 1980s. Further, adjustments in July 1983 and January 1984 actually increased the real value of benefits by 4–5 percent. Complicated program rules determine the precise level of benefit allowed for a given recipient.

In addition to federal SSI payments, which are uniform across the country, many states supplement SSI. For individuals living independently, 26 states and the District of Columbia provide supplemental assistance, ranging from $2 to $384 per month depending on the state. These supplemental payments are generally not indexed to inflation; in only six states have supplemental payments been adjusted to meet or exceed inflation. Some states that supplement SSI attune the level of supplementation to the going rate for a room in a boarding or lodging house. This practice has helped disabled individuals to maintain themselves in the community as long as they maintain SSI eligibility. All but seven states—Arkansas, Georgia, Kansas, Mississippi, Tennessee, Texas, and West Virginia—supplement living expenses for SSI recipients living in protective, supervisory, or group living situations. These payments also assist disabled people to maintain housing in the community. The level of supplementation varies by state.

The relevance of SSI to homeless people lies primarily in the fact that it is targeted to people with disabilities that prevent them from "engaging in gainful employment." Many homeless people fall into this category. From 1975, the first full year of SSI operation, through 1988, the proportion of recipients in the disabled category has grown from 45 percent to 66 percent. In 1988, two out of three SSI recipients were disabled; one out of two was disabled and under 65 years of age (4:695). With federal SSI payments and state supplements, many of these disabled individuals can remain in the community, either in independent situations or in supervised living arrangements.

Although most studies of the homeless population put the proportion suffering from severe mental disorder at about 25–35 percent (3:154), only 4 percent get SSI (1:43). In all likelihood, far higher proportions of the mentally disabled homeless population are eligible for federal SSI and state supplements to assist with housing. In 1987, nonelderly disabled people comprised 52.4 percent of SSI recipients. Of these nonelderly disabled, 24.1 percent (12.6% of all SSI recipients) were disabled by mental disorders other than retardation; 26.9 percent were disabled by mental retardation (4:695). In numerical terms, about 415,000 individuals suffering from mental illness received SSI in 1987. To put this in perspective, these mentally disabled SSI recipients are about 24 percent of the approximately 1.7 million people who, the National Institute of Mental Health estimates, are chronically mentally ill (10).

The biggest problem for SSI for the disabled in the 1980s was the period of accelerated case reviews that the Department of Health and Human Services (HHS) decided administratively to undertake in March 1981. These case reviews disqualified large numbers of disabled SSI recipients and stopped their benefits. Among those hardest hit by the process were those disabled by reason of mental illness. Under pressure, HHS eventually stopped these reviews until a more reasonable set of criteria could be developed which did not prejudice the outcome for many individuals with clear incapacities (11:82–89). During the period of these reviews, it seemed to many professionals who worked with this population that the risk of homelessness went up for mentally disabled beneficiaries who were dropped from the rolls (11:112–113).

Countering the "anti-mental" mood of the executive branch in the early 1980s, congressional action from 1983 onward has directed the SSI program to actively promote enrollment of eligible homeless people. Specific measures include prerelease arrangements for people leaving psychiatric facilities; emergency "while-you-wait" payments for clearly eligible new enrollees; exclusion of the cash value of food and shelter assistance by nonprofit organizations from the calculations that determine benefit levels; provisions for continued receipt of benefits during short hospital and shelter stays (up to three and six months, respectively); and demonstration projects to do outreach and on-the-spot enrollment in localities frequented by homeless people (4:686–688).

FOOD STAMPS

The Food Stamp Program (FSP) is designed to ensure that poor households can purchase food adequate to meet the U.S. Department of Agriculture's criteria for a nutritionally adequate low-cost diet. The rules establishing eligibility and benefits are very complex. The FSP distributed $11.3 billion worth of coupons in 1987 to 20.6 million individuals in 5.9 million households (4:1107).

The FSP has changed dramatically over the years, reaching its present form only in 1979, when a requirement for purchase was eliminated. Food stamps have been indexed for inflation since 1973 and have been available in all states since 1975.

Between 1979 and 1983, the year of maximum enrollment, FSP participation rose from 15.9 million to 21.6 million individuals, an increase of 36 percent. However, because 1983 was also the peak year in this decade for people in poverty, the FSP increase does not represent an increase in the percentage of poor people served by the program. In both 1979 and 1983, 61 percent of poor people participated in the FSP (this proportion fluctuated up and down during the intervening years). Since 1983, participation has dropped by 12 percent, to 19.1 million in 1987. The percentage of poor people served dropped slightly, to 59 percent (again with intervening fluctuations) (4:1120).

Average per person monthly food stamp benefits increased 12 percent between 1979 and 1983, from $44.00 to $50.00 (in constant 1988 dollars). Benefits then declined by 5 percent through 1987, to $47.40. Legislative changes increased benefits 5 percent beyond normal inflation adjustments in 1988, to $49.80—enough to compensate for the decline in value of food stamps since 1983 (4:1126).

Owing to legislative changes in 1981 and 1982, about 1 million people (about 5%) lost FSP eligibility, and the remainder suffered some loss of benefits (4:1121). The Food Security Act of 1985 (PL 99-198), the Stewart B. McKinney Homeless Assistance Act of 1987 (PL 100-77), and the Hunger Prevention Act of 1988 (PL 100-435) liberalized benefit and eligibility rules, but the net effects in terms of program participation are not known. The Hunger Prevention Act of 1988 also took the historic step of authorizing across-the-board increases in the maximum benefit over and above any inflation adjustments. These increases will benefit every household that receives food stamps.

Discussion

Clearly the decade of the 1980s saw an increase in poverty. This increase continues a trend that began in the 1970s for many households. The primary causes of this increase are changes in market income (people do not make as much from working), changes in means-tested benefits (fewer people get benefits, and some remaining recipients get lower benefits), population growth, changes in social insurance programs, and changes in federal tax policy.

In general, as poverty increases in the face of stable or increasing housing costs, one would expect to find households paying increasing proportions of their income for housing and foregoing other essential purchases. This shift happened in the 1980s (12:1–11). Another strategy people may use when possible is to increase household income, either by sending another worker into the labor force or by doubling up in housing so that more earners share the same rent; this also has happened (13). Very poor people who live with others are significantly less likely to become homeless than are individuals with a similar income who live alone (8:59). Virtually all people who eventually become homeless have tried these strategies on the way to homelessness.

Most people, including most very poor people, do not become homeless, even in the face of all the income and program shifts that happened in the 1980s. For example, New York City has a very unaffordable housing market, many poor female-headed families who receive AFDC, and in the common perception, many homeless families. Yet analysis indicates that only 3 percent of the city's welfare families become homeless and seek emergency housing in any given year (14). Nevertheless, preliminary analyses show that higher poverty rates, along with higher rents and lower vacancy rates, are significantly associated with increased numbers of homeless people in U.S. cities (15). In other analyses, higher cost of living, higher unemployment rates, lower rental vacancy rates, absence of a general assistance program, and a higher proportion of one-person households all predicted higher rates of homelessness (16:chap. 9). One may hypothesize that, as poverty increases, not only do low-income single individuals find it harder to pay for housing on their own but the relatives and friends with whom they might share housing are also stretched to the limit and less able to help out. Thus, increasing poverty and the decreasing effectiveness of safety-net programs strain all low-income households and reduce the personal and financial resources available to avoid homelessness.

Note

This chapter is an early report of a study, the full report of which appears in Burt MR, *Over the Edge: The Growth of Homelessness in the 1980s.* New York: Russell Sage Foundation and Urban Institute Press, 1991.

References

1. Burt MR, Cohen BE. *America's Homeless: Numbers, Characteristics, and the Programs That Serve Them.* Washington, D.C.: Urban Institute Press, 1989.
2. Burt MR, Cohen BE. Differences among homeless single women, women with children, and single men. *Social Problems 36(5):*508–524, 1989.
3. Rossi PH. *Down and Out in America: The Origins of Homelessness.* Chicago: University of Chicago Press, 1989.
4. House Committee on Ways and Means. *Background Material and Data on Programs within the Jurisdiction of the Committee on Ways and Means.* Washington, D.C.: Government Printing Office, 1989.
5. Klein BW, Rones PL. A profile of the working poor. *Monthly Labor Review 112(10):*3–13, 1989.
6. Litan RE, Lawrence RZ, Schultze CE. Improving America's living standards. *Brookings Review 7(1):*27, 1988-89. Cited in House Committee on Ways and Means, *Background Material and Data,* p. 512. See ref. 4.
7. Blackburn ML, Bloom DE, Freeman RB. The declining economic position of less-skilled American males. Paper presented at Russell Sage Foundation seminar, New York City, N.Y., November 1989.
8. Sosin MR, Colson P, Grossman S. *Poverty and Pathology: Social Institutions and Social Change.* Chicago: Chicago Community Trust, 1988.
9. Peterson RA, Weigand B. Ordering disorderly work careers on skid row. In Simpson RL, Simpson IH (eds.), *Research in the Sociology of Work: Unemployment.* Greenwich, Conn.: JAI Press, 1985.
10. Steering Committee on the Chronically Mentally Ill. *Toward a National Plan for the Chronically Mentally Ill.* Publication (ADM) 81-1077. Washington, D.C.: U.S. Department of Health and Human Services, 1980.
11. Burt MR, Pittman KJ. *Testing the Social Safety Net.* Washington, D.C.: Urban Institute Press, 1985.
12. Leonard PA, Dolbeare CN, Lazere EB. *A Place to Call Home: The Crisis in Housing for the Poor.* Washington, D.C.: Center on Budget and Policy Priorities and Low-Income Housing Information Service, 1989.
13. Mutchler JE, Krivo LJ. Availability and affordability: Household adaptation to a housing squeeze. *Social Forces 68:*241–261, 1989.
14. Weitzman BC. Pregnancy and childbirth: Risk factors for homelessness? *Family Planning Perspectives 21(4):*175–183, 1989.

15. Quigley JM. *Does Rent Control Cause Homelessness? Taking the Claim Seriously.* *Journal of Policy Analysis and Management* 9:88–93, 1990.

16. Burt MR. *Over the Edge: The Growth of Homelessness in the 1980s.* New York: Russell Sage Foundation and Urban Institute Press, 1991.

CHAPTER 17

The Shortage of
Low-Income Housing: The Role
of the Federal Government

Roberta Youmans, B.A.

The shortage of housing that low-income people can afford is a major, if not the major, cause of the current epidemic of homelessness. This chapter will discuss the federal government's influence on the supply of housing suitable for low-income households, and will describe and assess the various federal programs relevant to low-income housing.

Although housing conditions for the nation as a whole have improved since 1940, inequality in housing has increased, and the poorer segment of the population has not benefited significantly. The National Low Income Housing Information Service has estimated that there are twice as many very-low-income households looking for housing as there are units affordable at 30 percent of their income (1). The only way many very poor households can make ends meet is to obtain some type of federal housing assistance.

Three types of federal intervention are specifically related to the supply and affordability of low-income housing. The first type includes interventions that directly increase or decrease the number of low-income housing units; the second includes various subsidies to decrease the amount of rent or mortgage that low-income tenants or owners have to pay; and the third consists of tax measures that have a considerable effect on the housing supply.

Federal policies can be roughly divided into two groups, according to their effects: those that tend to increase the supply of affordable housing for low-income people, and those that tend to have the opposite effect. To some extent, this dichotomy is an oversimplification, since some policies increase the supply of low-income housing for some low-income people but decrease it for others. Not infrequently, the latter have very low incomes. Furthermore, in some instances regulations, administrative rules, or other modifications have radically changed the impact or even the intent of a program.

ROBERTA YOUMANS

Policies That Increase the Availability and/or Affordability of Low-Income Housing

The major types of federal housing program that increase the availability and/or affordability of low-income housing are provided either through the Department of Housing and Urban Development (HUD) (Table 17.1), or, in rural areas, through the Farmers Home Administration (FmHA) (Table 17.2). The impact of these programs depends on (a) what they do to make housing available, (b) what they do to make housing affordable, (c) what portion of the population in need can be served, and (d) the likelihood that these programs will be diverted for the use of higher-income groups.

Governmental programs provide either funds for the actual construction of units or income subsidies to enable tenants to find housing on the private market. The oldest and perhaps most successful construction program is the public housing program, enacted by Congress in 1937. Since its inception, approximately 1.4 million housing units have been constructed in cities, suburbs, and rural areas (2:Q-1). From 1974 to 1985, the Section 8 program facilitated the construction or rehabilitation of rental units for almost a million households (3). In rural areas, some 464,000 rental units (inclusive of Farm Labor Housing Loans and Grants) were constructed through the FmHA (communication from Art Collings, Housing Assistance Council). The Section 8 Certificate and Voucher programs do not make any units available, but they provide recipients with a guarantee of funds with which to obtain private units.

Almost all of the federal rental housing programs decrease the housing cost burden of the participants. Tenants in public housing and Section 8 programs pay the highest of (a) 30 percent of their adjusted gross income, (b) 10 percent of their gross income, or (c) the welfare shelter allowance. Tenants of these programs also get an allowance for utilities, the amount of which is then deducted from the rent. Unfortunately, as a way to save costs, many Public Housing Authorities (PHAs) set these allowances at an artificially low level, thereby forcing tenants to pay a much higher percentage of income toward their total housing costs.

Tenants who receive vouchers may pay more than 30 percent of their income for rent, depending on the method used to calculate the subsidy. Tenants with Section 8 certificates may only move into units that rent at levels below the so-called fair market rent. These rents are based on the slightly-below-average cost of rental housing in HUD-established areas. Voucher recipients may rent units at any price, but they pay any increase above 30 percent of their income out of their own pockets. In some cases, voucher holders may pay less than this, but in New York City, as of April 1987, fully 39 percent of all voucher holders were paying more than 30 percent of their income for rent (4). A recent change will permit some Section 8 certificate holders to pay more than 30 percent of their income, too.[1]

TABLE 17.1   FEDERAL LOW-INCOME RENTAL HOUSING PROGRAMS SUPPORTED BY HUD

Name of Program (year enacted)	Funds		Target Population		
				Tenant's	
			Category, or	Share of	
			Income as % of	Rent as %	Obligation
	Used for	Paid to	Median	of Income[a]	(years)
Public Housing (1937)	New construction, acquisition, substantial rehabilitation	Local public housing authority	All <80%; most <50%	30%	40
Section 202[b] (1959)	Low-interest loans, Section 8 subsidies attached to building	Nonprofit sponsors of housing	Low-income elderly (>62) or handicapped	30%	20
Section 8 —New construction and rehabilitation (1974)	Operating subsidy (maximum approved contract rent minus tenant's share)	Private owner of project constructed or rehabilitated for this program	All <80%	30%	5–20[c]
—Moderate rehabilitation (1978)	Same as 1974 program	Private owner of building who undertakes moderate repairs for this program	All <80%	30%	15
—Existing certificates (1974)	Operating subsidy (fair market rent minus tenant's share)	Private landlord (subsidy stays with tenants when they move)	All <80%	30%	5[d]
—Vouchers (1983)	Income subsidy to tenant (payment standard for area based on fair market rent minus 30% of tenants' monthly income)	Private landlord (rents are not capped)	Very-low-income or previously HUD-assisted families	30%	5

[a]Income for purposes of calculating rent in the HUD-assisted housing programs is adjusted by deducting from the household's gross income $480 per dependent per year; $400 for any elderly family; medical expenses >3 percent of income (for elderly families only); and child care expenses when necessary to enable a family member to be gainfully employed or to further education.

[b]All section numbers refer to the United States Housing Act of 1937 as amended.

[c]Owners of some Section 8 New Construction and Substantial Rehabilitation projects have the opportunity to opt out of their obligation to serve low-income families at five-year intervals. The 1987 and 1990 housing bills provide guidelines and protection for these tenants.

[d]Until the late 1980s, the term for the Section 8 certificates was 15 years. To reduce long-term budget costs of housing programs, this was reduced to 5.

TABLE 17.2   FEDERAL LOW-INCOME HOUSING PROGRAMS SUPPORTED BY FmHA

Name of Program (year law passed)	Funds — Used for	Funds — Paid to	Target Population — Category and/or Income as % of Median	Target Population — Recipient's Payment	Obligation to serve target population (years)
Section 502:[a] homeownership loans (1961)	Construction or purchase of new or existing housing	Interest subsidy paid on behalf of borrowers	40% of funds available for those under 50% of median	Subsidized (with 1% rise as income increases)[b]	33, or until house is sold
Section 515 (1962)	Loans for construction or rehabilitation of rental housing or cooperatives	Private, public, and nonprofit groups or individuals	Families, elderly, handicapped or disabled individuals with incomes <80%	Tenants pay 30% of income,[c] or basic rent	20, in most cases
Section 514/516: farm labor loans (1961) and grants (1962)	Loans/grants to build decent, safe, and sanitary housing for migrant, seasonal, or year-round farm laborers	Individuals, associations of farmers, or partnerships	Farm laborers (no income restrictions)	Rents based on operating costs or 30% of income	20, in most cases

[a]All sections refer to the Housing Act of 1949 (PL 81-171) as amended.

[b]Loans are made by FmHA at market rate of interest based on the federal government's long-term borrowing costs and subsidized for low-income families through the Interest Credit Program. Interest Credit enables the borrowing rate to be as low as 1 percent, but the rate varies according to the borrower's income and the amount of the loan. Borrowers who have received interest credits since October 1, 1979, are subject to "recapture" of part of that assistance when they sell or transfer their homes.

[c]Income for purposes of calculating rent in the FmHA programs is adjusted as in the HUD programs. (See Table 17.1, note a.)

Although Congress declared long ago that all families should be provided with decent housing, federal assistance for this is now provided to a small fraction of those in need. Approximately 6.6 million households were receiving assistance through the programs of HUD (2:B-2) and FmHA (personal communication from Art Collings, 1991) at the end of 1990. However, only one-quarter of all renters with incomes below the poverty level live in subsidized housing. There is some question as to whether these programs serve those who are truly in need. The eligibility guidelines for assisted housing set higher maximum income levels than do those for other income support programs.

Although most new households moving into assisted housing have incomes below 50 percent of the area median, some may earn as much as 80 percent. Some PHAs or private owners have been known to skip over the poorest households in order to rent units to those able to pay higher rents. Congress has directed PHAs and owners to give preference when selecting their tenants to households that are displaced, are living in substandard housing, or pay more than 50 percent of their income for housing.

This already limited supply of affordable housing may shrink as the federal subsidies expire or when projects designed for poor people are diverted to higher-income use. The Section 8 certificates, funded in the mid-1970s, as well as the first vouchers, began to expire in 1990. Congress has agreed to renew these subsidies with five years of "in kind" assistance, but the cost of doing so may be a reduction in the number of new families served (2:F-1–F-3;5). Additionally, public housing units are being demolished, some because they were built long ago and are now in need of repairs, others because they are now located on prime real estate (6). Other older HUD-insured projects (Secs. 221[d][3] and 236 of the U.S. Housing Act of 1937, and subsequent amendments) which now house households of low and moderate income, are in danger of being lost when their 20-year regulatory periods expire and owners prepay their mortgages. Finally, owners of Section 8 projects may opt out of their obligation to serve low-income households at five-year intervals.

Until the enactment of the Housing and Community Development Act of 1987 (7), most of the tenants displaced by any of the aforementioned activities received vouchers. That legislation mandated a one-for-one replacement for most public housing units sold or demolished (7:Sec. 121), although there are some loopholes in the act (6:Sec. 3). It also provided a temporary solution to the prepayment/opt-out problem to stem the tide of this loss (7:Secs. 201–235 and 262). Many FmHA rural rental housing units were also in danger of being lost. The 1987 act provided a permanent solution to this problem (7:Secs. 241–243). Several of its provisions were modified in the HUD Reform Act of 1989. Finally, in 1990, Congress enacted permanent legislation to preserve units for low- and moderate-income families (8) through actions regarding prepayment (8:Title VI) and opt-outs (8:Sec. 544).

The need to preserve each and every existing low-income housing unit is critical in light of the fact that so very few units are being added to the nationwide inventory. Tables 17.3 and 17.4 dramatize this situation. Between 1977 and 1980, HUD funds were reserved for an average of 293,308 units annually, and in 1990 the number shrank to 65,714. Similarly, between 1977 and 1980 FmHA funds were reserved for an average of 96,162 units annually, and in 1990 the number shrank to 41,036. Spending on HUD Public Housing and Section 8 funding dropped from $32.2 billion in 1981 to about $8.1 billion in 1990, while FmHA-subsidized loans dropped from about $3.5 billion in 1981 to about $1.9 billion in 1990.

TABLE 17.3   SUBSIDIZED HOUSING UNIT RESERVATIONS, 1976–1990

	1977–80 Average	1981–84 Average	1985–90 Average	Actual 1990
HUD PROGRAMS[a]				
Section 8				
—New Construction or Substantial rehabilitation	110,808	18,048	0	0
—Elderly (202)	21,502	14,814	11,992	6,717
—Handicapped (202)	0	0	0	2,165
—Moderate Rehabilitation	15,115	12,177	6,559	1,233
—SRO Moderate Rehabilitation[b]	0	0	0	2,165
—Existing	91,373	49,114	21,395	28,842
—Vouchers	0	3,526	41,015	22,622
Subtotal Section 8	238,798	97,679	80,961	63,744
Public Housing				
—Conventional	48,619	11,928	5,841	293
—Indian	5,891	2,896	2,698	1,677
Subtotal Public Housing	54,510	14,824	8,539	1,970
Total Section 8 and Public Housing	293,308	112,503	89,500	65,714
FmHA PROGRAMS[c]				
Section 502: homeownership loans	62,686	53,264	29,051	24,268
Section 515: rental or coop loans	32,030	27,635	20,118	16,063
Section 514/516: farm labor housing	1,446	592	546	705
Total FmHA	96,162	81,491	46,715	41,036

Source: Dolbeare C, *Familiar Themes: The Administration's FY 1992 Assisted Housing Budget.* Special memorandum, Low Income Housing Information Service. Washington, D.C.: National Low Income Housing Coalition, February 1991, p. 9.

[a]Section numbers for HUD programs refer to the United States Housing Act of 1937.

[b]This special Section 8 moderate rehabilitation program was authorized in the Stewart B. McKinney Act of 1987 and is used to rehabilitate or construct single-room occupancy facilities for homeless individuals. It is the only moderate rehabilitiation program still under way.

[c]Section numbers for FmHA programs refer to the Housing Act of 1949 (PL 81-171).

Policies Having Dual Effects

UNIFORM RELOCATION ACT

The Uniform Relocation Assistance and Real Property Acquisition Policies Act of 1970 (URA) was enacted to provide uniform compensation to people forced to relocate by direct federal agency action or by state or local governments receiving federal funds (9). The benefits made available to eligible tenants by the act include moving expenses, replacement housing or rental assistance payments, down payments, advisory services, and development of replace-

TABLE 17.4 SPENDING ON HOUSING

Year	HUD Public Housing and Section 8[a] (in millions of dollars)	FmHA-subsidized Loans[b] (in millions of dollars)
1981	32,200	3,470
1982	18,908	3,454
1983	14,280	2,952
1984	14,088	2,886
1985	11,747	2,834
1986	10,456	1,985
1987	8,935	1,990
1988	8,635	2,210
1989	7,851	1,865
1990	8,115	1,928

Source: HUD data from the Low Income Housing Information Service (1981–89) and from U.S. House of Representatives, *Conference Report on HUD-Independent Agencies Appropriations Bill, HR 2916* (Report no. 101-297). FmHA data provided by Art Collings from FmHA 205 Reports, FmHA MPH Division and AMAS Reports.

[a]Includes recapture and carryover balances.

[b]Includes Section 502 Homeownership Loans, Section 515 Rural Rental Housing Loans, and Section 514/516 Farm Labor Housing Loans and Grants.

ment housing from project funds if comparable replacement housing is not available. Homeowners are also reimbursed for the loss of their homes. However, the original act did not provide coverage to people displaced by programs that have been enacted since 1970. Furthermore, the courts have interpreted the language of the act very narrowly, often denying URA benefits to displaced tenants. Many poor tenants who lost their homes for the greater good of society undoubtedly became homeless as a result.

In April 1987, Congress finally amended the URA, after a process of almost six years (10). The new law now provides benefits to those who are displaced by any of 16 federal programs, whether it is the government or private individuals who do the displacing. Most of the inequities previously highlighted in court cases have been addressed. However, people displaced by federally assisted code-enforcement programs are those most likely not to receive the benefits of this act.

The benefit levels themselves are inadequate. In 1970, each displaced tenant household received a maximum of $4,000 in replacement housing payments to enable it to find a new place to live. In 1987, the payment was increased to a maximum of $5,250. If the increase had been proportional to the increase in the Consumer Price Index, displaced households should have received over $11,000 (according to a conversation with Bureau of Labor Statistics staff, mid-1987).

Therefore, the URA may in some instances help displaced people to find adequate housing, but in other instances it may leave them without available or affordable housing, while facilitating their displacement.

COMMUNITY DEVELOPMENT BLOCK GRANTS

The Community Development Block Grant (CDBG) program, enacted by Congress in 1974, has also often facilitated the displacement of low-income households. Many participating communities use their grants to repair rental units. Unfortunately, many units, once repaired with these funds, are no longer affordable to their current tenants. The General Accounting Office (GAO) surveyed 73 CDBG communities and found the potential for displacement to be strong. Most communities said they controlled rehabilitation, but others allowed rent increases of 5–50 percent. Most communities limited postrehabilitation rents to the Section 8 rent limits, but even those rents are not affordable to low-income tenants without subsidies. San Diego reported that average rents increased by a staggering 26 percent and that within two years more than half of the affected clients had vacated their units (11:3). Thus, although the CDBG has been used to provide low-income housing or shelters, units rehabilitated with its help have often turned into higher-rental ones, decreasing their affordability, displacing low-income people, and reducing the stock of low-income housing.

The Urban Development Action Grant (UDAG) program, which was popular with city officials, has also been known to displace households. The 1987 National Affordable Housing Act required that households displaced by either of the two aforementioned programs be provided with affordable replacement housing for five years (8:Sec. 509). The UDAG program was subsequently eliminated due to its often costly nature.

LOSS OF UNITS FROM THE FEDERALLY ASSISTED HOUSING STOCK: THE PUBLIC HOUSING HOMEOWNERSHIP DEMONSTRATION

The loss of units from the federally assisted housing stock makes a significant contribution to the reduction in availability of low-income housing. Some of these units are lost at the expiration of the required "low-cost" period, as described previously. Others are lost when projects have been allowed to deteriorate to the point of no return. Still others have been lost when HUD foreclosed on properties and sold them without subsidies.[2] Sometimes the federal government facilitates the loss of units by either waiving regulations or by directly promoting the loss, as in the Public Housing Homeownership Demonstration.

This demonstration, initiated by HUD in November 1984, was designed to test the ways in which lower-income families could purchase their existing public housing units (13). HUD chose to implement this program with very few guidelines. The department will continue to pay the remaining debt service on the units, but it will not provide operating subsidies. Tenants are not to be involuntarily relocated in connection with the demonstration. Those who do not wish to or are unable to purchase their units may be eligible for Section 8 certificates or vouchers.

Critics of the program contend that the best of the public housing stock will be sold, leaving the least desirable units for the poorest tenants (14). Others insist that replacement housing should be available and that it should not be of the voucher variety (15). Peggy Earlsman, attorney for tenants not wishing to purchase their units in the Paterson, New Jersey, demonstration sites, sums up the criticism: "The City of Paterson has a major housing shortage for lower-income people. The waiting list for public housing is extremely long; the taking of applications has been suspended since June of 1983 due to the length of the list. I have clients who have been on this list for over eight years. The City of Paterson Public Housing Authority has a suspended waiting list of 2,400 eligible families for Section 8; at present there are only 428 certificates available. The City has estimated that 36% of the City's approximately 138,000 residents are eligible for the 428 available Section 8 certificates. It is very infortunate that, given the desperate housing situation, public housing is being sold" (16). It should be noted that many public housing tenants who entered the program with low incomes presently have incomes greatly in excess of income limitations. These are the families most likely to purchase their units, thereby depriving low-income and very-low-income families of the opportunity to rent such units in the future. In fact, the income of the participants in the demonstration was approximately 2.5 times higher than the average income of those remaining as renters (17:137). The Housing and Community Development Act of 1987 authorizes a new public housing homeownership program, albeit with improved tenant protections and resale restrictions (7:Sec. 123). This program is being phased out and replaced by the HOPE program (9:Title IV-A).

ILLEGAL FORECLOSURES

In the HUD and FmHA single-family programs, the law requires that foreclosures not be effected without consideration of foreclosure avoidance by assignment of the mortgage to HUD or moratorium relief through FmHA. Thousands of foreclosures have been effected by the government in defiance of its obligation to provide foreclosure relief. The Veterans Administration housing program does not even have a statutorily mandated foreclosure relief program for homeowners who default on their loans for reasons beyond their control. Thus, many people have lost their homes because of illegal foreclosure by government agencies, and many of them were probably unable to find comparable housing.

TAX INCENTIVES

No discussion of federal housing assistance is complete without a review of the housing tax expenditure side of the equation—those revenues not received by the federal government as a result of special tax breaks for investors. In 1990, the federal government was expected to spend approximately $15 billion for direct housing outlays for poor people through HUD. It "spent" almost $68 billion on federal tax relief through the homeowners' deduction of mortgage interest and property taxes, and other investor deductions (18:8 and 11).[3]

Furthermore, these incentives are most valuable to those with higher marginal tax rates, the income class that could most easily afford to buy homes without such incentives. And the incentives for homeownership are much weaker for households in the lower tax brackets, whose income levels also make homeownership more difficult. Analysis of 1980 housing expenditures shows that the bottom quarter of all households received only one-eighth of all housing subsidies, while the top quarter got two-thirds (19). Capping these deductions or converting them to tax credits, which are more favorable to those in lower tax brackets, would go a long way toward equalizing housing assistance. In the Omnibus Budget Reconciliation Act of 1987, Congress took a very small first step in this regard by limiting deductions to homes with a value of $1 million or less (20:Sec. 10102).

Congress also altered the way in which many housing-related tax benefits are provided. The Tax Reform Act of 1986 (21) swept away incentives based on accelerated depreciation and replaced them with a new low-income housing tax credit. Owners can qualify for credits if their developments satisfy one of two set-aside requirements: (a) 20 percent of the units will be occupied by people with incomes of 50 percent or less of the area median; or (b) 40 percent of the units will be occupied by people with incomes of 60 percent or less of the median. The units must be maintained as low-income units for 15 years and in some cases up to 30 years, and credits are only permitted for units actually occupied by poor families. Rents in the low-income units are set at 30 percent of the qualifying low income. Each state receives an annual allocation of credits based on population, and states allocate the credits to owners (21:Sec. 252[a]). The National Council of State Housing Agencies reports that since its inception the tax credit program has produced approximately 316,000 units of low-income housing annually (22). The tax credit has been extended and modified and is now set to expire in 1991 (23).

Assessment of Federal Housing Policies

First, it should be stated that federal housing programs *have* been successful. A variety of programs have assisted and are currently assisting millions of families in attaining decent, safe, and sanitary housing that they could not obtain otherwise. Certainly, some of these programs need to be modified and re-designed in order to be more equitable, but they should also be expanded to serve additional families.

However, in recent years, as poverty rates have increased, funds for assisted housing have not kept up with the need. For every family now receiving aid, there are four who are unable to partake in such benefits. Since housing is not an entitlement program, in which almost everyone who meets the criteria receives assistance, many low-income families wait for years to receive their share of federal housing.

Waiting-list data vary by city. According to a 1982 study by the Council of Large Public Housing Authorities (CLPHA), the weighted average length of time on waiting lists for 12 authorities surveyed was 29 months for families and 25 months for elderly people. The longest wait was for families needing two or three bedrooms. Tenants in Miami had a 10-year wait. In New York City, applicants who were on the emergency list waited three to six months; those who merely had priorities had to wait up to 2 years; nonpriority applicants faced an indefinite waiting time (24). A more recent survey by CLPHA reports that there are twice as many families on the waiting list in Houston as there are units; and in New York City 93,000 families are waiting (25). These statistics, staggering as they are, underestimate the need, because many PHAs close their lists when there is no likelihood that applicants will be housed within a reasonable amount of time.

Since 1980, as mentioned previously, not only has the number of families assisted been reduced but the method of financing them has also been altered. Instead of subsidizing the actual construction of low-income housing, the Reagan administration and then the Bush administration have fostered a shift to housing allowances through an expansion of the Section 8 Certificate and Voucher programs. In 1980, funds were reserved for about 155,000 new project-based subsidies (i.e., built or rehabilitated units with which the subsidy stays) and only about 36,000 Section 8 Existing certificates (26:6). In 1990, by contrast, only some 12,000 new units were project-based, and some 51,500 are paid by vouchers or certificates (including units that may opt out or prepay) (18:n. 23). The voucher concept assumes that an adequate supply of housing exists. But in many markets, the only housing that exists is beyond the means of most poor families, even with the help of this subsidy.

In November 1989, President Bush announced a series of initiatives to address the housing needs of the nation. These proposals can only be characterized as modest. The centerpiece of the plan is Homeownership Opportunities for People Everywhere (HOPE) programs which will foster the sale of public housing units to the tenants. Some funds under HOPE would also be made available to nonprofit organizations and tenants for the acquisition of distressed, government-owned multifamily and other single-family properties for homeownership purposes. Congress authorized a modified version of the HOPE program in late 1990 and will most likely provide partial funding for such in fiscal 1992 (8:Title IV), since the House has appropriated $500 million in FY 1992 and the Senate has appropriated $440 million.

Congress has recently authorized HOME (8:Title II), a major new housing block grant program, for which the House has appropriated $500 million in FY 1992 and the Senate $2 billion. These HOME funds can be used by state and local governments and not-for-profit organizations for a limited amount of new construction, rehabilitation, and tenant-based assistance (27). However, only a small portion of the units will be targeted to very poor or homeless households, due to the lack of deep project-based rental subsidies.

Many states and municipalities are doing more than they claim they can to alleviate the low-income housing crisis (28,29). Charitable organizations are working hard, too. However, there is a critical need for federal intervention, including (a) rent subsidies where the supply of housing is adequate, and financial aid for construction where warranted; (b) dual protection for those who are displaced—strong requirements that prohibit the destruction of low-cost units financed with federal funds, and payment of adequate relocation expenses when relocation is unavoidable; (c) preservation of the existing supply of public and other HUD- and FmHA-assisted housing to protect tenants as well as the federal investment; and (d) a revision of the tax laws to ensure equitable distribution of housing assistance between the rich and the poor. Finally, welfare hotels burgeoning with homeless families should be viewed as a symptom, not a solution.

Notes

1. Section 543 of the National Affordable Housing Act of 1990 (PL 101-625) permits certificate holders to pay more than 30 percent of their income if the family notifies the Public Housing Authority (PHA) that it is interested in renting a unit that costs more than the fair market rent and the PHA determines that the rent is reasonable considering the family's other expenses.

2. Further information on the loss of HUD-assisted rental units can be found in a publication by S. Johnson and the National Clearinghouse for Legal Services (12).

3. Housing outlays included rental housing subsidies only, and tax expenditures included those for homeownership, rental, and rehabilitation.

References

1. Dolbeare C. *Rental Housing Crisis Index*. Washington, D.C.: National Low Income Housing Coalition, National Low Income Housing Information Service, 1986.

2. U.S. Department of Housing and Urban Development. *Congressional Justification for 1992 Estimates*, pt. 1. Washington, D.C.: HUD, 1985.

3. U.S. Department of Housing and Urban Development, Office of Housing. Preliminary tabulations for September 30, 1985.

4. Sole H. Memorandum to Joseph Shuldiner, general manager, New York City Public Housing Authority, May 12, 1987.

5. Departments of Veterans Affairs and Housing and Urban Development, and Independent Agencies Appropriations Act of 1991, PL 101-507; 104 Stat. 1361, November 5, 1990.

6. National Housing Law Project. *Public Housing in Peril.* Berkeley, Calif.: NHLP, January 1990.

7. Housing and Community Development Act of 1987, PL 100-242; 101 Stat. 1842.

8. *National Affordable Housing Act,* PL 101-625; 104 Stat. 4079, November 28, 1990.

9. *Uniform Relocation Assistance and Real Property Acquisition Policies Act of 1970,* 42 USC 4601.

10. *Surface Transportation and Uniform Relocation Act of 1987,* PL 100-17, 101 Stat. 132.

11. U.S. General Accounting Office. *Rental Rehabilitation with Limited Federal Involvement: Who Is Doing It? At What Cost? Who Benefits?* GAO/RCED-83-148. Washington, D.C.: GAO, July 11, 1983.

12. Johnson S, and the National Housing Law Project. *Preserving HUD-assisted Housing for Use by Low-Income Tenants: An Advocate's Guide.* Chicago, Ill.: National Clearinghouse for Legal Services, 1985.

13. Public Housing Homeownership Demonstration: Notice of funds availability and solicitation of applications. *49 Federal Register* 43028, October 25, 1984.

14. Silver H. Statement on HUD's Public Housing Homeownership Demonstration Program. In House Committee on Government Operations, Subcommittee on Employment and Housing, *Homeownership Demonstration Program,* pt. 2. Hearing, 99th Cong., 2d sess., April 10, 1986.

15. Wise S. Statement on HUD's Public Housing Demonstration Program. In House Committee on Government Operations, Subcommittee on Employment and Housing, *Homeownership Demonstration Program.* Hearing, 99th Cong., 1st sess., July 9, 1985.

16. Earlsman P. Letter to Barney Frank, Chairman of the Subcommittee on Employment and Housing. In House Committee on Government Operations, Subcommittee on Employment and Housing, *Home Ownership Demonstration Program,* pt. 2. See reference 13.

17. Rohe W, Stegman M. Public Housing Homeownership Demonstration assessment. Report submitted to the U.S. Department of Housing and Urban Development, April 1990.

18. Dolbeare C. *Familiar Themes: The Administration's FY 1992 Assisted Housing Budget.* Special memorandum, Low Income Housing Information Service. Washington, D.C.: National Low Income Housing Coalition, February 1991.

19. Dolbeare C. *Low Income Housing Needs.* Washington, D.C.: National Low Income Housing Coalition, December 1987.

20. *Omnibus Budget Reconciliation Act of 1987,* PL 100-203.

21. *Tax Reform Act of 1986,* PL 99-514, Sec. 42 of the Internal Revenue Code.

22. Aponte A. The Low Income Tax Credit. Testimony before the House Committee on Ways and Means, on behalf of the National Council of State Housing Agencies, April 10, 1991.

23. *Omnibus Budget Reconciliation Act of 1990,* PL 101-508.

24. Shapiro B. *Survey of Waiting Lists of Selected CLPHA Members and Other PHAs.* Report no. 82-8. Boston: Council of Large Public Housing Authorities, December 1982.

25. Sherwood W. *Survey of Development Needs.* Washington, D.C.: Council of Large Public Housing Authorities, January 1991.

26. Dolbeare C. *The 1988 Low Income Housing Budget.* Special memorandum, Low Income Housing Information Service, Washington, D.C.: National Low Income Housing Coalition, April 1987.

27. State and Local Housing Strategies (Title I) and the HOME Program (Title II). *Housing Law Bulletin 21(January–February)*:1–7, 1991.

28. Nenno M. *New Money and New Methods: A Catalog of State and Local Initiatives in Housing and Community Development*. Washington, D.C.: National Association of Housing and Redevelopment Officials, September 1985.

29. Council of State Community Affairs Agencies. *State Housing Initiatives: A Compendium*. Washington, D.C.: COSCAA, June 1986.

CHAPTER 18

Homeless-making Processes and the Homeless-Makers

René I. Jahiel, M.D., Ph.D.

Homelessness does not occur in a social vacuum. In general, the events that make people homeless are initiated and controlled by other people whom our society allows to engage in the various enterprises that contribute to the homelessness of others. The primary purpose of these enterprises is not to make people homeless but, rather, to achieve socially condoned aims such as making a living, becoming rich, obtaining a more desirable home, increasing efficiency at the workplace, promoting the growth of cultural institutions, giving cities a competitive advantage, or helping local or federal governments to balance their budgets or limit their debts. Homelessness occurs as a side effect. Yet it is a consequence of these enterprises, and therefore the discourse on homelessness must be broadened to reach into those areas of housing, income production, health care, and family life where the events and people contributing to homelessness are situated.

A new set of questions arises: (a) What social processes make people homeless? I refer to them as "homeless-making processes" in order to convey the meaning that the end result of these processes is to make some people homeless. (b) What social pressures build or magnify these processes? I refer to them as "pressures toward homelessness." (c) Who are the people and which are the institutions that initiate or carry out these processes and pressures? I refer to them as "homeless makers" in order to convey the meaning that their actions make some people homeless. (d) What are the stakes of the homeless makers in homeless-making processes and the pressures toward homelessness? (e) What resistance to antihomelessness programs might be anticipated from homeless makers and other societal actors, and how might it be overcome?

The last three chapters, as well as the monographs on homelessness cited in chapter 1, have discussed the first two questions as they relate to homeless people. In this chapter, the first four questions are discussed in relation to the homeless-makers. This change of focus is necessary not only for a full understanding of the place of homelessness in our social order but also for the development of effective strategies to prevent homelessness (these strategies, along with the fifth question, are discussed in chapter 21). As long as it is posited that homelessness is the result of individual failures or pathology, one can consider an approach to prevention targeted only to the individuals at risk of becoming homeless. However, if individuals' failures or pathology only make the individuals vulnerable to homeless-making processes that are societally determined and that, as shown in chapter 20, require that part of the population be homeless, the social processes themselves and the prime movers in these processes must become the target of intervention.

As shown in chapters 15–17, the growth of homelessness in the 1970s and 1980s required a complex interaction among factors associated with several economic or social sectors of our society. The object of this chapter is to make a synthesis of the contributions of our society to homelessness in these various sectors and to lay the groundwork for the discussion of prevention policies in chapter 21. The five sectors shown in Table 18.1—housing, employment, public assistance, health care, and family—are discussed in sequence. In each instance, the homeless-making processes and the evidence for their contributions to homelessness are briefly reviewed, and some of the pressures toward homelessness which contribute to these processes are identified and used as guides to the homeless-makers and to their stakes in the various pressures. In the final part, the interaction among homeless-makers is discussed with regard to the distribution of responsibilities for homelessness.

The Housing Sector

Homeless-making Processes

In the housing sector, there are two general homeless-making processes: displacement, and failure to find affordable housing. In addition, failure to find *appropriate* housing plays a role for those with special housing needs (e.g., mentally ill and/or alcohol-abusing people; families with children, and elderly or disabled individuals).

DISPLACEMENT.   Displacement is the loss of one's home against one's will. At the individual level, displacement may be physical (destruction of housing unit due to fire, decay, or condemnation), contractual (landlord's refusal to renew a lease), economic (rent increase or conversion to condominium or cooperative), or due to intimidation (harassment of tenants to make them flee) (1,2). A given household may be displaced several times in the same neighborhood or a different one (3).

Displacement studies are difficult to perform because of the complexity of the process and barriers to availability of data. An initial approach is to account

TABLE 18.1 HOMELESS-MAKING

HOUSING SECTOR

HOMELESS-MAKING PROCESSES
Displacement; failure to find affordable housing; failure to find supported housing (for people with special needs)

PRESSURES TOWARD HOMELESSNESS
Insufficient production of low-income housing; loss of low-income housing by abandonment, warehousing, gentrification, and loss of public housing); rising price of housing; competition for low-income housing by middle-class renters; high interest rates

HOMELESS-MAKERS
Landlords; developers; banks; insurers; business; not-for-profit institutions; upper- and middle-income households; international interests; government

---

EMPLOYMENT SECTOR

HOMELESS-MAKING PROCESSES
Exhaustion of financial resources due to unemployment; failure of wages to keep up with cost of living; failure to find employment after migration

PRESSURES TOWARD HOMELESSNESS
Market factors; intentional cyclical unemployment; redistribution of income within corporation or private business; pressures affecting workers' bargaining with employers; decreased effectiveness of unemployment insurance; ineffectiveness of approaches to reemployment

HOMELESS-MAKERS
Business and corporations; financial interests; professionals; contractors, and high-level employees; government

---

THE PUBLIC ASSISTANCE SECTOR

HOMELESS-MAKING PROCESSES
Denial of public assistance; inadequate level of public assistance benefits

PRESSURES TOWARD HOMELESSNESS
Changing attitudes toward the poor; political isolation of poor people; inadequate public assistance programs; inflation

HOMELESS-MAKERS
Conservative interests; middle classes; government

THE HEALTH, MENTAL HEALTH, AND SUBSTANCE ABUSE SECTORS

HOMELESS-MAKING PROCESSES
Economic impact of illness or disability; discrimination; expulsion because of behavior; running away because of refusal or inability to adapt to residential setting

---

(continued)

TABLE 18.1 *(Continued)*

THE HEALTH, MENTAL HEALTH, AND SUBSTANCE ABUSE SECTORS

PRESSURES TOWARD HOMELESSNESS
High cost of illness care; lack or inadequacy of income protection during illness or disability; insufficient support services in the community; lack of adaptation of services to clients with chronic health, mental health, or substance abuse problems; insufficient supported housing and supported work services; discrimination against chronically ill, mentally ill, or substance-abusing people by landlords and community

HOMELESS-MAKERS
Health care and social work institutions and professionals; landlords and employers; community members; government

---

THE FAMILY SECTOR

HOMELESS-MAKING PROCESSES
Running away; being thrown away; long-term homeless-making processes (see text)

PRESSURES TOWARD HOMELESSNESS
Violence, abuse, or fear thereof, or other family conflicts; failure of home to meet emotional needs; separation or divorce; economic burden posed by an individual to the household; inequality within the family regarding title to the home; foster care–related processes

HOMELESS-MAKERS
Family or household members (spouse, parent, child, or other in household); social workers, educators, and other professionals; governmental policy makers and administrators

---

for the number of households displaced in a given neighborhood. Marcuse identifies four processes: (a) direct last-tenant displacement; (b) direct chain displacement (several households displaced successively from the same housing unit); (c) exclusionary displacement (when a change imposed on a vacated unit makes it impossible for a new household to move in, though the unit would have been accessible to that household before the change); and (d) displacement pressure, an epidemic process whereby displacement of households from a neighborhood induces other households to move out (2). Marcuse added up all the losses of housing due to physical destruction, conversion to nonresidential use or higher-cost residences, and chain displacement, to estimate that 41,000–100,000 households, that is, 2–5 percent of households, were displaced yearly in New York City from 1970 to 1981 (2). Displacement may affect yearly as many as 2.5 million Americans (4). Studies such as Marcuse's provide an indicator of the number of people who are put at risk of homelessness by displacement, but they do not show how many of them become homeless during a given period.

Population-based studies of displacement (i.e., finding and following up the people who have been displaced in a given population) might provide a prospective approach to quantifying the homelessness-inducing effect of displacement. However, such studies are usually performed in three steps: compiling a list of people who have left a given set of addresses (i.e., people who have been displaced *or* have left of their own accord) from the Polk or the Haynes directories, two household-by-household directories available in most public libraries; finding their new addresses; and contacting them for information (5:16–26). Since the new addresses are used in the second step, this method selects against people who become homeless after displacement, and therefore it cannot be used for prospective studies of the number of people made homeless by displacement. Modification of this approach to include data on homeless people identified by name who used to reside in the study neighborhood might be worth considering if such data could be obtained from the agencies that serve homeless people in a given geographical area. Even so, migration out of the study area would be expected to leave out a significant part of the displaced population.

For the present, it is necessary to rely on retrospective approaches, such as interviews of homeless people. These studies show that displacement is an important precipitating factor of homelessness (chapter 4).

FAILURE TO FIND AFFORDABLE HOUSING.   The precipitating factor, displacement, is complicated by the environmental factor, lack of affordable housing. Many displaced people cannot find new homes because there is no housing that they can afford. Further, many more people are at risk of economic displacement because their income gives them only a tenuous hold on their domiciles. The usual way to gauge the size of that at-risk population is to compare the distribution of housing costs and household incomes in the domiciled population of the United States. Such data are available from annual surveys by the Department of Housing and Urban Development (6) and the Bureau of the Census (7), respectively. From these data, Dolbeare (8) has prepared tables showing the fraction of households with a given income who have to spend a given percentage of their income on housing costs (Table 18.2). Using such data, and assumptions about the maximum fraction of income that poor people can afford to spend on housing, the Ford Foundation estimated that in 1983 the housing affordability gap—the difference between the number of poor households and the number of units affordable to them—was 14 million (9). An alternative method, the market-basket approach, was devised by Stone (10). The household budget that corresponds to the minimum standard of living (derived from inflation-adjusted budgets published until 1977 by the Bureau of Labor Statistics for families of various sizes and compositions) is used along with the family's income to determine how much the family can spend on housing. For instance, in 1980 a family of four needed an income of $17,500 to be able to spend 25 percent of its income on shelter. Below an income of $11,000, it would not have been able to spend any money on shelter (10).

TABLE 18.2   PERCENTAGE DISTRIBUTION OF RENTERS AT GIVEN INCOME LEVELS,
BY PERCENTAGE OF INCOME SPENT ON HOUSING

Percentage of Income Spent on Housing	Yearly Household Income (in dollars)				
	0–6,999	7,000–14,999	15,000–24,999	>25,000	Total
>60	55.2	7.8	0.8	0.1	18.1
35–59	23.8	36.7	10.1	1.5	20.0
25–34	12.4	31.1	27.9	7.9	20.5
<25	8.6	24.5	61.3	90.5	41.2
Total	100.0	100.1	100.1	100.0	99.8
N^a	8,481	8,829	6,755	5,857	29,915

Source: Data from Dolbeare CN, *Low Income Housing Needs*. Washington, D.C.: Low Income Housing Coalition, December 1987.

[a]*N*, number of households in thousands.

Conversely, Dolbeare found that in 1985, 9.9 million domiciled households (11.1% of all U.S. households) were below the income level to cover any consumption needs other than housing (8:3).

These studies identify a large pool of people at economic risk of homelessness. However, they do not show how many will become literally homeless. Some of the people resort to illicit or other unrecorded earnings; others get financial support from their families or go into debt, sometimes for many years; still others manage by drastically reducing the quality of housing and other consumption at a cost to their health; and some double up or move to shelters or the streets. Again, one must rely on retrospective surveys of homeless people, which show that inability to pay for housing is one of the most important factors cited as causes of homelessness (chapter 4).

FAILURE TO FIND SUPPORTED HOUSING.   It is now generally agreed that some people need support in order to fulfill the financial and other responsibilities necessary to maintain a home. Among them are some frail elderly people and chronically mentally ill or substance-abusing people, as well as some single-parent families. Provision of supported housing for these groups is still at the demonstration level and only meets a small fraction of the need (chapter 11).

PRESSURES TOWARD HOMELESSNESS

INSUFFICIENT PRODUCTION OF LOW-INCOME HOUSING.   The current rate of construction of low-income housing is insufficient to compensate for the loss of units (chapter 15), and the federal subsidy needed by the private sector to produce low-income housing has decreased throughout the 1980s (chapter 17). For instance, in New York City, Stegman found that in 1987 there was a unmet need for 231,000 low- or moderate-income housing units because of limited private-market construction and decreased federal subsidies (11).

ABANDONMENT.   Abandonment is the withholding of funds or services needed to maintain housing. It may take place at the housing-unit level when the landlord stops maintaining the building, or at the neighborhood level when a reduction in public services is followed by fires or other destruction of housing. New York City lost 275,097 units because of destruction in 1970–81 (2).

WAREHOUSING.   Warehousing means keeping a housing unit vacant even though there is a demand for it. Buildings may be warehoused in anticipation of selling at a higher price. Housing units may be left vacant for a long time rather than decreasing the rent.

GENTRIFICATION.   Gentrification is defined in several ways (12,13). In general, it is a neighborhood change associated with a rise in property and land value, and a replacement of poor households by richer ones and/or new business or cultural establishments. At the housing-unit level, it is marked by attempts to force tenants out, by rent increases, and by conversion to cooperatives or condominiums. At the neighborhood level, it is marked by destruction or renovation of low-income buildings. In New York City, gentrification accounted for the loss of 10,000–40,000 units yearly in 1970–81 (2).

CONVERSION OF PUBLIC TO PRIVATE HOUSING.   Conversion of low-income public housing to private housing, usually accessible to middle- or moderate-income households, is another cause of loss of low-income housing which affects to a greater or lesser extent most federally supported low-income housing and is expected to become more widespread in the 1990s, as described in chapter 17.

The factors discussed in the previous four paragraphs cause a loss of low-income housing in the United States estimated by different analysts at 200,000–1 million units per year during 1975–85 (14). Furthermore, not only does the loss and insufficient production of low-income housing cause a direct decrease in the number of low-income units, but it also contributes to a rise in price of all housing according to the law of supply and demand.

THE RISING PRICE OF HOUSING.   Rents and associated housing expenses increased during the 1970s and 1980s (chapter 15). The rise in the ratio of rent to renter's income which occurred between 1970 and 1980 was not only due to the general improvement of housing, the movement of upper-income renters to homeownership, or the declining real income of renters; there was also an actual increase in real rent (chapter 15). This increase has affected the poor disproportionately. The National Association of Home Builders found that real (inflation-adjusted) rents for low-income households increased by 10 percent from 1974 to 1983, while those of households earning more than $30,000 per year did not increase (15:12).

COMPETITION BY MIDDLE-INCOME RENTERS FOR LOW-INCOME HOUSING. The increased cost of homeownership during the 1980s prevented some 1.6 million moderate-income households from buying houses, and they entered the rental housing market instead (16:260). As the price of housing increased, these households and other middle-income renters entered the competition for low-income rental housing, thereby not only increasing the demand (and therefore the price of rent) but also providing tenants whom many landlords found more desirable than low-income households. In 1983, only 54 percent of units renting below $250 per month were occupied by low-income renters (17:6).

HIGH INTEREST RATES. The high interest rates used in the late 1970s and early 1980s to combat inflation had deleterious effects on low-income households: (a) they pushed up rents to make up for landlords' increased mortgage costs; (b) they prevented young middle-class households from buying their own homes, thereby contributing to increased demand and prices in the rental market; and (c) they drove some low- or moderate-income owners who had variable-rate mortgages into forfeiture.

THE HOMELESS-MAKERS

LANDLORDS. There is a competitive asymmetry of tenant and landlord in the housing market, especially in the instance of "professional landlords" (those holding at least five housing units). Gilderbloom and Appelbaum (18:45–107) point out that renters are more numerous, concerned with only one housing unit, weakly if at all organized, and poorly informed; professional landlords are fewer, often have large holdings, and have formal as well as informal organizations and good sources of information, which allow them to know precisely what the market will bear. Their informal networks promote cooperation in the setting of rents determined by the tenants' income and/or ability to pay an increasing amount of their income for rent. Movement within the housing market is much more constrained for tenants than for landlords. Housing is a basic necessity for tenants; moving entails significant economic and non-economic costs; discriminatory practices close off large segments of the rental housing market to families with children or racial minorities; and many tenants are limited to rental housing, as they cannot afford to buy houses or condominiums. Landlords have much more freedom to shift their investments in housing or to wait for customers who will pay the set rent. Professional landlords are "relatively sophisticated investors, who approach rental housing much as they would any business investment" (18:84). Because of the relatively noncompetitive nature of the housing market for landlords and the existence of informal landlords' networks to keep rents high, policies that would raise tenants' incomes or increase the amount of available housing might not, by themselves, solve the problem of affordability, as the landlords would continue to push the rents upward (18:106–107).

During periods of economic expansion and rising real estate values, when there is actual or potential demand for commercial units or middle- or upper-income residential units, landlords have an opportunity to increase their profits with such units. Low-income neighborhoods, where the value of land is going up fast in anticipation of or during gentrification, give landlords opportunities for big and fast profits, through a variety of mechanisms described by Hartman et al. (5:27–39). Housing speculation—buying units, spending little to improve them, and reselling them soon at higher prices—becomes a significant source of profits, dwarfing those achieved through the collection of rent. The practices of "flipping" (purchase and quick resale in succession of several housing units) and "pyramiding" (borrowing money to buy housing units and then using them as collateral for future acquisitions) amplify these profits. The conversion of rental units to condominiums or cooperatives quickly brings a large amount of money to landlords. The replacement of apartment buildings by commercial or office buildings that command much higher rents or by higher-income apartment buildings is another way for landlords to increase their profits.

A small proportion of landlords use illegal methods to achieve similar ends. Some, "who are really 'disinvestment speculators' . . . may buy buildings with very little cash down . . . make no repairs, pay no property tax, get behind in fuel and utility bills, and just collect rent money—using some to pay off the loans and pocketing the rest . . . [eventually] they simply walk away from their buildings" (5:62). Under pressure to quickly empty out or destroy buildings so that they may be turned into more profitable investments, some landlords engage in criminal acts against tenants (19:24–34). For instance, Manhattan district attorney Robert Morgenthau charged, in a successful lawsuit against landlords, that "the conspirators installed drug addicts, prostitutes, thieves and other criminals in vacant apartments to commit burglaries and assaults against tenants, cause flooding, set fires, dump garbage and create bedlam. . . . While appearing to perform legitimate functions, such as collecting rent, it was agreed that [the superintendent] would fail to provide heat and other legitimate services. At the same time, he would lament to the tenants the deterioration of the building, its crime wave . . . urging them to move out. If the tenants complained or refused to move, the plan called for the conspirators to burglarize, ransack and destroy the tenants' apartments" (20:402). Arson, sometimes resulting in the loss of lives, is another common criminal action, used in part to collect insurance (in the vernacular, "selling out to the insurance company") and in part to clear a site for new housing (5:42–43).

When the economy enters a recession, this does not mean greater opportunities for low-income renters. Landlords do very little if any new construction or rehabilitation in such times, unless they are supported by governmental investment. While gentrification may be interrupted, there is a trend for middle-income renters who are doing poorly to move into low-income housing, thus displacing low-income renters.

Profit is the common thread of these various actions. In their dual role as entrepreneurs who organize and manage housing units for profit and as speculators who buy and sell housing units for quick profit, landlords, as a group, promote rising rents as well as all forms of displacement.

FINANCIAL INSTITUTIONS.   Financial institutions include banks (which gain interest on their loans and a claim on the property in case of default), developers (who get a fraction of the real estate profits), and insurance companies (who get premiums that exceed benefits paid). These "financial entrepreneurs" have two notable features: their contribution is essential, since the U.S. housing market has depended heavily on borrowing since early in the century (21); and they have a stranglehold on U.S. housing, because the decline in governmental funding for housing has removed the only alternative support (chapter 17). They contribute to nearly all phases of homelessness pressure in the housing sector. They withhold their funds ("redlining") when real estate values decrease and investment risks increase after abandonment by landlords and local government. On the other hand, Meyerson proposes that the initial development in abandonment may be a decreased supply of capital, as financial institutions shift investment away from housing in response to economic changes that make other types of investment more attractive (22). A similar situation occurs with respect to gentrification. An area that is already being gentrified may be attractive to financial institutions. Alternatively, according to Smith, financial institutions may initiate gentrification when there is (a) a rent gap (i.e., ground rent of the land significantly lower than its potential ground rent) (23) and (b) an economic situation whereby investment in housing is more attractive than other investment (24). In either instance, as rational economic actors, they tend to disinvest from low-income housing and to invest in high-income housing or commercial buildings, which bring higher returns. Their upward pressure on interest, development fees, or insurance premiums contributes to the rise in rental and homeownership prices. Their downward pressure on risk taking tends to favor middle-income households that compete with lower-income ones for the same units.

BUSINESS.   Business interests may exert pressures toward homelessness through their role in the supply of as well as the demand for housing. With regard to supply, the builders' push for profits tends to increase the cost of housing, especially when their own costs are rising. Large builders (those completing more than 100 houses annually or most apartment buildings) do the majority of housing construction in the United States and often have their own mortgage companies. They may support gentrification, but they may under appropriate conditions be receptive to building low-income housing, since their size allows economies of scale and is suitable to mass production of units (25).

On the demand side, large corporations need real estate for headquarters and office buildings as well as shared resources such as convention centers. Hotels, restaurants, newspapers and media, health facilities, and retail shops are among the industries with a major claim on real estate in cities and suburbs. They contribute to the replacement of lower-income housing by commercial buildings that command higher rents and increase ground value.

NOT-FOR-PROFIT CORPORATIONS.   In several cities, not-for-profit corporations such as universities, medical centers, museums, churches, and various other mission-oriented organizations have played a major role in replacing low- or moderate-income housing by their own buildings and displacing the former occupants. For example, in New York City, New York University has displaced occupants of low- and moderate-income housing and small business over several decades in at least 14 full city blocks south and east of Washington Square. The space has been used for classroom buildings, a library, a student center, a sports center, student housing, a high-rise cooperative, and four middle- to upper-income rental buildings for faculty and staff.

UPPER- AND MIDDLE-INCOME HOUSEHOLDS.   Middle- and upper-income households may contribute to a shortage of affordable housing and displacement of low-income households in at least five ways: (a) middle-income households compete with low-income households for some low-income housing, thereby decreasing the supply for the poor and driving up the price; (b) middle- and upper-income households are a pool of potential customers for conversion of low-income rental housing into high-priced rental housing, cooperatives, or condominiums; (c) as a neighborhood gains in middle- and high-income population, stores, professional offices, and other commercial establishments may be attracted to it, causing further displacement of low-income residents; (d) middle- and high-income households make demands for municipal and county services which may compete with those of low-income neighborhoods, contributing to abandonment of the latter; and (e) middle- and upper-income households may resist the movement of low-income households into "their" neighborhoods, with the aim of maintaining its "quality."

INTERNATIONAL INTERESTS.   There has been in the past decade a marked penetration of the U.S. economy by foreign interests from Japan, other Asian countries, Western Europe, Canada, Australia, and some Latin American countries. Multinational corporations have invested in high-priced real estate, often outpricing U.S. bidders and contributing to a rise in the price of real estate (26). Foreign businesses and upper-income families have made increasing demands on real estate in cities such as New York, Washington, Miami, Los Angeles, and Seattle, and in many other cities, large or small. Furthermore, the illicit drug traffic, a multi-billion-dollar industry, brings in money that is laundered and invested in high-priced real estate.

LOCAL GOVERNMENTS.   Local governments often facilitate pressures toward homelessness via tax abatements on gentrifying property, such as the J-51 program in New York City (19:16–23); zoning regulations; "planned shrinkage" (27) or "triage" (28), which lead to decreases in building code enforcement, waste collection, police and fire protection, and other services in low-income neighborhoods and contribute to fires (29) and neighborhood abandonment; razing of housing to make room for highways; and joint projects with the private sector, such as building convention centers.

Local governments may also add to pressures toward homelessness by what they do not do, for instance, by failing to stop the demolition or conversion of single-room occupancy hotels (SROs); failing to impose *moderate* rent control (in distinction to stringent rent control); failing to regulate conversion to condominiums or cooperatives so that tenants who cannot afford to convert do not lose their homes; failing to pass or enforce antispeculation laws to prevent flipping; failing to prosecute landlords who harass tenants; failing to intervene in areas where arson is increasing; and failing to introduce or implement anti-eviction programs. Many local governments have taken appropriate action on these problems, but only after much low-income housing has been lost.

Explanations of local governments' decision making stress the plurality of interest groups that compete for influence; the predominant influence of business and financial interests; and government officials' assessment of expected outcomes (30,31). A predominant role of business and financial institutions is consistent with the cities' need for growth (32), competition with other cities (33), and striving to ward off bankruptcy (34), as well as with elected officials' dependence on business and financial interests for election or reelection and for the successful outcome of policies. For these reasons, local governments tend to side with business, banking, and real estate developers to a greater extent than with other groups in matters such as downtown development, gentrification, rent control, tax abatements, and distribution of capital and services among different areas of the city. Some local governments have opposed these trends, However, as stated earlier, these programs have often come late. In some instances, as in Cincinnati, they have encountered such business resistance that they have failed (35). In other instances they have not had the magnitude needed to counteract the dominant forces of displacement and high housing prices (chapter 21).

STATE GOVERNMENTS.   State governments' activities are primarily in the area of regulation and financing of low- or moderate-income housing initiatives by the private and municipal sectors. The numerous approaches that have been used have been reviewed (36) and analyzed (14:65–90). State governments are subject to pressures similar to those acting on local governments (chapter 21).

THE FEDERAL GOVERNMENT AND THE FEDERAL RESERVE BOARD.   The housing programs of the federal government have been reviewed in chapter 17. In brief, while federal programs in housing have been successful, they have not kept up with the need, and the federal government has contributed to the shortage of affordable housing in the last two decades via its failure to provide public housing on the scale needed; the failure of subsidy programs such as Section 8 and vouchers (chapter 17) to meet the need for low-cost housing; tax policies that favored housing speculation, especially before the 1986 tax reform, and that continue to favor homeowners over renters; its failure to develop policies that would stop the escape of low-income public housing to the private sector upon termination of the obligated period or upon foreclosure; and its lack of policies to prevent foreclosure or eviction from public or federally subsidized property (chapter 17). The Federal Reserve Board contributed to the increased price of housing because of its support of very high interest rates in the 1970s and early 1980s. Even when inflation abated, in the second half of the 1980s, there was no improvement in the low-income housing situation because of hysteresis in the system: the Federal Reserve Board and the banks were slow to decrease interest rates, and landlords resisted lowering rents or converting business buildings to residential use even in the presence of high vacancy rates. Later, the 1990 recession was associated with decreased new construction and increased competition for low-income housing by middle-class people.

The Employment Sector

HOMELESS-MAKING PROCESSES

· There are three main employment-related homeless-making processes. Unemployment continues to the point where financial resources are exhausted. Low wages fail to keep pace with the cost of housing and living. Workers leave an area in search of employment elsewhere and fail to find it.

EXHAUSTION OF FINANCIAL RESOURCES BY UNEMPLOYMENT.   The unemployment rate has remained at more than 6 percent of the labor force during much of the 1980s (37) despite economic recovery after the recessions of 1980–82; therefore, the country has been suffering from a structural unemployment problem along with the cyclical ones of the recessions of 1981–82 and 1990–91. In addition to those listed in unemployment statistics, there are workers who have given up looking; and youths, women, and immigrants who want to enter the labor market but cannot find jobs. Many workers have had recurrent periods of unemployment and have had to settle for new jobs paying far less than the old ones. Workers not covered by insurance because they resigned or left (as opposed to being discharged) or were in noncovered jobs (e.g., in day labor or in the underground economy); workers who remain unemployed at the end of their benefit period; or workers who have high expenses during the period covered by insurance are at increased risk of homelessness. It is difficult to follow these groups as cohorts to find out how some of their members become homeless. Telephone inquiries to major research projects on unemployed worker cohorts revealed that those who became homeless would have been lost to follow-up. However, surveys of homeless people show retrospectively that loss of a job or failure to find a job was one of the most common factors cited as a cause of homelessness (chapter 4).

THE FAILURE OF WAGES TO KEEP UP WITH THE COST OF LIVING.   The increase in the number of low-paying jobs and the failure of the minimum wage to rise during the 1980s have been discussed in chapters 15 and 16, respectively. A low-paying job is seldom mentioned specifically as the principal cause of homelessness in surveys of homeless people. However, low wages may have been one of the underlying causes when reasons such as "unable to pay rent" or "not enough income" were given (chapter 4). Comparing monthly income at the minimum wage with the lowest available monthly rental shows that without supplementation, the income would have not been enough to pay the rent in most states (C. Dolbeare, personal communication, 1989).

FAILURE TO FIND A JOB AFTER MIGRATION TO A NEW AREA.   This factor is mentioned by homeless people at hearings or in surveys (chapter 4).

PRESSURES TOWARD HOMELESSNESS

MARKET FACTORS.   Factors such as changes in production that decrease the need for workers with certain skills; changes in consumption or financing that decrease output and cause layoffs; competition by foreign companies or workers; and relocation of companies were discussed in chapter 15. These factors, which cause cyclical, structural, and frictional unemployment (37), are distinct from the ones discussed below.

INTENTIONAL CYCLICAL UNEMPLOYMENT.   Defined by Isabel Sawhill as "a slowing of the economy with a resulting shortage of jobs—designed to discipline the inflation process" (38), intentional cyclical unemployment resulted from governmental and Federal Reserve Board antiinflationary policies in the late 1970s and early 1980s, which led to an unemployment rate of 10 percent by 1982. Since then, economic policies have maintained unemployment at a critical level—the nonaccelerating inflation rate of unemployment (NAIRU)—to achieve optimal control over inflation. The United States' NAIRU is currently estimated at 5–7 percent (39:27–34). Analyzing the trade-off between inflation and unemployment in the United States, Piven and Cloward suggest that it is slanted in favor of greater unemployment because "from the perspective of capital, . . . inflation is less successful than unemployment as a strategy to maximize profits" (40:23).

PRESSURE ON WAGES FROM REDISTRIBUTION OF INCOME. One of the features of the redistribution of wealth (from poor to rich) which occurred in the United States during the 1980s (39:19–25;41,42) was an increase in corporations' profits and in the incomes of their executives, while workers' wages remained low.

PRESSURES AFFECTING THE ABILITY OF WORKERS TO BARGAIN WITH EMPLOY-ERS. The ability of labor unions to resist these changes was lessened by the decreasing size and changed composition of the unionized workforce and a drive by the Reagan administration to weaken labor through deregulation policies and rulings of the National Labor Relations Board (NLRB) on collective bargaining (41:31–35). Furthermore, Piven and Cloward point out that the cuts in income maintenance programs during the 1980s exerted pressure on workers to take lower wages that they would not have accepted when the alternative of sufficient income maintenance existed (40:26–37).

THE DECREASED EFFECTIVENESS OF UNEMPLOYMENT INSURANCE. From the early 1970s to the late 1980s, both the duration of unemployment insurance and the proportion of unemployed workers receiving insurance have markedly decreased (chapter 16).

THE INEFFECTIVENESS OF APPROACHES TO REEMPLOYMENT. With regard to cyclical unemployment, there have been no large-scale programs to reemploy workers, as public works programs did during the Depression of the 1930s. This approach was precluded in part because of the policy of intentional unemployment of the early 1980s, discussed above. With regard to structural unemployment due to foreign competition, there has been no strong attempt to protect American workers. Again, this is in conflict with attempts by business to use the cheapest source of labor, which often means foreign workers. Structural unemployment due to inadequate competence of unskilled workers might be countered by education and training programs or apprenticeships. Although there has been much talk about such programs, they have not been implemented on a significant scale. Finally, frictional unemployment might be lessened by more effective organization to match company needs and worker expertise.

HOMELESS-MAKERS

CORPORATIONS AND BUSINESS. The massive mobilization and organization of corporations and business in the 1970s, described in detail by Edsall (43:107–140), greatly strengthened the political power of business and especially of large corporations, and consequently resulted in the election of probusiness administrations in the federal government and many state governments, as well as deregulation and labor policies that allowed business to markedly increase its profits. The "supply-side" theory's prediction that these changes would eventually provide economic benefits to all social classes was not borne out, as the increased power and freedom of corporations and business people were used to keep wages and employment down to maximize profits.

FINANCIAL INTERESTS. Banks, stockbrokers, insurance companies, and speculative investors generally had joint political interests with industrial corporations and business and gained political power along with them. The increase in corporations' debts and the rise in the capital and interest they pay to their creditors is another factor that tends to bite into profits and keep pressure on workers' wages. The takeovers or leveraged buyouts of companies which have increased considerably in the 1980s often squeeze wages or bring about layoffs in the interests of efficiency (39:153–168).

PROFESSIONALS, CONTRACTORS, AND HIGH-LEVEL EMPLOYEES. A host of professionals or managers (e.g., lawyers, accountants, computer experts, information specialists, advertisers, architects, decorators, physicians, health administrators, engineers, scientists, planners, administrators, and quality control or personnel specialists), working as employees or contractors, have had increasing leverage within companies, and their remuneration has tended to rise faster than that of lower-income workers.

GOVERNMENT. The federal government and the Federal Reserve Board have played a homeless-maker role in the various ways noted above: antiinflation programs that increased unemployment, deregulation that increased the power of business vis-à-vis labor; the weakening of labor unions by the NLRB; and the limiting of workers' options by cuts in income maintenance programs. In addition, federal, state, and local governments have contributed to pressures toward homelessness by terminating public employment programs and inadequately funding job retraining and vocational rehabilitation programs (chapter 11).

The Public Assistance Sector

HOMELESS-MAKING PROCESSES

The public assistance sector has contributed to the homelessness of two groups of people: those who had been on public assistance until support was interrupted or became inadequate, and those who lost their income and sought public assistance but failed to get it, or got insufficient assistance. Both groups became homeless because of the processes discussed in chapter 16: denial of public assistance and inadequate level of payments.

PRESSURES TOWARD HOMELESSNESS

CHANGING ATTITUDES TOWARD POOR PEOPLE.   There has long been a distinction between the poor people who are "deserving" and those who are not (44,45), but the dividing line between these two categories has moved back and forth. During the 1960s, the War on Poverty was launched, at significant expense to the federal and state governments, to improve the economic status and opportunities of a vast number of poor people as well as their participation in community and political decisions. From the mid-1970s on, a marked change in attitude occurred in the nation. A large mass of poor people, especially black unemployed men, and families headed by women, came to be seen as an "underclass"—unwilling to conform to mainstream society's norms of work, marriage, and behavior; unaccepting of education; and prone to criminal behavior, drug use, and abuse of welfare. This changed attitude was reflected in four highly influential publications, where it was argued, first, that welfare programs could be scaled back for greater efficiency and no additional support was needed (46); then, that poor people are poor because they refuse to work or do not work as hard as they should, and that the federal welfare policies of the 1960s had a deleterious effect on work, family, and behavior (47,48); and finally, that government should enforce the social obligations of poor people rather than support their dependency (49). In the late 1970s, when decreased productivity and inflation were biting into the real income of the middle classes, and corporations and business were actively looking to government for economic support or relief, considerable backing for retrenchment of welfare programs developed among the public and certain elites, clearing the way for new governmental policies.

Two other factors may also have played a role in the rising opposition to welfare. First, a number of poor people did engage in the activities ascribed to the underclass—crime, drugs, flouting of education, teenage pregnancy, and neglect of parental responsibility, as well as manipulation of the welfare system. A significant part of the public attributed these features to the entire population of poor, predominantly minority, neighborhoods.

Second, there was a broad movement, encouraged and probably prompted by the newly organized corporate and business community, to give greater value to one's self-interest and personal economic success. Reagan's influence with the masses sustained this value change. Helping less fortunate others was deprioritized and remains so, despite President Bush's campaign appeal for a "kinder, gentler America."

THE POLITICAL ISOLATION OF POOR PEOPLE. Since the Great Depression, there had been an alliance of dependent poor people, workers, and the Democratic party. Edsall describes how this alliance broke down in the 1970s, as union leadership and the rank and file of labor increasingly dissociated themselves from the dependent poor, and as the Democratic party moved toward a more conservative position (43:23–66). Thus the Democrats were unable to resist successfully two waves of retrenchment—in 1978 and, especially, in 1981, with the passage of the Omnibus Budget Reconciliation Act of 1981 (PL 97-35) (chapter 16)—and many Democrats participated in these moves, as they identified them with their own electoral prospects. The liberal philosophy that had brought the lower- and middle-income groups and the Democratic party together was deemphasized as the "L word" was shunned.

A second factor may well have been the growth of interest groups in the political arena. As various interest groups became more sophisticated and politically powerful, they became less dependent on political coalitions, and in some instances found it more favorable to "go it alone." This was particularly true of "deserving" poverty groups, such as the aged or the developmentally disabled, who thus avoided identification with the "undeserving" poor. The latter were poorly organized because of their lack of access to financial and organizational resources. Although they had many organizations, these were limited to particular sectors or groups (e.g., the Low-Income Housing Coalition and the Coalition for the Homeless), and they were not as effective in attacking the root causes of the problem as they might have been as part of a broad coalition representing poor people.

GOVERNMENTAL POLICIES. In response to the changed attitude toward poverty and the new constellation of political pressure groups, the federal government between 1978 and the mid-1980s enacted policies that severely limited eligibility for and benefits of support programs (chapter 16), relenting only in the second half of the decade with some measures to remove barriers to access.

INFLATION. Inflation had been severe in the 1970s, and it continued at a lower rate in the 1980s. Because most benefits other than Social Security were not indexed to the rate of inflation, public assistance payments lost in real value and became insufficient to meet minimum living and housing needs (chapter 16).

HOMELESS-MAKERS

In the public assistance sector, responsibility for pressures toward homelessness is dispersed through much of society. I would group the prime movers in the following categories.

CONSERVATIVE INTERESTS. The term *conservative interests* is used here to refer to corporate, financial, professional, and business groups and that part of the general public that is responsive to conservative ethical-social values and religious mass-appeal organizations. This combination of groups provided the financial and technical resources as well as the voting block necessary to bring itself to power in the 1980s and to actively promote policies that weakened public support programs and thereby weakened the poor and helped redistribute wealth to the rich.

THE MIDDLE CLASSES. Another component of the public (which overlapped in part with the first) consisted of people mobilized to defend their own quality of life, which they saw as imperiled by inflation and the resulting financial squeeze during the 1970s. They gave impetus to the revolt of the taxpayers, which started in the late 1970s and was marked by decreased local taxes on property (e.g., Proposition $2\frac{1}{2}$ in Massachusetts and Proposition 13 in California) and on income (federal income tax reduction during the Reagan administrations, and some state income tax reduction). It reduced state and federal governments' incomes, thus contributing to cuts in domestic programs.

GOVERNMENTAL POLICY MAKERS. Policy makers contributed to inflation in several ways during the 1970s, for instance, by financing the Vietnam War without raising taxes, by failing to devise an energy policy that would have provided cheaper alternatives to oil, and by implementing tax policies that favored speculation in real estate and inflation in the real estate market. They failed to resist the public pressure about tax reduction or to educate the public about the long-term effects of tax reduction on poor people. In the 1980s, they embraced without sufficient evidence supply-side policies that boomeranged, causing a rising budget deficit, and shifted support to defense programs and away from public support programs.

GOVERNMENTAL ADMINISTRATORS. There is evidence that some government employees went beyond what was required by law, regulation, or administrative edict in denying public assistance benefits, especially in the instance of SSI for chronically mentally ill people during the first half of the 1980s (chapter 16). In addition, public assistance administrators may be very reluctant to provide disability benefits to people disabled by alcoholism or other substance abuse. Finally, outreach to provide eligible people with information or assistance in the complicated processes needed to obtain public assistance is still inadequate despite attempts to improve it (chapter 16).

The Health, Mental Health, and Substance Abuse Sectors

HOMELESS-MAKING PROCESSES

Physical or mental disorders, disability, and substance abuse are associated with the following homeless-making processes: exhaustion of financial resources, exposure of the affected individuals to housing discrimination, and mood or behavior changes that may lead the affected individuals to run away from home or to be thrown out by landlord or family.

PRESSURES TOWARD HOMELESSNESS

HIGH COST OF MEDICAL CARE AND INSUFFICIENT INCOME PROTECTION DURING ILLNESS. The high cost of medical care, which has been exhaustively documented in numerous reports and newspaper articles, exerts pressure toward homelessness by its demands on the affected individual's finances. Most homeless people have no private health insurance (chapter 4), and a majority of them do not even have Medicaid (chapter 11).

INADEQUATE SUPPORT SERVICES. Case management or other support services are necessary to allow certain people with severe chronic mental illness or alcoholism to earn or manage money or to avoid expulsion or running away. Advocacy may also be needed to overcome discrimination. These services have not been available or accessible at the level of intensity and appropriateness needed to serve the population at need (chapter 11).

THE LACK OF SUPPORTED HOUSING AND SUPPORTED WORK. Supported housing is a relatively new concept, which became popular in the mid-1980s to prevent recurrence of homelessness, following demonstrations by the Robert Wood Johnson Foundation and the Department of Housing and Urban Development. It was incorporated in the 1989 revision of the McKinney Act and in some substance abuse program demonstrations in the late 1980s and early 1990s. However, as discussed in chapter 11, funding for supported housing or supported work is grossly inadequate, and only a small part of the need can be met.

DISCRIMINATION. Discrimination is a major factor in preventing the relocation of homeless people in general, particularly those with chronic mental illness, overt substance abuse, AIDS, or tuberculosis. Community opposition readily becomes organized when a site in the community is proposed. Adverse zoning regulations contribute to this pressure toward homelessness.

HOMELESS-MAKERS

HEALTH AND SOCIAL WORK INSTITUTIONS AND PROFESSIONALS. Individuals with chronic mental disorders or substance abuse problems have not been high in the priorities of health and social work professionals working in the community. Factors such as poor prognosis, resistance to treatment (chapter 8), and loss to follow-up have been cited as barriers to services. However, recent ethnographic (chapter 8), clinical (chapters 12,13), and methodological (chapter 24) research suggests that the failure to understand the realities of the environment in which these individuals live, to appreciate their point of view, and to modify methods and techniques (which were validated with other populations and may be inappropriate in the prehomeless and homeless environment) may constitute a much more important barrier.

GOVERNMENTAL POLICY MAKERS. A major responsibility for making chronically mentally ill and substance-abusing people homeless belongs to policy makers who did not provide enough funding, resources, and flexibility of approach to give these people the support and advocacy needed in the community after discharge from institutions. The responsibility belongs to the entire government rather than only to those concerned with the specific policies, since the latter often advocate within the government only to lose in the competition for governmental funds. While the other governmental policies that compete with antihomelessness policies are both legitimate and necessary, the ultimate governmental decision makers bear responsibility for a balance of effort which has not given enough support to antihomelessness policies.

COMMUNITY RESIDENTS. When they organize to refuse homes for homeless people in their community, local community residents play a homeless-making role.

The Family Sector

HOMELESS-MAKING PROCESSES

RUNNING AWAY. People who run away from their homes include women and their children, women alone, children, youths, and elderly people. In most instances they do so because of actual or threatened physical, sexual, or mental abuse, or severe neglect or incompatibility.

BEING THROWN AWAY. The same groups may be thrown away rather than leave of their own volition. A woman with or without work skills who lives with a man often becomes homeless when the latter ends the relationship (chapter 20); a youth may be thrown out when conflicts within the family reach a breaking point. A young child may be abandoned when the family feels totally out of resources or is dominated by drugs.

LONG-TERM PROCESSES.   Studies of the life histories of homeless adults reveal a high prevalence of very deficient family life in their childhood and youth. A history of childhood in foster care has been found with high frequency (chapter 4). Many homeless women with children have moved from one friend to another without having ever had a family home of their own (chapters 4 and 20). Thus, lack of a home with one's family during childhood may be a long-term homeless-making process.

PRESSURES TOWARD HOMELESSNESS

FAMILY CONFLICTS.   Family conflicts are part of chains of pressures, some going back to the parents' childhood, some relayed by external financial or other pressures, some resulting from substance abuse or other pathology on the part of parent or children, some due to family members' incompatible aims. They are aggravated by modalities of behavior, for instance, violence as a learned behavior, deficient or absent communication among family members, unsatisfactory sexual relations, repression of dissent within the family, or dissimulation or dishonesty. Another contributing factor might be a change in household composition, when stepparents replace natural parents, or when a succession of boyfriends or girlfriends move in.

INEQUALITY WITHIN THE FAMILY REGARDING TITLE TO THE HOME.   In many if not most instances, the husband has the rights to the apartment or house, so that a runaway wife cannot claim the home back from the husband and has the choice of either moving back to a threatening situation or being without a home.

FOSTER CARE–RELATED PRESSURES.   The foster care, or family service, system has come under considerable criticism. Funding for the social workers who monitor the family services tends to be insufficient, so that each social worker has a roster of cases which is too large. The family service providers constitute a heterogeneous group, some of whom view foster care only as a way of making money and may be exploitative and unwilling or unable to provide the nurture expected from a family. There is often delay in investigating abuse or neglect and in taking action about it. Children and youths often have several successive family providers. Except in those instances in which a special bond of affection develops, foster children who reach adulthood are released into the society at large without homes to go back to if things go bad. Thus, the defects of the foster care system create pressures toward homelessness by not allowing the normal internalization of the concept of a home and by failing to provide a stable home when foster children leave the system.

HOMELESS-MAKERS

FAMILY MEMBERS.   Family members who have throwaway or runaway children bear responsibility for the pressure toward homelessness resulting from the unresolved conflicts or actions at home. However, they often have no help in dealing with these problems.

SOCIAL WORKERS, EDUCATORS, AND OTHER PROFESSIONALS.   Professionals from various disciplines have been alerted to the role they must play in the discovery and resolution of child abuse. Their role in the prevention of homelessness of runaways or throwaways has not been similarly highlighted. Educators, social workers, and other professionals, as well as police officers, may often be aware of problem families yet take no action.

GOVERNMENTAL POLICY MAKERS AND ADMINISTRATORS.   Governmental policy makers may aggravate family-related homelessness pressures by insufficient funding for the social services needed and for the crisis intervention services that may have to be mobilized to address a crisis that is causing a risk of imminent homelessness. Administrators often play a role by their laxity in enforcing adequate monitoring or their lack of flexibility in responding to imminent crises.

Homeless People as Their Own Homeless-Makers

Many would argue that, notwithstanding these social forces, the people who become homeless are ultimately responsible for their own fate. This does not mean that they "choose" it but, rather, that their own decisions or actions or health status are the fundamental causes of their becoming homeless. Few would argue that these factors do not increase their vulnerability. However, two arguments may be advanced to affirm the role of society. First, studies of homeless people indicate that in a majority of instances external factors over which the individual had little control contributed to the loss of the home (chapter 4). Second, macrolevel studies suggest that the dynamics of the housing and job markets and the welfare system, which determine the ratio of low-income households to the affordable housing units available, are such that a certain proportion of our population has to be homeless (chapter 20).

A more subtle argument is that homelessness is a contemporary component of the subsistence strategy referred to by Hufton in studies of the eighteenth-century poor as economies of makeshift (50). Hopper, Susser, and Conover describe four characteristics of the economies of makeshift of contemporary poor populations: "their strictly ad hoc character; mobility; resort to public relief, parochial charity or begging; and participation in the underground economy" (51:213–214). The use of public shelters, like that of other sites where homeless people seek refuge, is part of a set of strategies that people use "as a way of managing upon duress. It is both a circumstance forced upon them and one that allows—indeed requires—some maneuvering on their part" (51:215). Thus, the decision to go homeless is determined in part by the social pressures that make it necessary to use economies of makeshift.

Discussion

The thesis of this chapter is that one cannot attain a full understanding of homelessness without accounting for the benefits that it brings to those who set in motion the events that cause it. The link between homeless-making processes and the homeless-makers is located at the level of the pressures toward homelessness. It is there that the events that bring profit or other gratification to the homeless-makers set the stage for the homeless-making processes. With a few exceptions, especially in the family sector, the homeless-makers are generally quite remote from the people who become homeless, because they move in different social circles; their actions that initiate pressures toward homelessness often take place long before the latter have been translated into homeless-making processes.

Therefore, students of homelessness must extend their investigations upstream, to the proximate homeless-making processes and beyond, to the pressures toward homelessness, and the homeless-makers. This may be done retrospectively using interviews of homeless people to delve into the sequences of events which brought about homelessness. However, this approach is inefficient and limited, because the homeless-makers are remote from the homeless in social distance and there is usually a long time interval between the homeless-makers' actions and the loss of the home. A stronger approach would consist of document- and interview-based prospective studies of individuals or agencies who are likely to be homeless-makers, combined with prospective studies of the populations subjected to the pressures toward homelessness which they generate.

HOMELESS-MAKING NETWORKS

The impact of the homeless-makers is augmented by their involvement in several chains or networks that, in effect, build coordinated pressures toward homelessness. These networks are usually not of a conspirational nature. Rather, they reflect a concordance of interests. There are horizontal networks involving a single group of actors, for instance, the informal networks of professional landlords discussed earlier. There are vertically connected networks within industries. For example, the contribution of the construction industry to the cost of housing reflects the profits of the manufacturers of raw building materials, the architect, the builders, and various ancillary industries as well as workers' wages. There are more complex networks. For instance, according to Beauregard (52), gentrification requires the production of potential gentrifiers, gentrifiable housing, and people who can be displaced; and the intervention of financial interests, landlords, and local governments who see gentrification as increasing revenues, improving the city's competitive position, or helping to forge alliances with local corporations. Logan and Molotch (53:50–98) describe the organization of interest groups in a "growth coalition" for expansion of a city's real estate which often leaves out the more marginal groups. Networks can also cut across several sectors. For instance, the network of banks and other financial interests in a city may cause pressures toward homelessness through interventions that decrease the quantity of low-income housing and exert pressures on companies to decrease their expenses, for instance, by dismissing workers. Local government incorporates a large horizontal network when its various departments exert homelessness pressures in the sectors of housing, employment, welfare, health care, and family services.

INVESTMENT AND DISINVESTMENT

Characteristically, many of the actions that build pressures toward homelessness represent investments—economic investments (e.g., capital investments), political investments (for elected government officials as well as the appointed bureaucracy), cultural investments (for universities and other cultural institutions), or quality-of-life investments (for gentrifying households). The same actions also represent disinvestments—economic disinvestments (of people who become unemployed, lose their welfare allowances, have their income reduced, or have to pay a higher fraction of their income for rent; or in neighborhoods that are abandoned, and areas that lose their industrial base); political disinvestment (in people whose political power is decreased by displacement from their neighborhoods or by their struggle with poverty); disinvestment in the development of individuals (e.g., the loss of education suffered by homeless children, or the harmful effects of inadequately supervised and assessed foster care). This coupling of investment and disinvestment may be causally related to a "zero-sum society" (54) or to the "new politics of inequality" (43), or to both. One of its correlates is that poverty is only a mediating factor of homelessness, and that deeper causes must be sought in the disinvestment of one part of our population, coupled to investment in another part.

THE QUESTION OF RESPONSIBILITY

A response to the above description of the investment-disinvestment process might be: "What else is new? We are in a competitive society." Not entirely so.

Our society does not allow certain forms of competition that are gravely injurious to others, such as crime, violence, and slavery. I would maintain that the competition that results in severe poverty and homelessness is of such a nature, because of the harm that these states do to human beings. Homelessness is a profoundly degrading experience, it exposes one to violence and disease, and it is associated with increased mortality.

This brings us to the question of responsibility. It is difficult to assign responsibility to a large network of individuals, especially when homelessness is not the immediate result of its actions but a side effect. Homelessness is, in part, the result of the greed of the homelessness makers, but greed has become almost part of our culture. Decreased altruism, relaxation of constraints to competition, and a much greater acceptance, even lionization, of greed have characterized the 1980s. Under such conditions, the responsibility of the individual becomes diluted in the norms of the time. While greed is to be opposed and fought in view of the harm it does, such opposition may not be effective until a major cultural change has occurred in the nation. This is not impossible, since such changes have occurred in almost every decade since the 1950s. The failures at the end of the 1980s and in the early 1990s of some real estate and banking enterprises associated with excessive greed may help promote a reconsideration of greed.

In the meantime, there is one segment of society responsible for all the people, and accountable for the end results of actions under its jurisdiction: that is, government. Therefore one can, and should, accuse the government of the United States, at all its levels and with only few exceptions, of having allowed and contributed to the misery, degradation, trauma, disease, and in some instances death of a large number of people in its population. It is hoped that the federal government, as well as state and local governments, will use their power to overcome the pressures toward homelessness current in our society.

References

1. Grier G, Grier E. *Urban Displacement: A Reconnaissance.* Washington, D.C.: U.S. Department of Housing and Urban Development, 1978.

2. Marcuse P. Abandonment, gentrification, and displacement: The linkages in New York City. In Smith N, Williams P (eds.), *Gentrification of the City.* Winchester, Mass.: Allen and Unwin, 1986, pp. 153–177.

3. LeGates R, Hartman C. The anatomy of displacement in the United States. In Smith, Williams (eds.), *Gentrification of the City,* pp. 178–200. See ref. 2.

4. LeGates R, Hartman C. *Displacement.* Berkeley, Calif.: Legal Services Anti-Displacement Project, 1981.

5. Hartman C, Keating D, LeGates R, with Turner S. *Displacement: How to Fight It.* Berkeley, Calif.: National Housing Law Project, 1986.

6. U.S. Department of Housing and Urban Development. *Annual Housing Survey: Gener-*

al Housing Characteristics for the United States and Regions. Washington, D.C.: Government Printing Office, 1983.

7. Bureau of the Census. *Current Housing Reports, Annual Housing Survey, 1983,* pt. C, *Financial Characteristics of the Inventory for the United States and Regions, 1983.* Ser. H-150-83. Washington, D.C.: Government Printing Office, 1983.

8. Dolbeare CN. *Low Income Housing Needs.* Washington, D.C.: Low Income Housing Coalition, December 1987.

9. Andrewes N. *The Challenge of Affordable Housing: A Perspective for the 1980s.* New York: Ford Foundation, 1986.

10. Stone ME. Housing and the economic crisis: An analysis and emergency program. In Hartman C (ed.), *America's Housing Crisis: What Is to Be Done?* Boston: Routledge and Kegan Paul, 1983, pp. 99–150.

11. Stegman MA. Housing. In Brecher C, Horton RD (eds.), *Setting Municipal Priorities, 1988.* New York: New York University Press, 1987, pp. 197–219.

12. Nelson KP. *Gentrification and Distressed Cities: An Assessment of Trends in Intra-Metropolitan Migration.* Madison: University of Wisconsin Press, 1988.

13. Gale DE. *Gentrification, Condominium Conversion, and Revitalization.* Lexington, Mass.: Lexington Books, 1984.

14. Schwartz DC, Ferlauto RC, Hoffman DN. *A New Housing Policy for America.* Philadelphia: Temple University Press, 1988.

15. National Association of Home Builders. *Low- and Moderate-Income Housing: Progress, Problems, and Prospects.* Washington, D.C.: The Association, 1986.

16. Senate Committee on Banking, Housing, and Urban Affairs. *A New National Housing Policy: Recommendations of Organizations and Individuals about Affordable Housing in America.* Committee Print no. 100-58. 100th Cong., 1st sess., Washington, D.C.: Government Printing Office, 1987.

17. National Housing Task Force. *A Decent Place to Live.* Washington, D.C.: The Task Force, 1988.

18. Gilderbloom JL, Appelbaum RP. *Rethinking Rental Housing.* Philadelphia: Temple University Press, 1988.

19. Rosenberg S. *Single Room Occupancy Hotels: Standing in the Way of the Gentry.* New York: Coalition for the Homeless and SRO Tenants Rights Coalition, 1985.

20. *People of the State of New York* v. *Lender, Lambert, et al.* New York State Supreme Court, New York County, 1984. Cited in Rosenberg, *Single Room Occupancy Hotels,* p. 60. See ref. 19.

21. Stone ME. Housing and the dynamics of U.S. capitalism. In Bratt RG, Hartman C, Meyerson A (eds.), *Critical Perspectives in Housing.* Philadelphia: Temple University Press, 1986, pp. 41–67.

22. Meyerson A. Housing abandonment: The role of institutional mortgage lenders. In Bratt, Hartman, Meyerson (eds.), *Critical Perspectives in Housing,* pp. 184–201. See ref. 21.

23. Smith N. Toward a theory of gentrification: A Back to the City movement by capital, not people. *Journal of the American Planning Association 45(4):* 538–548, 1979.

24. Smith N. Gentrification and uneven development. *Economic Geography 5:*139–155, 1982.

25. Schlesinger T., Erlich M. Housing: The industry that capitalism didn't forget. In Bratt, Hartman, Meyerson (eds.), *Critical Perspectives in Housing,* pp. 139–164. See ref. 21.

26. Drennan M. Local economy and local revenues. In Brecher, Horton (eds.), *Setting Municipal Priorities,* pp. 15–44. See ref. 11.

27. Starr R. City's housing administration proposed "planned shrinkage" of some slums. *New York Times,* February 3, 1976.

28. Marcuse P, Medoff P, Pereira A. Triage as urban policy. *Social Policy 12(3):*33–37, 1982.

29. Wallace R. Fire service productivity and the New York City fire crisis, 1968–1979. *Human Ecology 9(4):*433–464, 1981.

30. Pecorella RF. Fiscal crises and regime change: A contextual approach. In Stone CS, Sanders HT (eds.), *The Politics of Urban Development.* Lawrence: University Press of Kansas, 1987, pp. 52–72.

31. Elkin SL. *City and Regime in the American Republic.* Chicago: University of Chicago Press, 1987.

32. Molotch H. The city as a growth machine. *American Journal of Sociology 82:* 309–330, 1976.

33. Peterson PE. *City Limits.* Chicago: University of Chicago Press, 1981.

34. Brecher C, Horton RD. Introduction. In Brecher, Horton (eds.), *Setting Municipal Priorities,* pp. 1–3. See ref. 11.

35. Swanstrom C. Urban populism, uneven development, and the space for reform. In Cummings S (ed.), *Business Elites and Urban Development.* Albany: State University of New York Press, 1988, pp. 121–151.

36. Council of State Community Affairs Agencies. *State Housing Initiatives: A Compendium.* Washington, D.C.: COSCAA, 1986.

37. Johnson GE. What do we know about the unemployment problem to know what, if anything, will help? In Bawden DL, Skidmore F (eds.), *Rethinking Employment Policy.* Washington, D.C.: Urban Institute Press, 1989, pp. 37–57.

38. Sawhill IV. Rethinking employment policy. In Bawden, Skidmore (eds.), *Rethinking Employment Policy,* pp. 9–36. See ref. 37.

39. Krugman P. *The Age of Diminished Expectations.* Cambridge, Mass.: MIT Press, 1990.

40. Piven FF, Cloward RA. *The New Class War.* New York: Pantheon Books, 1985.

41. Edsall TB. The Reagan legacy. In Blumenthal S, Edsall TB (eds.), *The Reagan Legacy.* New York: Pantheon Books, 1988, pp. 3–49.

42. Phillips K. *The Politics of Rich and Poor.* New York: Random House, 1990.

43. Edsall TB. *The New Politics of Inequality.* New York: W. W. Norton, 1984.

44. Katz MB. *The Undeserving Poor: From the War on Poverty to the War on Welfare.* New York: Pantheon Books, 1989.

45. Axinn J, Stern MJ. *Dependency and Poverty: Old Problems in a New World.* Lexington, Mass.: Lexington Books, 1988.

46. Anderson M. *Welfare: The Political Economy of Welfare Reform in the United States.* Stanford, Calif.: Hoover Institution Press, 1978.

47. Gilder G. *Wealth and Poverty.* New York: Basic Books, 1981.

48. Murray C. *Losing Ground: American Social Policy, 1950–1980.* New York: Basic Books, 1984.

49. Mead L. *Beyond Entitlement: The Social Obligations of Citizenship.* New York: Free Press, 1986.

50. Hufton O. *The Poor of Eighteenth-Century France, 1750–1789.* Oxford: Clarendon, 1974.

51. Hopper K, Susser E, Conover S. Economies of makeshift: Deindustrialization and homelessness in New York City. *Urban Anthropology 14(1–3):*183–236, 1985.

52. Beauregard RA. The chaos and complexity of gentrification. In Smith, Williams (eds.), *Gentrification of the City,* pp. 50–98. See ref. 2.

53. Logan JR, Molotch HL. *Urban Fortunes.* Berkeley: University of California Press, 1987.

54. Thurow, LC. *The Zero-Sum Society.* New York: Basic Books, 1980.

PART IV

Interventions Directed at the Social Environment

CHAPTER 19

The Role of Legal Aid Organizations in Helping Homeless People

Gary L. Blasi, M.A.

Homelessness is not often thought of as a legal problem. Certainly few homeless people view as among their most urgent needs access to a lawyer or the courts. And advocates for homeless people generally tend to focus on the most evident and critical problems of providing shelter. On the other hand, in many communities in America, it has been lawyers and judges who have brought the reality of homelessness to the public consciousness, and it has often been lawyers and judges who have compelled reluctant government officials to take action, however inadequate (1). Moreover, in many cases, the predicament of individual homeless people stems directly from the illegal acts of others, such as illegal evictions or the denial of welfare or other benefits. To the extent that homeless people have, either collectively or individually, any hope of legal redress, they must generally look to the legal aid system. That system has, like many of the other institutions on which poor people depend, responded with uneven results.

One of the basic tenets of American society is that we are all equal before the law. The further belief that equality before the law requires meaningful access to a complicated judicial system has motivated and sustained a legal aid system that provides some level of legal assistance to the poor in virtually every community in the country. However, the level at which legal aid organizations are funded generally results in only the appearance of access to the judicial system. In Los Angeles, for example, legal services organizations are able to provide one attorney for every 16,000 eligible clients. Legal aid organizations confront many demands for assistance of many different kinds. Decision makers in legal aid organizations suffer from many of the same biases and stereotypes about the homeless which afflict people in many other settings. The result is often that homeless poor people lack access to even those charged with the obligation to help enforce their rights. Happily, this is not always the case. The experience of advocates in New York, Los Angeles, and other cities suggests that advocacy and litigation on behalf of homeless people, both individually and collectively, can lead to significant systemic changes and concrete benefits to individuals. Moreover, that same experience suggests that litigation on behalf of homeless people often leads to changes that benefit all poor people.

The biography of almost every homeless person or family reflects a confluence of individual tragedies and the failure of institutions. There is a strong imperative in the American culture to attribute homelessness to personal failure. So long as the illusion persisted that all homeless people were the "traditional" homeless—alcoholic and mentally ill people—there arose no reason to raise public policy beyond treatment. However, in the early 1980s it became increasingly clear that many homeless people were suffering from no disability beyond poverty. For all the sophisticated social scientific studies of the "causes" of homelessness, there are some facts that do not require statistical analysis. For instance, people who have no income have difficulty paying rent.

Some Areas for Advocacy

INCOME MAINTENANCE PROGRAMS

The various components of what remains of the "social safety net" are operated by bureaucracies with budgets fixed by politicians. Every state operates a program called Aid to Families with Dependent Children (AFDC), funded in part by federal dollars and intended to provide for poor family units with dependent children. The federal government, with state participation, funds the Social Security Disability Insurance and Supplemental Security Income programs, intended to provide for aged and disabled poor people. In virtually every state, there are income maintenance programs of last resort, known variously as "county relief," county welfare," or "general assistance." Many of these programs are so complex that even legal services attorneys are familiar only with the regulations that govern the operation of one or two of the many programs, yet it is often the details of those regulations, rather than any broad public pronouncement, which determine whether people are aided in a way that allows them to secure shelter.

It is sometimes useful to think of each of the welfare programs as a kind of Rube Goldberg machine, with dozens of valves regulating the flow of people into and out of the system. It is those regulatory valves that often determine whether homeless people are aided or left in the street. Moreover, there are often two distinct regulatory schemes: the one that exists in the regulations on paper, and the one that exists in the actual practice of welfare workers confronted with enormous caseloads. In virtually every program in every jurisdiction, there are regulatory valves by which the bureaucracies keep homeless people out of the system intended in principle to aid them. Some of them are subtle, others are not.

RESIDENCE OR ADDRESS REQUIREMENTS.   It requires no particular genius to deduce that homeless people are generally without addresses, yet virtually every welfare program has, or has had until recently, a requirement that recipients have an address. This "catch-22" is presented quite clearly to the homeless person seeking aid. He or she receives no assistance without an address and can obtain no address without assistance. While this may seem perfectly ridiculous to the untrained mind, government attorneys, welfare bureaucrats, and even appellate court judges (2) have no difficulty with this concept.[1] Legal challenges to address requirements have met with some success. Address requirements have been eliminated in recent laws on food stamps and Medicaid (chapter 11).

IDENTIFICATION REQUIREMENTS.   One of the facts of life on the street is that it is hard to maintain one's possessions. Homeless people are often the victims of muggers and lose their identification papers with their wallets or purses. Yet many welfare programs require some kind of documentary identification before even emergency assistance is provided. Thus, the homeless individual who has lost all money along with his or her identification is told to obtain a birth certificate, a process that requires money, information, and time, often weeks or months. Investigations by advocates in Los Angeles revealed that the practice of the County Welfare Department was to vary the identification requirements of the General Relief Program as a means to control intake. When the number of homeless people applying for help increased, welfare workers began to insist on certified copies of birth certificates rather than other, more easily obtainable, documents. Investigation also revealed that the stringent identification requirements were directly responsible for the denial of aid to thousands of homeless applicants. And it was this practice that was the subject of the first (and successful) lawsuit on behalf of the homeless people of Los Angeles County (4).

ACCESS FOR MENTALLY DISABLED PEOPLE.   Many homeless individuals with mental or developmental disabilities are denied assistance as a consequence of their inability to complete application and recertification processes. The application forms, the complex tasks that must be performed to receive or maintain assistance, and the miserable physical conditions and long waits in welfare offices are all as certain an obstacle to a homeless person who is mentally disabled as a staircase is to a homeless person confined to a wheelchair. From a legal point of view, mental and physical disabilities are indistinguishable. Section 504 of the Rehabilitation Act of 1973 (29 USC Sec. 794) forbids such discrimination in programs funded with federal dollars. What is more difficult than establishing the illegality of officials' discriminatory practices is devising solutions or remedies that are meaningful to homeless people. There is, of course, a wide range of disabilities among mentally disabled homeless people.

While assistance in obtaining a regular source of income may solve the problem of shelter for some, those with more severe disabilities may require assistance in the form of money management and ongoing casework (chapter 12). And it is those kinds of significant changes in the entire method of administering aid programs which judges are most reluctant to order.

Shelter and Last-Resort Housing

PREVENTING EVICTIONS.   Preventing an individual from becoming homeless is obviously to be preferred to securing emergency shelter after the individual has been forced to the streets. Virtually every legal aid organization provides some level of legal assistance to people facing eviction. However, it is also the case that the vast majority of eviction cases are brought for nonpayment of rent. Where the nonpayment of rent is not the consequence of unhabitable conditions or other illegal actions on the part of landlords, the most any attorney can do is to enforce procedural rights that may delay eviction.

PRESERVING LAST-RESORT HOUSING.   The experience of many communities, particularly New York City, has led advocates to the conclusion that the provision of emergency shelter is not enough. Unless the longer-term housing needs of homeless people are met, the shelters become housing. It is clear that to address the problem of homelessness over the long term, steps must be taken to save what remains of our last-resort housing. There are a number of roles that legal aid organizations can play and have played in helping to preserve housing.[2] These roles may include contesting evictions of current residents; providing technical assistance to community groups intent on acquiring or rehabilitating housing; providing technical assistance in local legislative activity; and taking direct legal action. Whether direct legal action can help in preserving housing depends primarily upon whether the forces responsible for the threatened destruction include those of government. There are very few examples of legal challenges to the operations of the private real estate market which lead a developer to bulldoze a single-room occupancy hotel (SRO) and replace it with an office building. Government agencies, however, are in general subject to more stringent controls, which may require the provision of replacement housing and relocation assistance to displaced tenants and the preparation of environmental reviews. To the extent that federal funds are used, there may be additional requirements that the project benefit low-income people. However, it is likely that in most cases, legal action can be only a complement to community activity and community action to preserve housing.

CREATING AND PRESERVING EMERGENCY SHELTERS.   As many church and community groups have found, there are obstacles to the creation and operation of emergency shelters beyond the lack of money or other resources. There are often legal obstacles. For example, local zoning laws were generally drafted before emergency shelters existed. Depending on interpretation, zoning laws may restrict new emergency shelter facilities to manufacturing or industrial zones where there are no suitable buildings or resources. It is a rare neighborhood that welcomes an emergency shelter. When the city of Los Angeles sought to relocate an emergency shelter in the heart of Skid Row, the necessary zoning variance was opposed by business owners who operated various kinds of industrial plants in the area. Nor is it an accident of geography that one of the largest shelters in New York City is located on Ward's Island in the East River.

The processes by which variances in zoning laws can be obtained are complex. Much the same can be said about local building codes and ordinances. Like zoning laws, the building codes used as models in most communities do not envision emergency shelters as a type of housing. And like zoning laws, building and safety codes are often used by interests hostile to the operation of shelters in particular areas. Here again, legal expertise can be indispensable.

Approaches to Advocacy

There is often a tension in legal services work between those who want to emphasize "service" cases (i.e., cases representing individuals with individual problems) and those who favor an emphasis on "impact" cases (i.e., cases that have an impact on common problems of many people). The handling of individual clients' cases is certainly gratifying in that the results obtained for a particular human being over time can be seen. However, legal service advocates who handle only service cases often see themselves as dispensers of Band-Aids in a disaster, overwhelmed by the numbers of people needing help and compelled by the lack of resources to turn away many people with legitimate claims. Further, in the hierarchy of values in the legal profession, it is often those who litigate "impact" cases who are most respected by their peers, even if, in an objective sense, some of those "impact" cases assist fewer people than are helped by an attorney who competently handles individual legal problems for many clients. Most experienced legal services attorneys agree that the legal issues that affect poor people can only be effectively addressed by a combination of "impact" and "service" work. This is perhaps nowhere seen more clearly than in the legal problems of the poor and homeless.

INDIVIDUAL ADVOCACY

Those problems of homeless and near-homeless people which have a legal component are marked, as are their other problems, by desperation. A housed client who needs a birth certificate in order to apply for a driver's license is quite different from a homeless client who must have a birth certificate in order to obtain general assistance and the means to find even a Skid Row hotel room. A housed client facing a lawsuit for money damages or a welfare overpayment has a problem of an entirely different order than a homeless client facing a fixed, punitive penalty of ineligibility for welfare assistance. Legal aid agencies, like other service organizations, have not often responded appropriately to the urgency of the individual and collective legal problems of homeless people.

There are understandable, if not acceptable, reasons for this response, or lack of it. First, the very urgency of the client's need makes it difficult for him or her to deal with an intake and processing system that often relies on expected behavior that is difficult or impossible for homeless people—the keeping of appointments is difficult; correspondence by mail is impossible. Second, legal aid staff members suffer from some of the same stereotyping about homeless people as does the rest of society, regardless of their social and political views. To the conservative, homeless people are "bums," while to the radical, they are members of the "lumpenproletariat." Neither view suggests that the problems of homeless people are worthy of much effort. Third, those dealing with home-less clients find that there are severe limits to the effectiveness of purely "legal" work. While lawyers and legal workers may not want to do what they see as "social work," the fact is that often, without help or intervention in many areas, whatever legal assistance is offered is absolutely irrelevant. Finally, homeless people have severe problems in gaining access to legal services.

The first component of the complex of barriers to access to legal services for homeless people is the lack of information and understanding—both on the part of the homeless and on that of the providers who deal with food, shelter, and the like—about what kinds of problems may be properly seen as legal problems. The fact is that a substantial number of people are homeless as a result of the denial of legal rights. Virtually every county and state in the United States guarantees to indigent citizens some right to subsistence, generally through some kind of general assistance program. These rights often exist only on paper or are granted and denied at the whim of those empowered to do so. It is the primary function of the legal system to see that those rights that exist on paper find expression in reality. In addition to such broad areas, there are particular legal problems of great importance to homeless people. For example, homeless people are entitled by law to federal food stamps but are often denied them in practice. Homeless mentally ill people are often discriminated against by agen-cies that are obliged by law to furnish access. Therefore, it is important that those who work with homeless people in nonlegal areas begin to understand the legal aspects of homelessness and to urge local legal aid organizations to become involved.

For homeless people themselves, the problems of access to legal aid are less abstract. People who must wait in line for hours to eat cannot reasonably be expected to walk several miles to a legal aid office. Few legal aid organizations offer outreach services in areas where there are large numbers of homeless people. In Los Angeles, two poverty law agencies have tried to overcome this particular problem. The first, the Inner City Law Center, is physically located in the heart of Skid Row. Both volunteers and paid staff see clients on a walk-in basis three times a week. The offices of the Inner City Law Center have also served as a gathering place and communication center in the heart of one of the greatest concentrations of homeless people in the United States. The more traditional legal aid organization in Los Angeles, the Legal Aid Foundation of Los Angeles, has funded a Homeless Outreach Project, involving paralegals and lay advocates who work not in an office but on the streets. Under the supervision of attorneys, they go into the streets, welfare office waiting rooms, soup lines, and parks, and offer on-the-spot advice and advocacy, as well as referral. This program has been extremely successful, both in assisting clients and in gathering the information needed in support of "impact" litigation on behalf of homeless people.

SYSTEMIC APPROACHES

There are, obviously, limits to what can be achieved by means of advocacy for individual homeless clients. If an entire system refuses to provide legally required assistance, no amount of individual advocacy will achieve very much. It is for that reason that legal aid and public interest attorneys have filed legal challenges to systemwide denials of rights to homeless people. Attorneys for the homeless have used a number of different strategies. It is obvious that the best litigation strategy will depend in part upon local conditions. The tests of a good litigation strategy are whether the strategy has a good chance of success in court, and whether success in court will mean something in the reality of the streets. It is important that nonlawyers with extensive experience in the practical problems of homeless people be involved in the development of the strategy, for what looks like a significant victory to an attorney (e.g., a court decision that homeless people have a right to shelter) may be meaningless on the street (e.g., if the court decision does not say who is required to pay for that shelter).

The first and most critical step in devising a litigation strategy is a detailed factual analysis of the local system. It will sometimes be the case that the most successful strategy involves bringing a series of carefully targeted cases challenging a particular practice, rather than bringing one case seeking an order that will direct someone to provide adequate shelter for homeless people. This is so, in part, because it is much easier to convince a judge to correct one illegal practice than to convince him or her to replace the judgment and actions of an entire political body with his or her own. In any event, attorneys for homeless people must develop a detailed and comprehensive understanding of the local welfare and shelter system.

The possibility of successful litigation is probably greater if there is at least some kind of emergency shelter system already in place. Thus, New York City had in place a municipal shelter system and an ancient local law that obliged the city not to turn away homeless people. Los Angeles had an emergency shelter system consisting of a number of Skid Row flophouses in which homeless applicants for general assistance were placed and which were paid via a voucher system. In both instances, the existing system was a disgrace, but there was at least a system. In both cities, litigation has focused on compelling local government to expand and improve existing shelter systems. That is not to say that an existing shelter system is a prerequisite to successful litigation. As noted earlier, virtually every community has a law that requires someone to "relieve and support" poor people who are not otherwise supported. The point may be made that to "relieve and support" the poor means, at least, to provide the essentials of human existence, if it means anything at all.

A second, and very necessary, step in the litigation process is to recognize that the judicial system is in fact part of the political system. While cases may be decided on arcane legal principles, the result of a case often depends on a judge's assessment of community values and the community's desired solution to a problem. The task of educating the middle class and decision makers in the community about the reality of homelessness is as important to litigation as it is to legislation. If the local newspaper portrays homeless people as dangerous, predatory vagabonds who have voluntarily adopted homelessness as a lifestyle, the task of a lawyer asking a judge in that community for a court order is immeasurably more difficult.

The third critical element in bringing litigation on behalf of homeless people is developing methods to bring the ugly reality of the streets and alleys into the courtroom. Advocates for homeless people must understand the degree to which life on the streets is completely incomprehensible to most judges. In several lawsuits filed in Los Angeles, the principal means of communicating the reality of the streets was the filing of literally hundreds of affidavits of homeless people who had themselves been the victims of the challenged government action. These affidavits were all hand-written, taken down in welfare office waiting rooms, soup lines, and missions, by attorneys or others on the basis of interviews conducted on the spot. The most effective of these affidavits accurately portrayed the life of a full human being with a past, a family, dreams, hopes and fears, and described in detail the days, weeks, or months of homelessness (6).

Another way to bring the truth about homelessness into the court is by means of experts' affidavits and testimony. The experts may include academic researchers in sociology, medicine, psychology, and the like. Many advocates for homeless people have been gratified by the response from local university faculties and graduate students. If there are not already academic people who have done research in areas related to homelessness, it is likely that there may be people willing to explore these areas. In addition to academic experts, there are also people whose expertise derives from experience (e.g., mission workers, and emergency room doctors and nurses). Some of the most compelling affidavits filed in Los Angeles litigations have been those of emergency room nurses who have treated the medical consequences of homelessness (6).

AN INTEGRATED APPROACH

Advocates for homeless people have often found that after they left the courtroom with a legal victory, their struggles were just beginning. As in many other areas of the legal system, there is the reality of the courtroom, and then there is the reality of the street. Court orders are not self-enforcing. Vigilant monitoring is necessary to ensure that what was won in the courtroom is not lost in the welfare office or the shelter. That monitoring cannot effectively be done from behind a desk. It is necessary to go out into the streets, the welfare offices, and the shelters to talk with homeless people firsthand. It is also necessary to handle a significant volume of individual "service" cases of homeless people in order to ensure that rights that exist on paper are respected in practice. Legal advocates must maintain good communication with service providers who work with homeless people in various ways. And then, it is often necessary to go back to court.

In Los Angeles, an attempt was made to do all these things in a series of related large-scale law suits. The litigation teams included not only attorneys from the seven public interest law firms who worked on the litigation[3] but also paralegals and street advocates from the Homeless Outreach Project and advocates who handle individual service cases in the office. In this manner, the litigation team was able to develop strategies on the basis of complete information, obtain affidavits from hundreds of homeless people, maintain links to coalitions of community and service workers, and monitor the effectiveness of orders obtained in court.

Conclusions and Perspectives for the Future

The very fact of homelessness in the richest nation on earth raises contradictions that are moral, political, and legal. It is the fact that we have not as yet accepted homelessness as a society which creates the possibility for advocates for the homeless to effect meaningful change. In many ways, litigation on behalf of homeless people may be the most effective way to address problems that affect poor people generally. Homelessness is a starker and more dramatic fact than simple poverty. It is one thing to urge a judge or legislative body to increase the benefits given to welfare recipients, on whom much conservative venom has been vented in the public press or the media. It is another thing to ask the same judge or legislative body to ensure that homeless poor people have at least the absolute necessities of life, including shelter.

It is a sad commentary on American life that we have retreated so far from the goal of the 1949 Housing Act (42 USC Sec. 1450)—"a decent home and suitable living environment for every American family"—that advocates for poor people must organize, lobby, and litigate even for emergency shelters for people living on our streets, in alleys, cars, and all-night theaters. That is, however, our responsibility and our challenge. So long as we do not as a society regard homelessness as an acceptable feature of American life, there will be opportunities for advocates for the poor to make a difference. If homelessness comes to be regarded as an acceptable state for poor people, then we will have lost more than any of us can now measure.

Notes

1. But cf. *Nelson* v. *Board of Supervisors* (3).

2. An excellent, though now somewhat dated, guide as to how legal services advocates can assist in the preservation of SRO housing is given by Werner and Bryson (5).

3. The seven firms are the American Civil Liberties Union, the Western Center on Law and Poverty, the Inner City Law Center, Mental Health Advocacy Services, San Fernando Valley Neighborhood Legal Services, the Center for Law in the Public Interest, and the Legal Aid Foundation of Los Angeles.

References

1. Roisman FW. Establishing a right to housing: An advanced guide. *20 Housing Law Bulletin 39*, 1990.

2. *Adkins* v. *Leach* (1971) 17 Cal. App. 3d 771.

3. *Nelson* v. *Board of Supervisors* (1987) 190 Cal. App. 3d 25.

4. *Eisenheim* v. *Board of Supervisors*. Los Angeles County Superior Court, no. 479453, December 20, 1983.

5. Werner FE, Bryson DB. A guide to the preservation and maintenance of single room occupancy (SRO) housing. *Clearinghouse Review 15 (12):*999–1007, 1982.

6. Statement by Gary Blasi. In House Committee on Government Operations, *The Federal Response to the Homeless Crisis*. Intergovernmental Relations and Human Resources Subcommittee, 98th Cong., 2d sess., December 18, 1984. Washington, D.C.: Government Printing Office, 1985, pp. 1120–1211.

CHAPTER 20

The Growth of Homelessness:
An Aggregate Rather Than
an Individual Problem

Kay Young McChesney, Ph.D.

The homeless young mother with a baby in one arm and a toddler in the other, standing on a Los Angeles street corner, knows nothing of the macroeconomics of poverty and housing, yet her plight is the result of political and economic forces over which she has no control. Whatever the individual circumstances of her poverty, she is homeless, in the end, because of a combination of national political and economic choices that have resulted in homelessness on a wide scale in the United States for the first time since the Depression. This chapter will show how individuals facing aggregate market characteristics over which they have no control are affected by larger systems governing employment and the supply of housing. First, the argument that homelessness is a problem of aggregates, not individuals, will be presented. Second, empirical research that shows four types of homeless families will be summarized. Finally, some policy implications of the view that homelessness is the result of the macroeconomics of poverty and housing will be presented.

The macroeconomics of homelessness in the aggregate can be seen as a ratio (1,2). The numerator is the number of households living under the poverty line. These are the households that can afford only low-income housing. The denominator is the number of affordable low-income housing units in the housing stock. Using the federal government's standard rent: income ratio, these are the housing units that rent for 30 percent or less of the poverty line for a given household size. When the number of poor households exceeds the number of low-income housing units, a shortage of low-income housing exists. When the number of poor households far exceeds the number of low-income housing units, homelessness is the inevitable result. This concept is similar to that of the housing affordability gap, defined by Andrews as the number of poor households minus the number of housing units affordable to them. She estimated that the gap was 14 million housing units in 1983 (2:5). By 1985, according to another study, there were about 11.6 million low-income renter households competing for 4.7 million low-rent units, for a ratio of 2.5 times as many poor households as there were housing units they could afford (3). Given an acute shortage of low-income housing, when the number of households who can pay more for their housing is exhausted, and the number of households who can double up with families or friends is exhausted, the remainder are left without housing options and become homeless.

The Process of Becoming Homeless

How does the shortage of low-income housing affect poor people? How do people go from having a home to being homeless? These are process questions, the sort of questions that cannot be answered by cross-sectional data but require longitudinal ethnographic studies. However, few such studies have been done (chapter 8); therefore, the next best approximation is an open-ended retrospective review of how now-homeless households have lost their housing.

In an intensive interview study of 87 mothers living in shelters for homeless families in Los Angeles County during 1985–86, extensive retrospective histories of how the families had become homeless were taken (4,5). Analysis of the tape-recorded and transcribed interviews showed four types of families— unemployed couples, mothers leaving relationships, mothers receiving Aid to Families with Dependent Children (AFDC), and mothers who had been homeless teens (4,5).

The unemployed couples were primarily married couples with two or more children. In a typical family, the husband had previously worked full-time at a job that had enabled him to support the family, for example, as a construction worker, a welder, or a machinist. He had lost his job, had been unable to find a new one, and had run through his unemployment benefits. As their finances became increasingly precarious, these families were eventually evicted for nonpayment of rent. They doubled up with relatives if they could. Subsequently, still without work, they became homeless.

Before becoming homeless, the mothers leaving relationships had been supported by the male partners with whom they had been living. They had usually left their men, and thus their housing, suddenly. Many were victims of domestic violence, but some had been locked out or had left their men for other reasons. If they had somewhere to go, they doubled up for a day or two. More often, they went directly to the streets or the shelter, often ending up in a homeless shelter because the battered women's shelters were full. At this point, they needed temporary emergency housing. However, they had no money to get into new housing. Further, although they often had skills and work experience, they had no child care and thus could not go to work. Typically, they applied for AFDC while they were in the shelter, but because of high rents and move-in costs, their AFDC was not enough to get them into new housing.

The AFDC mothers had been supporting themselves on AFDC for several years before becoming homeless. They had become homeless because of "the squeeze"—their AFDC benefits remained the same while their rents rose steadily. (For example, by 1985 a typical mother with one child received $458 per month in AFDC benefits, while a typical inner-city one-bedroom apartment rented for $350 or more, leaving the AFDC mother with only $100 or so for all other expenses, including light, heat, and telephone.) Eventually, they missed a rent payment. Once behind, they were never able to catch up. They usually left their apartments under threat of eviction, doubled up if they could, and then ended up in shelters for homeless families. Once out of their former dwellings, they had no way of acquiring enough money to move into new apartments and they often lost their AFDC benefits as well for lack of an address.

Mothers who had been homeless teens were typically young women with only one child. They shared a history of having been severely abused as children and then having run away from home or from a subsequent foster placement. As teenagers, alone on the street with no way to support themselves, they often turned to subsistence prostitution. Eventually, they got pregnant and decided to keep their babies. Once their babies arrived, the mothers were eligible for AFDC, but AFDC was not enough to get them into permanent housing. For mothers who had been homeless teens, it had often been several years since they had lived in stable permanent housing. These young women often had extensive histories of doubling up—two nights with a friend, two months with a new boyfriend, a few days with another person they met on the street—but they were unable to stabilize themselves. They tended to have tried to live on the streets with their babies before arriving in the shelter.

Analysis of these four types of family histories of homelessness suggests some common elements. Becoming homeless is a process (chapter 8). Rather than a single event, it is a series of events, often occurring over several years, that culminates in the state of literal homelessness. Another thing these heads of household had in common was unemployment. They were poor because they were not working. For the unemployed couples, the loss of a job caused a rapid descent in poverty. Leaving their men had the same effect for the mothers leaving relationships. The AFDC mothers and mothers who had been homeless teens had been poor all along. However, all of these individuals once displaced from stable residences, faced the reality of the low-income housing ratio. The rental prices of available units cost more than they could pay. Further, the obstacle of high move-in costs (first and last month's rent plus cleaning deposit) was virtually insurmountable. Thus, once they ran out of people to double up with, they became homeless.

Discussion

Viewing homelessness from the vantage point of the housing ratio leads to two conclusions. First, if homelessness is the net result of the aggregate housing ratio, the only strategies that will be effective in dealing with it are those that decrease the number of poor households competing for affordable housing, or increase the number of low-income units they can afford.

Second, if homelessness is the net result of the aggregate housing ratio, it follows that homelessness is *not* caused by individual characteristics or behaviors. Whatever the specific reasons for nonparticipation in the labor market (for instance, having worked in a plant that closed, or having minor children and no child care), a person is ultimately homeless because there are not enough low-income housing units to go around. At most, personal characteristics operate as a selection mechanism. Given that the aggregate housing ratio decrees that some households will be homeless, those who are the least able to compete in the labor market are simply the most likely to lose their homes.

These conclusions have implications for policy. Most communities' first response to homelessness is to open emergency shelters. The implication of such a strategy is that homelessness is due to temporary displacement, and thus homeless people need only emergency shelter while they look for permanent housing. From the vantage point of the aggregate housing ratio, this logic is flawed. While emergency shelters provide short-term humanitarian relief to specific individuals and households, they reflect at best a Band-Aid approach. They do nothing to change either the numerator or the denominator of the housing ratio, and thus will have no effect on the total number of households that lack access to permanent, affordable low-income housing.

When communities find that in spite of the presence of emergency shelters, homelessness continues to increase, they often respond by developing transitional housing programs. There are two types of transitional housing programs. In some, homeless individuals are provided with housing for several months while being trained in "living skills" such as budgeting, shopping, and home management. The implication of such a strategy is that the program participants are homeless because they have "defects" in their personal characteristics or behaviors which can be "fixed" by program participation. In other programs, homeless people are merely provided with housing for several months while they look for permanent housing. The implication here is that, given enough time and a stable base from which to look, a household will eventually find permanent housing. Both types of programs may benefit specific households. However, from the vantage point of the housing ratio, neither will have much effect on homelessness. Assuming that graduates of transitional living programs are more competitive in the rental housing market, as they move into permanent affordable housing they will merely displace other poor households who would have occupied the same units. Thus, the long-term effect of transitional living programs on the aggregate housing ratio is to provide a few additional units of low-income housing through which poor people are forced to rotate at six-month intervals.

Does this mean that emergency shelter programs and transitional housing programs should be discontinued? Given the current crisis, emergency shelter is essential. It is also possible although not yet proven that as a result of living skills training received in transitional housing, a few households may do better once given affordable permanent housing. However, communities that choose to spend money on these short-term housing programs should be aware that the programs will not affect the aggregate housing ratio.

Further, there is a danger that having spent considerable sums of money on short-term "solutions," communities will falsely assume that they have dealt with the problem. The example of New York City can serve as a cautionary tale in this respect. In the early 1980s, the city adopted an emergency shelter approach rather than a permanent housing approach to deal with its growing number of homeless people. In 1981, there was a 25-percent increase in the number of families seeking shelter, but a family's average length of stay in the system was two months. In other words, the system was being used as temporary shelter. Meanwhile, the city did little to deal with the underlying problem—the growing shortage of low-income housing. By October 1984, the city was sheltering 3,100 families a night, with an average stay of 7.8 months. By the end of 1985, it was sheltering 4,100 families a night, and by November 1987, it was sheltering 5,200 families a night, with an average stay of 13 months. By 1987, it was spending about $305 million per year to house 28,000 people per night, including an average of $1,612 per month per family for hotel rooms without cooking facilities (New York City Human Resources Administration, personal communication, 1987). Had New York City chosen to put the same level of resources into building permanent, affordable housing by the end of the 1970s, the severity of its current low-income housing crisis might have been considerably moderated. Eventually, a $10.4-billion, 10-year program to build about 225,000 permanent units of low-income housing was announced (4), suggesting that New York City might have finally begun to attend to the structural roots of the problem.

Conclusion

In summary, I have argued that the root causes of homelessness lie in the macroeconomics of poverty and housing, rather than in the characteristics of homeless people. Consequently, only policies that increase the supply of affordable low-income housing or decrease the demand for such housing will prove effective as strategies to decrease the number of homeless people. Alternative strategies, such as the provision of emergency shelters or transitional housing programs, may benefit program participants but will have no effect on the underlying shortage of low-income housing.

As a nation, we have only ourselves to blame for the present low-income housing shortage. We find ourselves in the present crisis because we have ignored the macroeconomics of the low-income housing ratio. The responsible course is to acknowledge that homeless people are the victims of bad policy and poor planning, and to begin setting the low-income housing ratio right by building new low-income housing units and preserving existing low-income units, while providing the opportunity to work to all those who want it.

References

1. Dolbeare C. *Rental Housing Crisis Index*. Washington, D.C.: National Low Income Housing Coalition, 1986.

2. Andrews N. *The Challenge of Affordable Housing: A Perspective for the 1980s*. New York: Ford Foundation, 1986.

3. Leonard PA, Dolbeare CN, Lazere EB. *A Place to Call Home: The Crisis in Housing for the Poor*. Washington, D.C.: Center on Budget and Policy Priorities, 1989.

4. McChesney KY. Women without: Homeless mothers and their children. Ph.D. diss., University of Southern California, 1987.

5. McChesney KY. Homeless families: Four patterns of poverty. In Robertson MJ, Greenblatt M (eds.), *Homelessness: The National Perspective*. New York: Plenum, 1991.

CHAPTER 21

Toward the Prevention
of Homelessness

René I. Jahiel, M.D., Ph.D.

P reventing homelessness means three things: keeping it from occurring in the first place; providing homeless people with stable homes and incomes, along with needed services; and keeping homelessness from recurring. As shown in chapter 20, this requires intervention at the aggregate level, and as shown in chapter 18, such intervention must take into account the benefits that powerful groups derive from the factors that give rise to homelessness. Full prevention of homelessness is a major undertaking, expected to elicit strong resistance. It has not been attempted in the 1980s. This chapter does not provide a blueprint for this enterprise. Rather, it has three objectives.

First, it provides an assessment of the effort needed for, and the cost of, full prevention of homelessness in the short term, that is, in the next one to four years. To my knowledge, such an assessment has not been presented before, possibly because of the weakness of the available data. However, the existing data, unsatisfactory as they are, nevertheless allow a gross estimate of the range of magnitude of the parameters of homelessness. I shall draw upon the data presented in chapters 11 and 22 to make a gross estimate of the quantitative features of full prevention in the short term.

Prevention in the short term, especially if it is undertaken during a period of recession or depression, would have to take place within a "zero-sum economy" (1). This suggests that the groups who benefit from the factors giving rise to homelessness would have to lose some of their benefits, and therefore that significant resistance to prevention would be encountered. In the second part of this chapter, three scenarios for the short-term evolution of homelessness in the United States are presented. Their end results range from aggravation of homelessness to significant if not full prevention. The interactions of forces for prevention and forces for resistance to it are discussed in each instance, along with strategic considerations to promote prevention.

In the third and final part of the chapter, prospects for the long term, that is,

10–30 years down the road, are discussed. If at that time the economy is expanding a zero-sum situation could be avoided, and there might be less resistance to prevention. Additional approaches, which become feasible in the long term, are outlined.

Quantitative Aspects of Prevention in the Short Term

TARGET POPULATIONS

The target populations include literally homeless and doubled-up homeless people and low-income domiciled people who spend an excessive part of their income for housing. Three estimates of the number of people who are homeless on a given night are used, based on the data of Table 22.4. They are a low estimate of 679,000 (corresponding to the most restrictive assumptions), a middle estimate of 1,350,000, and a high estimate of 2,322,000 (corresponding to the least restrictive assumptions). They correspond to about 500,000; 1 million; and 1.7 million households, respectively. The estimated number of doubled-up people is 7.56 million, in 2.16 million households. (The ratio of people to households is larger for doubled-up people because it is assumed that most such people who have been enumerated belong to families.) Finally, it is estimated that there are 14 million households living in poverty whose housing expenses are more than 35 percent of their income (chapter 18).

RESOURCES

The resources needed are housing, income, and services. About 0.5–1.7 million housing units are needed for literally homeless households and about 2 million for doubled-up households. Income is needed to bring each household's income to the level where housing-related costs are 35 percent of income. As described in chapter 11, up to three-quarters of the literally homeless households may need services to improve their functional and health status and their quality of life.[1] There is not enough information to assess the service needs of doubled-up homeless people or domiciled poor people paying more than 35 percent of their income for housing.

FUNDING

Discussions of funding policies usually compare cost margins of alternative programs, including existing programs. This is consistent with the gradualistic approach in American policy making. However, when an unsolved problem, like homelessness, is of extraordinary magnitude, this procedure fails to present the policies in proper perspective. In this section I use a different approach, namely, I ask how much money would be needed to provide during one year a home, an adequate income, and needed services to the entire population that is literally homeless or doubled up on a given day in the United States. This does not mean that I am actually proposing some sort of crash program. Such a program would be not only unrealistic politically but also questionable with regard to uncertainties over its effectiveness and side effects.

The main objective of this exercise is to assess the cost of overcoming homelessness. There are so many unknown factors that the best one can do is to determine an order of magnitude. Further, the cost of the program would be greater if it were spread out over a number of years than if it were realized in one year. It should also be emphasized that I am not speaking only about costs to the federal government, as expenses would be shared between federal, state, and local governments and the private sector.

With these caveats in place, I will now discuss the quantitative aspects of financing the program. This will be done first by estimating unit costs of housing, income, and services, and then by estimating total costs for the population involved.

HOUSING. The 1988 cost for a new unit of public housing was $68,669, (2:76). If future operating and modernization costs are included, Congress would have to spend an additional $33,000 per unit, for a total of about $102,000 per unit (3). Comparison of the costs of new housing units under public housing or other programs such as Section 8 or Section 236 (chapter 17) have yielded differing estimates, some finding public housing cheaper (4), others more expensive (5), and still others within a narrow range (6). In New York City, the cost of major rehabilitation or reconstruction of warehoused units was estimated at $85,000 per unit for the "hard costs," plus $10,000 for the "soft costs" of city financing (7). A more recent New York City estimate of "hard costs" alone was $70,000–95,000 for rehabilitation and $65,000–85,000 for new construction, with an average of about $80,000 for hard costs per housing unit (D. Brown, personal communication, February 20, 1990). Hard and soft costs may be lower in other cities (although they might be even higher in a few cities). Taking these various factors into consideration, I use as my first estimate $80,000 per housing unit, assuming the current approaches to construction, development, financing, and utilization of housing.

Several suggestions have been made recently for radical changes that would markedly reduce the cost of low-income housing. A major proposal, developed by a group of policy analysts and presented by Hartman, would reduce cost by using nonprofit housing corporations funded by governmental capital grants, thus eliminating most private-sector profits (8). Sweat equity (the participation of future residents in construction, rehabilitation, or renovation of the buildings in which they would own or rent housing units) is another way to decrease costs. Several other approaches to less expensive housing have been described by HomeBase (9). A still different approach is to increase the number of households allowed to occupy a given public housing unit (10). A combination of such approaches might decrease the cost to $40,000 per unit.

Therefore, two cost estimates will be used in this chapter: $80,000 and $40,000 per unit. In addition, it will be assumed that the there is no attrition in the existing stock of low-income units, inclusive of public housing, Section 8 and other subsidized housing, and single-room occupancy hotels (SROs).

INCOME. By income, I mean cash from work or public subsidy, together with food stamps, housing vouchers, Section 8 certificates, and other "in kind" income. The income is computed on the assumption that housing expenses are 30 percent of income in an SRO or 35 percent in an apartment. Housing for a single homeless person would be a room in an SRO at about $300 per month; hence the yearly income needed is $300 × 12/0.3 = $12,000 (equivalent to an hourly wage of about $6.60 in year-round full-time employment at 35 hours per week). A literally homeless family would pay, on average, $525 per month for an apartment and utilities; hence the yearly income needed is $525 × 12/0.35 = $18,000 (corresponding to a year-round, full-time, 35-hour-a-week job at about $10 per hour). These estimates, which were developed in 1991, would change as the cost of housing changes. For households that are doubled up, or those that are domiciled but pay an excessive percentage of income for housing, I would follow Wright's approach of providing additional income to bring them up to the poverty line (11), along with income supplements or rent reductions determined by a "market basket" approach (12) or by the 35-percent guideline for rent and utilities as a percentage of income.

SERVICES. The services I considered here are those needed to improve functional status (e.g., job training, education, substance abuse treatment, physical and mental health care, counseling, and assistance in job search). A household that needs multiple services would be assigned a cost of $12,000 per year.[2] Households with no special service needs (most of which would be one-person households) would be assigned $3,000 for initial moving costs, help in finding jobs for their adult members, and health care until covered by an employer's group policy.

AGGREGATE COSTS FOR THE FIRST YEAR

THE LITERALLY HOMELESS POPULATION. The aggregate cost for the literally homeless population will be computed first, using the "middle" estimate of that population's point prevalence:[3]

- Number of homeless individuals: 1.3 million;
- Number of homeless households: 1.0 million;
- Cost for building or renovating housing: $80 billion (with current estimates),

or as low as $40 billion (with maximum use of proposed economies);
- Income for the 85 percent of households needing $12,000 each (i.e., one-person households): $10.2 billion;
- Income for the 15 percent of households needing $18.000 each (i.e., households of families with children): $2.7 billion;
- Services for the 75 percent of households needing $12,000: $9.0 billion;
- Services for the 25 percent of households needing $3,000: $0.75 billion;
- Total cost for the literally homeless population: $102.65 billion with current housing cost estimates, going down to as low as $62.65 billion with maximal use of proposed economies.

If the low estimate of the literally homeless population (about 650,000) is used, the funds needed would be about half of the above total: $51.3 billion to $31.3 billion. If the high estimate of the literally homeless population (about 2.3 million) is used, the costs would be about $185 billion to $113 billion.[4]

THE DOUBLED-UP HOMELESS POPULATION.   The aggregate costs are computed as follows:

- Number of doubled-up homeless individuals (rounded): 7 million;
- Number of doubled-up households: 2 million (assuming 3.5 people per household);
- Cost for housing: $160 billion, or as low as $80 billion with maximal economies;
- Income needed: $36 billion (at $18,000 per household);
- Services needed: $6 billion (at $3,000 per household);
- Total cost for doubled-up homeless population: $202 billion or as low as $122 billion with maximal use of proposed economies.

DOMICILED INDIVIDUALS PAYING AN EXCESSIVE PERCENTAGE OF INCOME FOR HOUSING.   An average yearly cost of $3,000 per household is assumed in order to bring the housing-related costs down to 35 percent of income for 14 million households. The aggregate cost would be $42 billion.

TOTAL COST.   The total cost for the three populations would range from $429 billion to $195 billion, depending upon assumptions about the cost of housing and the size of the literally homeless population, with a more likely estimate of $287 billion using intermediate assumptions.

POLITICAL IMPLICATIONS OF THE TOTAL COST

At first, the size of the total cost comes as a shock. However, it appears that the bill for the savings and loan crisis—which, presumably, we as a nation are prepared to pay—is at least of the same order of magnitude. Besides, a part of the total cost is already budgeted under current federal, state, and local programs; and the extra cost would be divided among public, private not-for-profit, and private for-profit sources. Finally, although the program has been presented, for the sake of simplicity, as a one-year thrust, it would in fact be spread out over a number of years, and so would the funding. Therefore, as Wright points out (11), the main obstacle is not economic but political (or cultural).

The political-cultural barriers to large-scale funding of antihomelessness programs in the present political climate are due in part to uncertainty concerning the answers to the following questions: Is the population involved worth the effort? Are homeless or near-homeless people retrievable as a functional social group? Won't all the effort and money go to waste if they remain a burden to society for years to come, if not for their entire lives? Even if most homeless people can be functionally reintegrated into society, is the effort and cost worth it, in comparison with alternate uses of the money—for instance in educational, environmental, or defense programs? How much money are the dominant economic groups and the general tax-paying public willing to give up in order to provide the necessary housing, income, and services to homeless and other very poor people? How much effort are homeless and other very poor people capable of devoting to political organization, and are they willing to do it? Attitudes regarding these questions determine to a great extent what strategies might be used to deal with the problem of homelessness in the United States.

Prevention Strategies in the Short Term

The prospects for prevention in the short term (i.e., in the next 5–10 years) hinge on two perspectives now contending in our society. According to one perspective, homelessness is an undesirable but tolerable condition. It falls in the same category as poverty, unemployment, or illiteracy, which are tolerated up to a point beyond which action must be taken to bring the level down. People who are homeless or at risk of homelessness compete with other groups for limited resources, the allocation of which is subject to cost-benefit analysis and considerations of the relative "worth" and power of the competing groups.

According to the other perspective, homelessness is in the same category as slavery or the abuse of elderly or retarded people in institutions—that is, it is a condition that cannot be tolerated. The abuse of poor or disabled people by depriving them of their homes must be abolished, irrespective of cost-benefit analysis and considerations of individuals' relative "worth" and power.

I discuss three scenarios for the evolution of homelessness and its prevention in the United States. They correspond, respectively, to the first perspective with a high tolerable level of homelessness; to the first perspective with a low tolerable level; and to the second perspective, aiming at abolition of homelessness.

Alford's concept of dominant, challenging, and repressed structural interest groups is used. According to that concept, "dominant structural interests are those served by the structure of social, economic, and political institutions. . . . Precisely because of this, the interests involved do not continuously have to organize and act to defend their interests; other institutions do that for them. Challenging structural interests are those created by the changing nature of society. Repressed structural interests are the opposite of dominant ones (although not necessarily always in conflict with them); the nature of the institutions guarantees that they will *not* be served unless extraordinary political energies are mobilized" (13:14).

SCENARIO 1

This scenario is driven by the dominant structural interests. It is predicated on a social order that encourages individual and corporate members of its high-income sector to increase their earnings and profits, with minimal restraints, and fails to provide sufficient protection to members of its low-income sector. The rich and middle classes, whose income and wealth are increasing, drive up the price of housing. Keeping the minimum wage and corporate taxes low helps to siphon company profits to the owners and executives instead of letting the profits "trickle down" to the employees as better pay, or to the government, which could use them for social welfare. With inadequate income from taxes, and with pressures for the outlay of money exerted by banks (national debt service, high interest rates, rescue of banks in economic difficulties) and by certain industries (e.g., defense, at the federal level; and urban renewal, at the local level), the federal, state, and local governments decrease their support for the poor by reducing, or at least not increasing, benefit programs (e.g., income programs, housing programs, and job retraining), thus driving the poor into still more severe poverty. As the pressures and processes that cause homelessness (chapter 18) intensify, and the ratio of poor households to affordable housing units (chapter 20) becomes more and more unfavorable to the poor, an increasing number of people are unable to keep their homes, and the rate of homelessness keeps increasing.

As the disparity between rich and poor increases and millions of people lose their homes and are forced into a degrading, damaging life, it becomes necessary, in a society based on ethical principles as ours is, to justify what is happening. This is done in a twofold manner. First, there is recourse to the concepts of freedom and responsibility for one's progress in life, two of the most basic tenets of our society. The rationale is that anyone has the freedom to succeed and that one's qualities of judgment, drive, and social behavior are what bring about success. All other factors in the life of "successful" people—the advantages they may have at the start, the ruthlessness with which they have suppressed others, the greed that sustained them in their quest, the opportunism they exhibited at the right time—are either disregarded or converted into positive qualities. Conversely, those who do not succeed are thought to have only themselves to blame. If they had exerted better judgment, had led a more moral life, had been better adjusted to their environment, their failure would not have happened. There is no mention of the social disadvantages of class or race that they may have been saddled with, of the economic situation in which they may have been trapped as a result of forces over which they had no control, of the damage done by victimization at the hands of more ruthless people, and of the handicaps created by various kinds of labels. Thus, the blame is put on the homeless people, in a classic "blame-the-victim" approach (14). This assuages the guilt that rich and successful people might have had concerning those they have pushed down on their way up, and justifies the advantages that they continue to receive. It negates the need for any change in the social system (see concluding paragraph of chapter 3). This attitude may become so ingrained in our society that homeless people may internalize it, believing that they are at fault for their own situation.

The second justification of this state of affairs is that homelessness is necessary to show people what happens when one does not work hard enough, conform, or play up to the powerful of the world. These two attitudes—blaming homeless people, and setting them up as a necessary example—lessen the investment that society might be willing to make to help them.

Yet the situation of homelessness is so horrible that many in our culture, with its Judeo-Christian roots, recoil at the idea of abandoning anyone to such a fate. This attitude, which might refuel attempts to help homeless people, is countered in several ways. First, it is asserted that people are homeless by their own choice. Second, an attempt is made to minimize the size of the homeless population, in two ways: the doubled-up households (the majority of homeless people; see chapter 22) are not counted as homeless; and the number of people who are homeless in the streets and shelters (the literally homeless) is presented as smaller than it actually is, either by relying on enumeration methods that yield a low number or by selecting the most conservative estimates (chapter 22). Third, some programs are started at a low funding level, well beneath what is needed, but they are given much visibility, creating the impression that something is being done. Finally, some programs that alleviate the hardships of homeless people, such as health care programs, are undertaken and presented as evidence that the government is helping, even though such programs do little to stem the rise of homelessness.

As the number of homeless people continues to increase and the spectacle of seeing them on the street disturbs local residents as well as foreign visitors, who carry it back home as part of their impression of America, a "put-away" approach is used. Chronically mentally ill individuals are institutionalized; elderly people are put in nursing homes; camps are set up away from the city for the rehabilitation of alcohol or drug abusers; people with AIDS are sequestered into special facilities; chronically homeless people are bussed to other areas; families are segregated into welfare hotels; shelters and barracks-type facilities grow in number and size and evolve from emergency facilities to community institutions. In this manner, a sort of "apartheid by income" is created, whereby the poorest in our society—the homeless—are separated from the rest of society and forced to lead a life with different and lower standards concerning home and social interaction, forming the newest and most oppressed underclass.

In the meantime, these developments stimulate the growth of a vigorous "homelessness industry" that includes shelter operators and personnel; food services; owners and operators of welfare hotels and various forms of housing *ad minima;* professional personnel; research personnel; a government bureaucracy dealing with administration, regulation, and evaluation; some private businesses providing services and goods to others in the "industry"; and last but not least, landlords, developers, insurance companies, and banks. As a result of this, the local, state, and national governments increase their spending on "the problem of homelessness," but the "solution" only creates jobs and income for several dominant groups in our society, including, ironically, some of those characterized in chapter 18 as homeless-makers.

SCENARIO 2

This scenario is driven by challenging structural interests, in Alford's nomenclature (13). In this instance, the most prominent challenging groups are local and state governments, along with coalitions of providers and advocates for homeless people. Government officials act to pull together special interests or even supersede them in order to prevent urban decline and maintain public order, while working together with local business (15, 16). For public officials, homelessness is a problem that must be addressed because of its harmful effects on the city. Advocates such as the National Coalition for the Homeless act as the principal representative groups for homeless people, sometimes together with providers. In general, the challenging structural interests act not in opposition but rather in interaction with the dominant business groups to bring those at risk of becoming homeless into the picture in the course of business activity and urban planning.

Unlike scenario 1, the challenging structural interest scenario is based on the premise that low incomes and the lack of affordable housing are at the root of the problem. However, scenario 2, unlike scenario 3, does not require significant structural changes in the economics of housing for poor people or in the power relationships of the repressed low-income groups in our society. Housing remains primarily a private, for-profit enterprise; corporate interests are not challenged; the safety net of welfare does not reach the level of social support achieved in several European countries; and direct governmental intervention, such as public works or public housing, is undertaken on a relatively small scale. Scenario 2 is predicated on the thesis that significant progress in the fight against homelessness can be achieved by incremental changes realized following compromise or accommodation with the dominant interests. Government plays an essential role in this process: it is the agent that mediates between challenging and dominant interests and ensures that changes occur incrementally and that their costs are assumed by the entire population rather than predominantly by business interests.

I will now briefly describe certain recent innovations or proposals that are compatible with scenario 2, before resuming the description of the scenario. Schwartz et al. list the approaches that state governments have taken in the 1980s. They include facilitating the purchase of single-family housing units by low- and middle-income households; inducing landlords and developers to provide more low-income housing; intervening in cases of imminent eviction; and providing shelters, transitional housing, and some permanent housing. State governments have given banks, developers, and landlords economic incentives to participate in such approaches. Before 1980, the main incentive was the issuance by states of tax-free bonds in order to loan the proceeds to builders and developers at interest rates below the prevailing ones. In the 1980s, new financing methods have been introduced, such as "interest-rate buydowns, deferred payment loans, lease-purchase contracts, shared appreciation and shared equity mortgages, sale and lease back arrangements, low closing cost buydowns, upfront capital grants as subsidy for rental projects, joint purchase rehabilitation loans, and special mortgage insurance programs . . . along with more typical kinds of housing assistance: direct low-interest loans, second mortgages, loan guarantees, rent payment guarantees, and direct subsidies" (17:66–67). A description of these approaches is given by the Council of State Community Affairs Agencies (COSCAA) (18) and the Council of State Housing Agencies (CHSA) (19).

In their housing program for America, Schwartz and colleagues call for a federal homeownership program creating 330,000 affordable units annually, a rental production program creating 370,000 low- and middle-income units, and rehabilitation of 140,000 units for frail elderly people, for a total of 840,000 units annually, financed in part during the first year by $10 billion of federal expenditures, and in subsequent years by federal contributions of $5 billion from general revenue and a housing trust fund, and $5 billion from personal income tax revenue, presumably generated by the success of the program (17). However, with building or rehabilitation costs at $60,000–80,000 per unit, the program would cost $50–67 billion, and it is not clear whether the state, local, and private sectors would be willing to undertake this expense. Yet the number of units planned would cover far less than the entire literally homeless population, even if all of it went to such homeless people. Actually, the program would set in competition a much greater number of households of domiciled low-income people and doubled-up homeless households, along with literally homeless ones, altogether totalling in the tens of millions. It is predictable that the first two categories, which are better risks, would get the major share of the plan.

Wright (11) proposes separate programs aimed at the episodically homeless and the long-term homeless. The premises on which programs for the former group are based is that most of them are in marginal economic circumstances that leave them at the mercy of economic events. Wright proposes several measures: (a) providing rent insurance for households within 150 percent of the poverty level who spend at least 40 percent of their income on housing; (b) expanding the range of workers covered by unemployment compensation; (c) increasing the duration of unemployment compensation payments to 40 months or more; (d) making employers aware of the economic hardships caused by large-scale layoffs and plant closings; (e) creating low-interest "bridge" loans for persons or families facing impending homelessness; (f) enacting more stringent regulations to protect from eviction households caught in a short-term economic bind; and (g) establishing a program of emergency "work relief" to help unemployed workers through a short-term period with publicly subsidized employment. Wright also recommends resuming federal intervention to subsidize some form of public housing. For the long-term homeless, who are mainly single, as well as for other single homeless people who have alcohol problems or mental or physical health problems, he suggests a system of rooming or boarding houses like SROs, with on-site social and health services.

Sosin et al. point out that "at any one time [homelessness] only affects a minority of those in need. These are very poor who have particular traits and are affected by a lack of supportive services or institutions in particular ways. Prevention often involves spending considerable sums for a larger group" (20:357). Along these lines, they suggest (a) work programs, including special programs targeted to homeless people and taking into account the need of many homeless people to acquire skills and self-esteem as well as to resume work habits; in such programs, work should be paid well enough to make housing affordable; (b) a substantial increase in the size of the welfare grants to make them comparable with the cost of housing; (c) an income maintenance emergency program to deal with crises; (d) advocacy and outreach in welfare, to provide poor people with all the benefits they are entitled to; (e) emergency financial aid to provide security deposits and help in housing search for households who are being displaced, as well as those who are already homeless; and (f) special programs for those with special needs, such as people with substance abuse problems or mental disorder (20:357–366).

At the 1991 Fanny Mae Housing Conference, Lindblom proposed a prevention program, including (a) prevention of eviction both by informing tenants of their rights and responsibilities and by giving eviction notices to tenants *and* an appropriate government agency with enough time to allow tenants to get legal assistance and the agency to provide mediation and/or cash assistance; (b) deducting rent money from monthly SSI or general assistance checks in order to pay the landlords directly; (c) maintaining or increasing the number of people in shared housing; (d) helping displaced households to find affordable housing; (e) providing homeless people with information, referral, and security deposits to facilitate the transition to housing; and (f) developing better prevention strategies following discharge from mental hospitals or emancipation from foster care. At a more fundamental level, he proposed (a) increasing the income of the very poor on public assistance with higher assistance payments, full utilization of benefit programs, removing barriers to eligibility due to work-derived income or sharing of housing, protecting against improper decertification, raising some income eligibility limits, and more readily including mental disorder or substance abuse as qualifying disabilities; (b) promoting federal macroeconomic policies that give more attention to unemployment and less to reducing inflation, along with new and expanded public employment programs; (c) raising the earned income tax credit to provide a wage supplement for every hour a poor person works; (d) creating more affordable housing by increasing availability of section 8 (including making households pay more than 30% of their rent), preserving SROs, promoting sharing of housing, creating new low-cost housing, and offsetting neighborhood resistance to the low-income tenants; (e) targeting the full housing rental subsidy to extremely low-income households; and (f) strengthening families (21).

Some of Lindblom's proposals are more compatible with scenario 1 than with scenario 2—for instance, deducting rent money from monthly assistance checks, promoting "shared housing" (i.e., doubling up), or requiring very low income people to pay more than 30 percent of their income for rent. In general, however, the proposals are in line with scenario 2, as they focus on poverty and housing but fail to give a quantitative appraisal of resources and funds needed to eliminate all or most of homelessness; and especially because they do not address the question of competition with other programs, nor strategic considerations regarding the pressures toward homelessness in our society. These remarks also apply to the other approaches described under scenario 2.

Thus, scenario 2, incorporating these approaches, reveals serious problems of implementation. Government staff members, working with advocates for homeless people, prepare legislation to enact and fund these approaches and guide it through the process of becoming law, with the support of influential politicians whose career would be helped by their association with a successful antihomelessness program. In anticipation of resistance to spending a large sum of money for homeless people, the staff prunes down the proposals. While the total cost of the program might require about $300 billion from the federal government and state and local governments for full implementation, the set of proposals submitted to the various legislative bodies amounts to less than $100 billion. Even so, the funds are cut further as the proposal goes through the phases of preparation of legislation, formulation of regulations, and administration, because of competition at each phase with more powerful interest groups (e.g., savings and loans, defense, infrastructure). By the time the programs are funded, they are down to one-fifth or less of the amount needed for full implementation. Further, the business people (e.g., real estate companies, employers of very poor people) who are needed to implement some of the program's projects do not participate to the extent needed because other, more profitable, enterprises compete for their time and money.

Thus, legislators and administrators must make hard decisions concerning who can be helped. In general, homeless families with children have priority, and consequently, the prevalence of homelessness of family groups decreases markedly. The prevalence of homelessness among other individuals decreases only slightly. In order to do something for the latter groups, the quality of shelters is improved by legislation and court action.

Public pressure for action decreases because there has been some improvement in the numbers and the situation of homeless people, and homelessness is not a bread-and-butter issue. Further, additional action might mean more taxes. Influential politicians lose some of their interest in the issue. Advocates for homeless people, who are already involved in this scenario, continue to press for more programs and money, but as long as there is some progress, they do not opt for the approaches of other scenarios. Homelessness remains a social problem that the society has learned to live with, given the balance of pressures toward homelessness and pressures toward its prevention.

In summary, neither of the first two scenarios' programs is likely to eliminate homelessness. Therefore it is necessary to turn to scenario 3, even though its strategy is far more difficult to implement.

SCENARIO 3

This scenario is driven by repressed structural interests. According to Alford's model, it can be successful only with extraordinary efforts (13). Two versions are given, with efforts at the micro or macro level, respectively.

MICRO LEVEL.   Interventions in the local environment aim to prevent or terminate homelessness by using approaches such as those listed by HomeBase, the San Francisco Bay Area advocacy organization for homeless people: (a) sweat equity rehabilitation and reconstruction of units; (b) limited-equity cooperatives; (c) nonprofit agency master leasing for shared housing; (d) mobile homes; (e) modular prefabricated housing; (f) SROs as permanent housing; (g) development of low-income housing by nonprofit organizations such as Habitat for Humanity; (h) nonprofit management of residential hotels; (i) density bonus, to allow extra units of low-rent housing to be built; (j) use of redevelopment agency funds to develop permanent low-income housing (9: Appendix to Step 8, pp. 1–13). These approaches, as well as more traditional use of Section 8, are implemented project by project, housing unit by housing unit. This is "advocate-intensive" and "consumer-intensive" work, requiring a lot of effort. Advocates, volunteers, and college students participate, and people at risk of becoming homeless may be energized or motivated to be self-advocates. Other areas of intense advocacy are the provision of transitional housing for people with mental health, substance abuse, or other problems; efforts to help homeless people to get their entitlements; and efforts to help homeless people to obtain training or retraining for work and to find adequately paid job opportunities.

MACRO LEVEL.   In this version of the scenario, important changes have to take place in the national economy. The objectives are to markedly reduce the homeless-making processes and pressures toward homelessness described in chapter 18. In the housing sector, the supply of low-income housing is increased by (a) resuming a significant program of public housing; (b) supporting with governmental capital grants nonprofit housing corporations, thus eliminating two of the main causes of high housing prices—profit for landlords or developers, and mortgage interest; and (c) supporting community-based nonprofit corporations organized by tenants (8). The stock of low-income housing can be kept from diminishing by strictly enforced regulations protecting SROs and other low-income housing; by improved municipal services to low-income neighborhoods; and by an active community of tenants trained in methods to resist displacement (22). In the employment sector, higher pay for low-income workers is realized by (a) increasing an inflation-adjusted minimum wage to a level adequate to pay for housing and basic life needs; (b) inducing business (e.g., via a tax credit that would depend upon the ratio of company profits to wages paid) to narrow down its profit margin in order to raise the salaries of the lowest-paid workers; and (c) giving employees a significant interest in the company, either as share-holders or as recipients of bonuses based on company performance. With regard to unemployment and welfare, households' income is safeguarded to protect their ability to pay for housing and basic living needs by (a) providing everyone with at least a minimal income through public support, negative income tax, or other means; (b) providing those who need it with a realistic program of vocational rehabilitation, coupled with needed social support (e.g., day care for the infants and young children of working mothers); and (c) instituting a vigorous outreach program to ensure that people get their entitlements. In the health sector, health security is achieved with (a) a national health program for all residents in the United States; (b) a national program of financial protection for loss of income sustained through illness or disability; and (c) a multiservice community support program (including, but not limited to, supported housing and client-oriented case management) for people with handicap-induced vulnerability. In the education sector, vulnerability to homelessness is prevented by (a) targeting education (including but not limited to, training in literacy and basic quantitative skills) to preparation for the job opportunities that will be available at graduation; (b) providing special education tailored to the needs of the individuals and linked to supported work in the community; and (c) designing effective antidrug education. In the family sector, the family contribution to homelessness is markedly reduced by (a) improving the quality of foster care and establishing a new program to help foster children make the transition from foster homes to homes of their own when they become adults; (b) providing early intervention to attack the underlying causes of chronic family conflicts and the environmental conditions that foster such conflicts; and (c) providing greater economic freedom to all members of the family, so that those who run away or are thrown out can establish new homes rather than becoming homeless.

In contrast to scenario 2, these objectives entail some structural changes, and they make demands on the homeless-makers rather than on those who become homeless or on third parties. Therefore scenario 3 must deal with the strong opposition that would be encountered in almost all, if not all, the involved sectors of society. This might be done as follows:

1. Local tenants' or poor people's initiatives, such as those described by HomeBase (see above), or programs of resistance to displacement would be supported by advocates and their successes made known to a wider public by community and national advocacy organizations, with special efforts exerted to identify, reach, and organize those population groups that would tend to benefit most from such initiatives. The results of innovative preventive programs by states, such as the negative income tax for the poor, would be assessed and information on such programs disseminated throughout the nation. At the same time, bills would be introduced in Congress for national programs along the same lines. An example is the bill introduced by Representative Dellums based on the proposal presented by Hartman (8). Academic researchers might play a very important role in this phase by doing empirical case studies or program evaluations and by providing statistics and other data to help in the formulation of legislative proposals. At the national level, the main purpose of this stage would be not to accomplish significant legislative changes but rather to provide models or instruments that would be used in public education and organizational work.

2. Leadership in grassroots movements, education of the public, the energizing effect of small local victories, and the provision of clear objectives would pave the way for organization of poor people to defend more effectively their own interests, one of which is prevention of homelessness. Although the difficulties encountered in attempting to organize poor people have been well documented, one should not forget past instances of the successful organization of major movements of poor people, such as the organization of labor into unions

early in the twentieth century and the organization of blacks into the civil rights movement in midcentury.

3. The current recession might be followed by a period of economic expansion in the mid-1990s. A period of economic expansion is more favorable to allocation of funds to poverty programs because, in contrast to the zero-sum situation that would exist in periods with little or no expansion, such allocation can be done without exposing the homeless-makers to significant losses. In the expansionary period of the mid-1980s, corporations and high-income individuals reaped unprecedentedly huge profits, some of them linked to pressures toward homelessness, as discussed in chapter 18. It is essential that this not occur in a new expansionary period. However, an ethical reaction against some of the excesses of the 1980s is likely to grow during the 1990s. A reaction against the lionization of greed in the 1980s has already started, following the collapse of real estate speculations, the savings and loan debacle, and the arbitrage scandals in 1988–90. The scholarly community may play an important role by exposing myths about homeless people and their blame-the-victim significance (chapter 3), and by educating the public about the pressures toward homelessness and homeless-making processes. The homeless-making processes are only side effects of the homeless-makers' actions. However, the citizenry has, through public awareness of environmental problems, become sensitized to the importance of policy regarding side effects and could be expected to be receptive to an extension of this approach to homelessness and other forms of severe poverty. For instance, legislation might require that potential side effects of profit that could cause pressures toward homelessness be strictly prevented. The ethical reaction against greed and the inequities that result from it would decrease the resistance of public and legislators to nonprofit enterprises and to greater governmental provision of capital grants, increased protection against unemployment, and increased real minimum wages. Here again, one could make an analogy with the history of labor organizing and the civil rights movement, both of which were associated with profound changes in public attitudes.

4. Finally, the movement for homeless and other very poor people would need to have a significant impact in the political arena. Two prerequisites are needed: first, organization of homeless people and other very poor people and their allies for voting and for forming coalitions around given candidates; and second, a realistic and well-phased legislative program at the state as well as at the federal level.

Prevention Strategies in the Long Term

In the long term, 15–35 years down the road, expected demographic changes and possible economic and political changes may have a marked impact on the prevention of homelessness. The main demographic change will be the aging of the post–World War II baby boom cohort, members of which will reach the age of 65 between 2010 and 2030. This may create a large increase in the number of dependent elderly people, and therefore, increased demand on the public support system, at the time when the cohort of people born during the relatively low-birthrate period 1965–80 reaches age 45 and the cohort of people born between 1980 and 2000 reaches age 30. These cohorts would have a major responsibility to generate funds for support of the large elderly cohort. At the same time, the youngest cohort would make significant demands on the social support system, if the prevalence of young adult unemployment and single-parent families stays at its present level. Society would be stressed in providing support for two cohorts, and prevention of poverty and homelessness may become much more difficult than it is now.

On the other hand, the lead time that is now available might provide an opportunity to develop economic and political strategies that could greatly facilitate prevention, if they are implemented *together*. The economic strategies would aim to increase the productivity of the U.S. work force over the next 20 or more years. Comprehensive educational and anti–substance abuse programs are necessary as an essential first step to increase productivity per worker. In addition, there must be improved prevention of mental and physical disability and better adjustment of the workplace to fit the needs of individuals with mental or physical handicaps, along with imaginative changes to improve their productivity. A second set of changes would involve improved workplace efficiency; the adjustment of profits and high salaries to an optimal point at which competitiveness improves; the growth of research and development; governmental support of key new industries; and a sophisticated international marketing strategy.

Alone, these economic changes would not ensure a successful campaign against severe poverty and homelessness. The increased output could be wasted in increasing the inequality between poor and rich, or in expensive defense or space programs. Therefore, steps are needed in the political arena to contain the forces pushing toward greater inequality or toward international conflict. The formation of a coalition of labor, poor people, and very poor and homeless people appears to be almost a prerequisite, and the Democratic party appears to be the natural sponsor for such a coalition. Further, this coalition would have to be supported by extensive community organization, and increased voter registration and voting of all involved groups, including homeless people. As stated earlier, a period of improved productivity and economic expansion would be more compatible with formation of a coalition of poor and salaried people than would one of economic contraction, in which smaller groups are forced into a defensive position and tend to fight for their own interests only. The coalition would gradually bring about housing policies such as capital grants to nonprofit housing corporations, which would decrease the housing affordability gap; as well as policies that would increase the purchasing power of all households to and beyond the minimum computed with the market basket approach. Finally, policies would also have to be developed to prevent potentially dangerous side effects, such as inflation, or to counteract their dangers for low-income people by methods such as indexing salaries and public support to the cost of living. This would require considerable planning and a highly coordinated approach, but the stakes are worth it.

Notes

1. The goods, services, and monies needed by homeless people during the year in which they make the transition from homelessness to the domiciled state may be divided into those needed by all homeless people and those needed only by homeless people with certain characteristics. The first category includes housing, meals, clothing, and basic health care expenses. The second category includes diverse items. Homeless households moving into apartments need funds for moving and for furnishing the apartments. Homeless families with children may need services related to education, health, and mental health, as well as various support services such as child care. Homeless people with chronic health problems (such as AIDS) may have large medical care expenses. Homeless people with mental disorder may require mental health services, supported living arrangements, and other services. Homeless people with substance abuse problems may require detoxification and various modalities of treatment. More than 90 percent of homeless people capable of working do not have full-time steady jobs, and they may need help in finding such jobs. Possibly as many as half of them need some job training, either because there are no openings for the kind of work they are trained to do and they have to be retrained in another line of work, or because they have never had adequate education and training for modern jobs. Some homeless adults who are illiterate or nearly illiterate or who are mildly retarded need basic or special education. Many homeless individuals do not have all the benefits they are entitled to and find it difficult to deal with bureaucracies; therefore, they need help from social workers.

It is extremely difficult to assess the distribution of total service needs in the homeless population. Survey data (e.g., those discussed in chapters 4, 5, and 11) present data about one or two service needs at a time. If one assumes that the different service needs are distributed independently of one another, then nearly all homeless people have special service needs. On the other hand, if most of the special service needs are concentrated in the population with mental disorder, substance abuse, or both, one deals with a subset of maybe 40 percent of the homeless adults who are not in family groups. In this chapter, it will be assumed that 70 percent (i.e., the midpoint between 40% and 100%) of homeless adults who are not in family groups have special needs and that all homeless families with children have special needs. Since the latter constitute 15 percent of households, and the former constitute about 60 percent of all homeless households (85% × 0.7), it is assumed that about 75 percent of homeless households have special service needs. This does not imply that the causes of homelessness reside primarily in the pathology of homeless people but, rather, that the vulnerability factors that mediated homelessness, the personal damage caused by the situation of homelessness, and the special efforts needed to resume life in the general community require various special services.

2. There is very little information on the cost of the multiple services needed by homeless people. The figure $12,000 (exclusive of meals and lodging) is given for the multiservices program of Small and Associates for adults who are homeless and substance abusers (chapter

11). For lack of other sources, I will be using this figure for the 75 percent of households that might need multiple services, as explained in note 1, above.

3. Population numbers are rounded to two significant figures.

4. With respect to the population that is literally homeless at some time during the year (annual prevalence), computations are much more difficult. It is not known what fraction of that population is doubled up during the same year, nor how many literally homeless households are served by a given housing unit during the year. Nor is there accurate information about the rate of decrease in the number of available low-income housing units during the year. Finally, it is not known what fraction of the 20- to 25-percent annual increase in demand for shelter is due to an increase in the number of homeless people (chapter 22). Because of these additional uncertainties, these computations are not attempted here.

References

1. Thurow LC. *The Zero-Sum Society.* New York: Basic Books, 1980.

2. Bratt RG. *Rebuilding a Low-Income Housing Policy.* Philadelphia: Temple University Press, 1989.

3. Stegman MA. *The Role of Public Housing in a Revitalized National Housing Policy.* Working Paper no. HP 19. Cambridge, Mass.: Massachusetts Institute of Technology, Center for Real Estate Development, 1988.

4. General Accounting Office. *Evaluation of Alternatives for Financing Low and Moderate Income Rental Housing.* Report to Congress, PAD 80-13. Washington, D.C.: Government Printing Office, 1980.

5. Urban Research and Engineering. *The Costs of HUD Multifamily Housing Programs.* Report prepared for the U.S. Department of Housing and Urban Development. Washington, D.C.: HUD Office of Policy Development and Research, 1982.

6. Bratt RG. *Mutual Housing Associations.* Washington, D.C.: Neighborhood Reinvestment Corporation, 1984.

7. Tobler E. The homeless. In Brecher C, Horton RD (eds.), *Setting Municipal Priorities, 1990.* New York: New York University Press, 1989.

8. Hartman C. *A Program to Provide All Americans with Decent, Affordable Housing.* Washington, D.C.: Institute for Policy Studies, 1988.

9. HomeBase. *A Place for Everyone: Community-Based Planning for the Provision of Housing and Services to Homeless People.* San Francisco: HomeBase, 1990.

10. Hoch C. *Using Existing Housing Stock as a Homelessness Prevention Measure.* Paper presented at the 8th meeting of the Homelessness Study Group, at the annual meeting of the American Public Health Association, Chicago, Ill., October 21, 1989.

11. Wright J. *Address Unknown: The Homeless in America.* New York: Aldine de Gruyter, 1989.

12. Stone ME. Housing and the economic crisis: An analysis and emergency program. In Hartman C (ed.), *America's Housing Crisis: What Is to Be Done?* Boston: Routledge and Kegan Paul, 1983, pp. 99–150.

13. Alford RR. *Health Care Politics: Ideological and Group Barriers to Reform.* Chicago: University of Chicago Press, 1975.

14. Ryan W. *Blaming the Victim.* New York: Random House, 1971.

15. Gur TR, King DS. *The State and the City.* Chicago: University of Chicago Press, 1987.

16. Elkin SL. *City and Regime in the American Republic.* Chicago: University of Chicago Press, 1987.

17. Schwartz DC, Ferlauto RC, Hoffman DN. *A New Housing Policy for America*. Philadelphia: Temple University Press, 1988.

18. Council of State Community Affairs Agencies. *State Housing Initiatives: A Compendium*. Washington, D.C.: COSCAA, 1986.

19. Council of State Housing Agencies. *Housing Initiatives of State Housing Finance Agencies*. Washington, D.C.: CHSA, 1987.

20. Sosin MR, Colson P., Grossman S. *Homelessness in Chicago: Poverty and Pathology, Social Institutions and Social Change*. Chicago: Chicago Community Trust, 1988.

21. Lindblom EN. Toward a comprehensive homelessness-prevention strategy. *Housing Policy Debate 2(3)*:957–1025, 1991.

22. Hartman C, Keating D, LeGates R, with Turner S. *Displacement: How to Fight It*. Berkeley, Calif.: National Housing Law Project, 1986.

PART V

Methodology

CHAPTER 22

The Size of the Homeless Population

René I. Jahiel, M.D., Ph.D.

Knowing the size of the homeless population is essential to planning effectively to provide housing, jobs, and public support to homeless people. Getting the necessary data is fraught with extraordinary difficulties. As yet, these difficulties have not been surmounted, but the causes of error have been pinpointed (1–3). In this chapter, I will discuss some key methodological issues before critically reviewing the history and results of studies of the size of various homeless populations in the 1980s and estimating the size of the homeless populations in the early 1990s.

Methodological Issues

THE DEFINITION AND CLASSIFICATION OF HOMELESSNESS

The population that is homeless on a given day can be cleaved in two ways to yield groups that differ considerably with regard to enumeration methods. The cleavage planes are those between doubled-up and literally homeless people, and between homeless people who use shelter or meal services and those who do not.

The term *the literal homeless* was coined by Rossi et al. (4) to refer to people who spend the night in shelters or on the streets. People who are temporarily in hospitals or jails, who squat, or who are in welfare hotels are usually included among the literally homeless. Literally homeless people may be enumerated by visiting the shelters, streets, or other sites where they are at night. However, there is no such access to people who are doubled up with other households, and indirect methods must be used for their enumeration.

Service-using homeless people may be accessed via the shelters, food services, or day centers that they use. Many literally homeless people use these services, but only a few doubled-up people do. Therefore, "literally homeless people" and "service-using homeless people" are categories that overlap markedly.

THE ACCURACY OF ENUMERATION

In considering the accuracy of enumeration, we must take into account investigators' ability to enumerate (via census or sample) *all* homeless people at the site or service under study, without including in the count people who are not homeless and without counting any given homeless person more than once.

Enumeration in shelters and other service facilities is at least a two-step process. The first step is to identify all the service facilities in the city or other geographic area under study. Shelters include not only general shelters for single men or women but also shelters restricted to families, youths, or battered women and children; detoxification centers; alcohol or drug treatment centers; residential centers for mentally ill people or AIDS patients which are used by homeless people; and small ad hoc shelters, for instance, in churches or synagogues. Food services include soup kitchens, pantries, meal services at shelters, and mobile meal services.

Since there is no national registry of facilities for homeless people, the facilities are usually identified with the help of "key informants," individuals who are presumably familiar with the local homeless population by virtue of their work as providers, advocates, police officers, governmental officials, and so on. The validity of this approach has been questioned, as will be discussed later. To try to identify all facilities, many investigators have used "snowballing," that is, one informant refers to other informants, and so on. This has been criticized because it may leave out facilities that are not part of the main network(s) (3). Aware of this problem, some investigators have used several rounds of identification of facilities by key informants, including at least one after the fieldwork is under way (5).

The second step is the enumeration of homeless people in the identified facilities or a sample thereof. Several pitfalls must be guarded against in interpreting the results of enumeration studies. Some facilities may not grant access. Homeless people must be enumerated directly, as opposed to counting the number of beds (the number of homeless people may be greater or less than the number of beds) or the number of meals served (one person may be served more than once). The timing of the enumeration is important, since at certain times of night the homeless people may not have arrived or may have already left. Finally, it must be ascertained whether domiciled people have been included in the count. This is generally not a problem in shelters, but it is a problem in meal services, which are used by domiciled as well as homeless people.

Enumeration on the streets also involves a two-step process. The first decision is whether to attempt a census (i.e., enumeration of all homeless people in a city or county) or whether to enumerate in a sample of areas and extrapolate the findings to the entire city or county. In the latter instance, the sample is usually stratified according to the expected density of the homeless population in the area predicted by key informants.

The second step is the identification and enumeration of homeless people on the streets. The term *the streets* includes a wide variety of sites: (a) the streets themselves (sidewalks, pavements, and alleyways); (b) parks, beaches, fields, woods, caves, riverbeds, or other uncovered areas, or areas under bridges or overpasses; (c) garages, toolsheds, construction sites, or other unoccupied work sites; (d) public or private buildings that let homeless people stay for the night, such as subway, bus, or train stations, airports, hospital emergency rooms, offices of agencies, coffeeshops, all-night theaters (for the price of an admission ticket), and so forth; (e) residential buildings' doorsteps, roofs, backyards, and courtyards, or (for squatters) empty apartments or houses; (f) underground tunnels or chambers; (g) parked vehicles and parking lots; and (h) moving vehicles (e.g., subways, buses, and trains).

The enumerators should familiarize themselves with the selected areas before the actual enumeration. Even so, it is difficult to make a complete enumeration. Some sites (for instance, the interiors of residential or business buildings, most underground tunnels or chambers, and moving vehicles) may be inaccessible to enumerators. Even in accessible sites, homeless people may be hard to see, since, for safety as well as privacy, they often find ways to make themselves inconspicuous. Further, they are often awake at night or sleep lightly, and may leave the area if they see enumerators, especially when the latter are accompanied by police personnel (1).

In general, the count is performed at night, when there are fewer domiciled people on the streets and the homeless people who use shelters have already left the street. However, the remaining domiciled people must be distinguished from homeless people. This is done in two ways, inspection or interrogation, either of which is prone to undercounting. Inspection relies on homeless people's typically unkempt appearance and tendency to carry their possessions with them. Homeless people who do not fit these stereotype tend to be left out. Interrogation means waking up or stopping people and asking them if they are homeless. Homeless people who do not want to identify themselves as such and say they are domiciled, who refuse to answer the question, or who leave before the enumerator has a chance to approach them are not counted.

Duplication (counting the same person twice) may also be a problem. This may occur when a homeless person meets the enumerators twice in the same area or when a homeless person spends part of the night in a shelter and part in the street and is counted in both places. Duplication is minimized by doing the counts during as short a period as possible, and by identifying homeless people by name and checking for duplicated names.

Key informants are used in facility-based counts to identify the facilities, and in street-based counts to classify locations according to the expected density of the homeless population. They may also be used as conduits to homeless people or to documents about homeless people. Roth et al. used as key informants the staff of religious or other voluntary organizations, community chests, welfare or children's services, mental health boards or health departments, hospital emergency services, cheap hotels and motels, the police, the media, and the like. They warned that "most homeless people are or can be nearly invisible to much of the formal service system . . . and that key informants were, by and large, unable to identify the characteristics of the overall homeless population in their community. Where they worked directly with segments of the homeless population, they tended to generalize the characteristics of that subgroup to the whole" (6:29–30).

Changes over Time

Over a period of a week to a month, homeless people often move between the streets, shelters, and hotels but move much less often between these sites and doubled-up accommodations (4,6,7). This suggests that a large part of the doubled-up population may be distinct from the street and shelter population.

The street-to-shelter ratio of homeless populations varies considerably with the season (4) and other factors. The range of street-to-shelter ratios reported between 1983 and 1985 was 0.35–2.74 (8). Thus, it is inadvisable to project the number of homeless people on the street from that in shelters, or vice versa, especially if no corrections are introduced for season, climate, and the availability of local shelter.

Point prevalence is the ratio of the number of people who are homeless in a given geographic area on a given night to the area's total population. *Annual prevalence* is the ratio of the number of people who have been homeless at some time during the year to the area's population. The prevalence of homeless people is usually given in numbers per either 1,000 or 10,000 total local population. The annual prevalence of homeless people may be obtained directly only for those who used shelters or other facilities during the year and whose names were recorded there.

The annual prevalence is sometimes extrapolated from the data on point prevalence as follows: From the point prevalence of homelessness on a given day and the number of people who have been homeless for stated durations on that day, the monthly incidence (the number of people who become homeless per month) is calculated. The annual prevalence is equal to the monthly incidence times 12, plus the number of people who have been homeless for one year or longer (4,9). However, this computation makes several assumptions, for instance, that both the monthly incidence and the duration of homelessness remain the same throughout the year, and that each person has only one episode of homelessness per year. The latter assumption is contradicted by the fact that recurrent homelessness is very frequent (7).

Changes in the size of the local homeless population over a period of years may be studied directly by repeat enumerations in the same area (10–12) or indirectly from serial studies of the demand for shelter (i.e., the number of people requesting shelter) as well as the unmet demand (i.e., the number of people turned away) (13–19). However, the latter approach provides data on only the demand for shelter. Changes in the demand for shelter do not necessarily reflect changes in the size of the homeless population, since an increase in the aggregate demand per shelter may be due to an increase in the demand for shelter per homeless person (e.g., because of a change in the number of shelters contacted by a homeless person during an episode of homelessness, or a change in the number of episodes of homelessness per person per year). Furthermore, this approach is not sensitive to changes in the number of homeless people who do not request shelter.

Point Prevalence: The Literally Homeless Population

ESTIMATES PROVIDED BY KEY INFORMANTS

The first national estimate of the homeless population done in the 1980s was based on telephone interviews of key informants in several U.S. cities and was conducted by the Community for Creative Non-Violence (CCNV) in 1982. It projected that there were 2–3 million homeless Americans at a given point in time (20). It came under severe attack for uncritical survey methodology and was represented as overstating the number of homeless people. Perhaps because of that, many subsequent researchers took pains to advance only "conservative" estimates, even if this led to underestimation.

The second national study was performed by the U.S. Department of Housing and Urban Development (HUD). It extrapolated various local estimates by key informants, including (a) the highest published estimates in 1980–83, (b) 500 interviews of key informants in 60 cities during January and February 1984, (c) a survey of 184 shelter operators in February 1984, and (d) the national shelter population multiplied by 1.78 to account for homeless people in the streets (21). The data set with the broadest base and the fewest a priori objections is the one derived from the 60 metropolitan areas. However, the validity of its results was attacked on several counts by expert witnesses at two congressional hearings (22,23). Apparently, the informants had provided estimates of the number of homeless people within city limits, but these figures had been divided by the populations of the Ranally Metropolitan Areas (RMAs) enclosing these cities, to obtain the homelessness rates in the RMAs. On average, each RMA has a population three times that of its principal city. Therefore, this error could have given rise to gross underestimation of homelessness rates. Furthermore, the study, which was done under pressure to obtain data very fast, was criticized for sloppiness (23). A third criticism was that contacts with key informants were made by "snowballing sampling." This may leave out entire groups of homeless people unknown to the particular informants selected (3).

Despite the wide publicity given to these criticisms, the HUD report was widely accepted by the federal government and was used to guide policy on homelessness. In addition, two secondary assertions it presented, which are also controversial, were widely used. These are the ratio of all homeless people to those in shelters, given as 2.7:1 by HUD (despite the evidence cited above that the fraction of homeless people in shelters varies widely); and the ratio of homeless people in metropolitan areas with a population over 250,000 to those in metropolitan areas with less than 250,000, given by HUD as 2:1 (24).

Tucker used the HUD study's data along with estimates for a few additional cities. In contrast with the HUD study, he used the population of the cities (not the RMAs) as denominator. He computed separate averages for small, medium, and large cities (25).

The National Alliance to End Homelessness used data from the HUD and Tucker studies for the principal cities of the RMAs. They found an average homelessness rate of 2.8 per 1,000 city population in these cities. Further, they assumed that the remainder of the RMAs and the nonmetropolitan areas had a homelessness rate one-third that of the principal cities, that is, 0.9 per 1,000 population (8).

Other estimates of homelessness rates have been given for a large number of cities in the Comprehensive Homelessness Assistance Plans (CHAPs) submitted by state homelessness agencies to HUD under Title IV-A of the Stuart B. McKinney Homeless Assistance Act (PL 100-77) (26); by the Council of State and Community Affairs Agencies, as reported by Schwartz and colleagues (27); and by various local studies (28–39).

THE ENUMERATION OF LITERALLY HOMELESS POPULATIONS

CENSUSES IN SHELTERS AND ON THE STREETS.   Eight census studies were performed at night in seven large cities with populations greater than 250,000: Phoenix (40); Pittsburgh (41); Nashville (42); Washington, D.C. (43); Boston (10); Omaha (44); and Birmingham, Alabama (45) (Table 22.1). The census was done at night by people familiar with the area's homeless population. There was no police escort (in Pittsburgh, police officers did the count in the course of their ordinary duties but did not escort enumerators). Homeless people were identified by inspection.

The uncorrected point prevalence ranged from 1 to 5 literally homeless people per 1,000 city population, with a mean of 2.7. Because the enumeration was by inspection, some domiciled people fitting the homeless stereotype may have been included, while homeless people who did not differ in appearance from the general population may have been excluded. Duplication, which was corrected for in the Pittsburgh study, may have contributed to some overcount-

TABLE 22.1   THE ENUMERATION OF LITERALLY HOMELESS PEOPLE
IN AMERICAN CITIES

City[a]	Year of Count	Number Homeless	City's Population (millions)	Rates of Homelessness (per 1,000)		
				×1	×1.5	×1.7
Cities in RMAS with Population Greater than 1 Million						
Phoenix (40)	1983	2,477	0.868	2.854	4.281	7.278
Pittsburgh (41)	1983	857	0.405	2.116	—	3.597
Washington, D.C. (43)	1985	2,562	0.628	4.082	—	6.939
Boston (10)	1986	2,863	0.566	5.058	—	8.599
Mean				3.528		6.603
Cities in RMAS with Population between 250,000 and 1 Million						
Nashville (42)	1983	914	0.469	1.949	2.924	4.970
Omaha (44)	1986	331	0.365	0.906	1.359	2.310
Birmingham (45)	1987	598	0.281	2.128	3.192	5.425
Mean				1.661	2.492	4.235

Note: The rationale for the correction factors is in the text.
[a]Numbers in parentheses are reference citations.

ing, but in general the design of the studies appears to preclude a large effect. A number of homeless people were not included because they were in inaccessible sites or avoided the enumerators. After extensive searches of sample areas in Washington, D.C., Robinson estimated that the counts should be multiplied by a factor of at least 1.7 to correct for undercounting in this type of enumeration (43).

In some cities (Phoenix, Nashville, Omaha, and Birmingham), counts were limited to the downtown area. This may cause a large undercount because, while the rest of the city has a much lower homeless population density, its area is much larger, so that the total homeless population that is missed is significant. For instance, Vernez et al. (9) found that the total homeless population in Alameda County's census blocks believed to have zero homeless population density was of the same order of magnitude as the total homeless population of the much smaller area composed of blocks with medium and high homeless population density.

In Table 22.1, counts from the cities in RMAs with more than 1 million population and those in RMAs with 250,000–1 million population are averaged separately. Three sets of estimates of the number of homeless people per 1,000 city inhabitants are given. They are derived, respectively, from uncorrected counts; counts multiplied by 1.5 (for those cities where counts were performed only downtown) to correct for homeless people in the rest of the city; and counts multiplied by 1.7, to correct for homeless people missed by enumerators. The

fully corrected mean homeless population densities are 6.603 per 1,000 and
4.235 per 1,000 in large and medium-sized cities, respectively.

STUDIES USING SAMPLING METHODOLOGY. In Chicago (4,46) and three
California counties (9), census blocks were classified by key informants according to expected homeless population density, and blocks with high expected
density were oversampled, while those with low or zero expected density were
either undersampled (Chicago) or omitted (California). Trained interviewers,
accompanied by police officers, approached people in the street at night to ask
them if they were homeless.

These studies of literally homeless people reported point prevalences ranging
from 0.357 per 1,000 (Orange County [9]) to 0.781 per 1,000 (one of the two
Chicago samples [4]). However, it has been argued that two fixed errors have
caused marked undercounting (1). First, a large number of homeless people in
the street may have refused to answer the interviewers or identify themselves as
homeless. Second, many homeless people may have left the block when they
saw interviewers arrive along with police officers. Appelbaum estimates that if
the homeless people missed because of these two errors had been included, the
count would have been double to quadruple the reported figure (1). It appears
that the shelter sample was also underestimated because several types of shelter
(e.g., battered women's shelters, youth shelters, and detoxification centers)
were not included. The California study is subject to similar criticism of its
street count, with the added problem that the areas expected to have zero
population density were not included in the study, although a check in one of the
counties showed that such areas may have up to 50 percent of the county's
homeless population (9).

THE ENUMERATION OF SERVICE-USING POPULATIONS

CENSUSES IN SHELTERS ONLY. A daily census of shelter or hotel accommodations for homeless people is available in several cities. For instance, in New
York City, the total number of people in facilities operated by the city was
27,459 in January 1988 (Table 22.2); at the same time, there were an estimated
1,000–1,500 homeless people in shelters operated by churches or synagogues
(47), for a grand total of some 28,750.

Momeni (48) attempted to estimate the total literally homeless population by
assuming a fixed ratio of homeless people in the street to those in shelters, using
HUD's 2.3 multiplier (21) or Freeman and Hall's 3.23 multiplier (49). As stated
earlier, this practice is unwarranted because of the large variance in that ratio in
different cities, seasons, or years (8).

SAMPLING IN SHELTERS AND MEAL SERVICES. Urban Institute researchers estimated the service-using homeless population of cities with 100,000 or greater

TABLE 22.2   THE NUMBER OF HOMELESS PEOPLE IN THE NEW YORK CITY
SHELTER SYSTEM

	Average Daily Number of Homeless People[a]			
		Homeless Families		Total[b] of
Year	Single Individuals	Families	Individuals	Individuals
1981	2,703	750	2,550	5,253
1982	3,752	1,088	3,699	7,451
1983	4,518	2,042	6,943	11,461
1984	6,110	2,943	10,006	16,116
1985	7,184	3,554	12,084	19,268
1986	8,805	4,183	14,222	23,027
1987	10,004	4,962	16,871	26,935
1988	9,939	5,153	17,520	27,459
1989	10,319	3,985	13,549	23,808

Sources: Data are from New York City Human Resources Administration.

[a]The figures refer to counts of single individuals in public shelters on one night in January and counts of families in public shelters on one night in June. Families were assumed to have a mean of 3.4 members. The count did not include the following: individuals or families in emergency shelters of churches or synagogues on winter nights (estimated at 500–1,500 persons); and single individuals or families who spent the night "on the street"; who were in transitional apartments, hospitals, or jails; or who doubled up with other households.

[b]Sum of the number of single individuals and that of individuals in homeless families.

population in March 1987 (5). They used a two-stage probability sample, with an initial sampling of 20 cities and then a random sample of 381 providers of services, including meal services, shelters with meals, and shelters without meals. The services were identified by a multicycle snowballing approach, with the last cycle when the researchers were in the field. A sophisticated sampling and weighting design was used (50). "Service use" was defined as use of a meal service or shelter at least once during the week of the study. There were 194,017 service-using homeless adults in U.S. cities with populations over 100,000, for a service-using adult homelessness rate of 3.17 per 1,000 population (5).

THE CAPTURE-RECAPTURE TECHNIQUE.   This method estimates the total service-using homeless population of a given geographical area by doing a series of at least two enumerations of the population using the services at a given time. The members of the population using the services are identified by name or other distinguishing features at each enumeration, and the size of the total service-using population is derived from the fraction of the homeless population common to the two enumerations (3). Cowan et al. listed several assumptions that must be satisfied, including homogeneous observation proba- bility, stationarity of the population in the area, and constant size of the population during the observation period, and they point out that since it is unlikely that homeless populations meet these assumptions, the results must be interpreted with caution (3). The method has been used only once in the United States, in four pairs of data from shelters in Baltimore, which yielded a shelter-using population of 874–1,022 among 760,000 Baltimoreans in 1986, corresponding to a rate of 1.15–1.35 per 1,000 (3).

Point Prevalence: The Doubled-up Population

An attempt to enumerate families doubled-up with other households in Boston was performed during one month in the fall of 1983. It yielded 981 unduplicated cases, that is, 1.75 families per 1,000 population, or 6.125 individuals per 1,000 population. Yet this study markedly underestimated Boston's doubled-up population, since (a) 3 out of 15 communities were not included; (b) four organizations refused to participate for fear of reprisals against their clients; (c) only families who had been in contact with service organizations were included; and (d) only families with children were included (10). The collection of data over a period of a month represents a slight deviation from point prevalence, expected to cause a slight overestimate.

In New York City, an indirect approach was used. The total residential water consumption was determined, and on the basis of the difference between the actual consumption and that expected if only the members of the household on record were in the housing unit, it was estimated that there were 69,000 families (i.e., 9.8 families per 1,000 population) doubled-up with other households at any given time in 1987 (51). Assuming a mean family size of 3.5, there would be 241,500 doubled-up individuals in New York City, or 34.3 per 1,000 population. Another estimate was 35,000 households doubling in public housing and 73,000 in private housing, for a total of 108,000 doubled-up households in New York City in the early 1980s (52). Assuming a mean family size of 3.5, there would be 378,000 doubled-up individuals in New York City, or 54.0 per 1,000 population.

Projections of National Point Prevalence: Literal Homelessness

Estimates of the national point prevalence of literally homeless or service-using homeless people reflect the relative accuracy of the local estimates and the assumptions used in extrapolating the national figure. The CCNV's projection of 2–3 million homeless people in 1982–83 was based on local estimates by key informants in several cities (20). It is not possible to ascertain the accuracy of the local figures; furthermore, the extrapolation did not take into account the presumed variation in different types of urban and nonurban areas. The estimate by Schwartz et al. of 600,000–1 million homeless people was derived from data presented in applications for funds by area planners who had obtained it from key informants, local surveys, or various secondary sources (27); again, there is no way of assessing the accuracy of the local estimates or of the extrapolation procedure used.

Three national estimates are based in whole or in part on HUD's 1984 60-city survey. They are those of HUD itself (21); of Tucker (who added estimates from a few more cities and corrected the denominator population that is likely to have been in error in HUD's computation (25); and of the National Alliance to End Homelessness (referred to hereafter as "the Alliance"). The Alliance's estimate was derived from HUD's and Tucker's data and used more sophisticated methods of weighing estimates from different types of urban and nonurban areas in performing the national extrapolation. It projected 368,000–736,000 homeless people in 1988 (8).

Burt and Cohen's data from samples of service-using homeless people in cities over 100,000 people were extrapolated to 679,231 homeless people in March 1987 (5).

The estimates yielded by the more recent studies (i.e., excluding the CCNV and HUD estimates) tend to cluster between 600,000 and 800,000. This has given credence to the proposition that literally homeless people do not number more than 1 million, even after allowance has been made for the growth of the population since the latest results. However, I will show in the next sections that this clustering is due to the use of similar assumptions in the studies.

CRITIQUE OF ASSUMPTIONS USED IN PROJECTIONS

The studies of the Alliance (8) and of Burt and Cohen (5,50) are the only ones that will be discussed, since they are the only recent studies that give all the details of calculations.

The Alliance (8) assumed first that HUD's national metropolitan figure of 210,000 was a correct estimate of the literally homeless population of the RMA's principal cities on a given night early in 1984. This corresponds to a rate of 2.8 per 1,000. Second, it assumed that the literal homelessness rate of the remaining RMA areas and nonmetropolitan areas was about one-third that of the principal cities, that is, 0.9 per 1,000, yielding an estimate of 145,000 literally homeless people outside the principal cities. Adding the two gave a national estimate of 355,000 (i.e., 1.5 per 1,000) in February 1984. The Alliance extrapolated the data to a lower bound of 368,000 and an upper bound of 736,000 in 1988, on the basis of assumed yearly average rates of growth of the homeless population of 1 percent and 20 percent, respectively.

Burt and Cohen (5,50) used as starting points the number of homeless adults who had used shelter or meal services in their sample of cities with more than 100,000 inhabitants at least once during a seven-day period in March 1987, and

RENÉ I. JAHIEL

they projected an adult, service-using homeless population of 194,017 in all U.S. cities with more than 100,000 inhabitants. Further, they raised that number by 15 percent to account for homeless children, and by another 33 percent to account for non-service-using homeless people, thus arriving at an estimate of 343,005 literally homeless people in cities with more than 100,000 population, that is, a rate of 5.6 per 1,000.

Finally, they assumed that the homelessness rate in the remainder of the metropolitan areas of cities with more than 100,000 inhabitants, in other metropolitan areas, and in nonmetropolitan areas was one-third that of the cities with more than 100,000 inhabitants, that is, 1.87 per 1,000. With this assumption, they calculated that there were 230,945 literally homeless people in these other metropolitan areas and 105,281 in nonmetropolitan areas, for a total literally homeless population of 679,231 in the United States in March 1987. Burt and Cohen did not attempt to extrapolate their estimate to future years (5,50).

Two critical assumptions have to be examined, one regarding the multiplier used to extrapolate from the homeless population of each RMA's principal city to that of the whole country, and the other regarding the yearly rate of growth of that population.

With regard to the first assumption, both the Alliance (8) and Burt and Cohen (5,50) assumed that the homeless population density outside of the principal cities was one-third that of the cities. This is based on very flimsy evidence, namely, the study of one suburban area, Fairfax County (8), which yielded a homeless population of density about one-third that of the area's principal city, Washington, D.C. Not only does this constitute a sample of $N = 1$, but the Fairfax County study has some unusual features. For instance, the fraction of homeless people in institutions (jails, hospitals, and treatment centers) was 30 percent (8), a much larger figure than that reported in other sites (4). It might thus be inferred that a considerable number of homeless people in the streets or fields of Fairfax County were missed in the count. Furthermore, Fairfax County is a rich county, with a primarily middle-class population, unlike many other peripheral areas of RMAs, some of which have very low median incomes. The other evidence advanced by both studies—comparison of homeless populations in wards of Washington, D.C., with high and low homeless population densities—is not relevant, as it concerns intracity comparison.

On the other hand, the estimates of the homeless populations in 82 cities of various sizes located in metropolitan areas of various sizes provided by HUD workers (21) and by Tucker (25) and reproduced in the report *Housing and Homelessness* (8:53–54) show a considerable heterogeneity of homeless population density within each category. The homelessness rate of the peripheral cities of an RMA was often of the same order as, or higher than, that of the principal city (e.g., Newark, 9.6 per 1,000, v. New York, 4.0 per 1,000; Santa Monica, 10.2 per 1,000, v. Los Angeles, 10.5 per 1,000) in 1984 (8). Secondary analysis of the 82-city data showed that large, medium-sized, and small cities had average homelessness rates of 4.5–4.8 per 1,000 population in RMAs with more than 1 million inhabitants, and 1.4–2.8 per 1,000 in RMAs of 250,000–1 million inhabitants; and medium-sized and small cities had average rates of 0.9 and 1.8, respectively, in RMAs with less than 250,000 inhabitants (Table 22.3). Thus, the homelessness rate appears to be more related to the size of the RMA than to that of the city within the RMA (Table 22.3). These findings are not compatible with the assumption that the homelessness rate in that part of the RMA outside its principal city is one-third that of the principal city.

With regard to the second assumption, the main source of information is the United States Conference of Mayors' annual survey of the demand for shelter in some 25 cities (19). There is considerable variance among cities. For instance, increased demand for shelter ranged across cities from 0 percent to 70 percent in 1989 (18). As discussed earlier, a change in the demand for shelter may be due to a change in the number of homeless people, in the relative number of homeless people who ask for shelter, or in the number of times a given individual asks for shelter. It is unlikely that any single factor is responsible for the entire 20-percent average yearly increase in demand for shelter during the period 1985–90, but there are no data to show how much each factor contributed.

ESTIMATED NATIONAL LITERALLY HOMELESS POPULATION USING ALTERNATIVE ASSUMPTIONS

Table 22.4 shows how different assumptions about the two parameters discussed above affect projections of the literally homeless population of the United States on a given night early in 1990. Three sets of nine estimates each were generated with the Alliance data (8), the Burt-Cohen data (5,50), and the seven-city data of Table 22.1 (10,40–45), respectively.

Inspection of Table 22.4 shows that the assumptions used in making national extrapolations are a much more important determinant of the variance of the estimates than is the source of the data. Indeed, when the same assumptions are used with data from the different sources, the estimates tend to converge. Therefore, decisions about the likelihood of particular estimates are actually decisions about the likelihood that the assumptions used are correct. Table 22.4 shows mean values of subsets of the 27 estimates, grouped on the basis of the assumptions used. At the low end, the assumptions are that the number of homeless people has remained stationary over the years and that the homelessness rate in the remainder of the RMA is one-third that in its principal city; with these assumptions, the mean estimated point prevalence is 526,000 literally homeless individuals on a given night of 1990. At high end, the assumptions are that the number of homeless people has been increasing at an average rate of 20 percent per year and that the homelessness rate in the remainder of the RMA is the same as that of the principal city; with these assumptions, the mean estimated point prevalence is 2,322,000 literally homeless individuals on the same

TABLE 22.3   MEAN NUMBER OF HOMELESS INDIVIDUALS PER 1,000 CITY POPULATION

City Population	RMA Population					
	>1 Million		250,000–1 Million		<1 Million	
	I[a]	II[b]	I	II	I	II
250,000	4.8	4.2	1.4	1.5	—	—
100,000–250,000	4.8	4.6	2.8	3.5	0.9	1.1
<100,000	4.5	3.9	1.7	1.6	1.8	1.7

Source: Calculated from data in National Alliance to End Homelessness, *Housing and Homelessness*. Washington, D.C.: The Alliance, 1988, pp. 53–54.

[a]I, mean obtained by dividing the total number of homeless people in the cities in a given category by the total population of the cities in that category. In the RMAs with more than 1 million people, there were 32 cities with more than 250,000 people, 5 cities with 100,000–250,000, and 4 cities with less than 100,000. In the RMAs with 250,000–1 million people, there were 9 cities with 250,000–1 million people; 14 cities with 100,000–250,000; and 6 cities with less than 100,000. In the RMAs with less than 250,000 people, there were 4 cities with 100,000 to 250,000 people; and 8 cities with less than 100,000 people.

[b]II, mean calculated by dividing the sum of the number of homeless people per 1,000 population for all the cities in the category by the number of cities in the category.

night. Thus, using the same data, with the same definition of homelessness, one can obtain a national estimate anywhere between these two extrema by using differing combinations of assumptions about the two parameters under consideration.

The Annual Prevalence of Literal Homelessness

There are few, if any, reliable estimates of the annual prevalence of literal homelessness. A rule of thumb used by many administrators is that the annual prevalence is twice the point prevalence. In the Rand study, annual prevalence was computed from data on point prevalence and duration of homelessness; the calculated ratios of annual prevalence to point prevalence were 5.8, 3.4, and 2.3 in Orange, Alameda, and Yolo counties, respectively (9). As discussed earlier, the assumptions made to allow this type of computation have not been validated empirically. Thus the multiplier used to compute annual prevalence from point prevalence may range from two to six. Applying these multipliers to the extrema of projected point prevalence would yield extrema of annual prevalence on the order of 1.5 and 12 million people who are literally homeless at some point in the year.

TABLE 22.4 ESTIMATES, USING DIFFERING PARAMETERS, OF THE POINT PREVALENCE OF LITERAL HOMELESSNESS IN THE UNITED STATES, SPRING 1990

Source of Data[a] and Year of Data Collection[b]	Multiplier for Growth over Time of Literally Homeless Population	Homeless Individuals (in millions), by Multiplier for Rest of Metropolitan Area		
		Low Multiplier	Middle Multiplier	High Multiplier
Alliance, 1984 (8)	1.00	0.355	0.596	0.877
	1.772	0.629	1.056	1.554
	2.986	1.060	1.779	2.619
Burt and Cohen, 1987 (5, 50)	1.00	0.679	0.909	1.140
	1.33	0.903	1.209	1.156
	1.73	1.175	1.573	1.972
Seven cities, 1985 (10, 40–45)	1.00	0.545	0.749	0.954
	1.61	0.877	1.206	1.535
	2.49	1.537	1.866	2.375
Mean of 3 cells with lowest multipliers	0.526			
Mean of 3 central cells		1.157		
Mean of 3 cells with middle yearly and high area multiplier				1.535
Mean of 3 cells with highest multipliers				2.322

Note: The determination of the multipliers for growth over time and for the remainder of the metropolitan area is discussed in the appendix to this chapter.

[a]Numbers in parentheses are reference citations.

[b]Most of the Alliance's data were collected in February 1984. Burt and Cohen's data were collected during one week of March 1987. The data from the seven cities (Table 22.1) were collected between 1983 and 1987; the mean date was early 1985.

Projections of the Doubled-up Homeless Population in the United States

The data from the Boston and New York studies summarized in the discussion on point prevalence (10,51,52) are the only ones based on actual measurements. Extrapolation to the U.S. population of about 240 million would yield a national point prevalence of 420,000 doubled-up families, or 1.47 million individuals, according to the Boston data; 2.352 million doubled-up families, or 8.2 million individuals, with the first set of New York data; and 3.696 doubled-up families or 12.94 million individuals with the second set of New York data (assuming a mean family size of 3.5). Since there is little or no information on the duration of episodes of doubled-up homelessness, or on the rate of growth of the doubled-up homeless population, it is not possible to extrapolate from these estimates to annual prevalence or to update the estimate. Furthermore, the assumption of a 3.5-person average doubled-up household is not backed by hard data. The average household size might be smaller than that figure if there is a significantly larger than expected number of single doubled-up individuals.

Estimates for Purposes of Planning

At a certain point, planners must shift from discussing ranges of values to estimating specific numbers of homeless individuals, households, and children. Estimates are in part subjective, being based on the planner's judgment about alternative assumptions and his or her decision to risk underestimating more than overestimating or vice versa. To conclude this chapter, I would like to give the estimates I would select and the reasons why.

THE MULTIPLIER FOR THE MEAN YEARLY INCREASE. I would select 10 percent, because increased recurrence of homelessness within the same year, increased demand by one person to several shelters, and increased demand by doubled-up people elicited by increased supply of shelter might contribute, along with increased prevalence of homelessness, to the reported 20-percent mean yearly increase.

THE MULTIPLIER FOR THE HOMELESS POPULATION IN THE REMAINDER OF THE RMA. I would make two alternative selections: 1.0, and 0.67. I selected the first figure because I believe that the concept of a homeless population localized in the principal city of the RMA is not accurate anymore. It does not take into account the facts that many peripheral cities have low-income and homeless populations as large as that of the principal city (e.g., Newark and New York), and that some middle-class peripheral cities have large homeless populations (e.g., Santa Monica) (8:53–54). I am using the second figure because it is the mean of the figure of 0.33 usually given for this correction and 1.0.

   I would also assume that 25 percent of homeless individuals are children (18), that the members of homeless families constitute 36 percent of homeless individuals (18), and that the average homeless family size is 3.5.

THE NATIONAL POINT PREVALENCE OF LITERAL HOMELESSNESS. Applying the above assumptions to data from Table 22.4 would yield the following range (corresponding to the 0.33 and 1.0 estimates for the multiplier for the remainder of the RMA, respectively):

• Homeless individuals, 1,157,000–1,535,000;

- Homeless children, 289,000–384,000; and
- Homeless households, 856,000–1,136,000.

THE ANNUAL PREVALENCE OF LITERAL HOMELESSNESS. I would select an annual-prevalence-to-point-prevalence ratio of 2.0:1.0, according to the consensus among homelessness service providers. This would yield:

- Homeless individuals, 2,314,000–3,070,000;
- Homeless children, 578,000–768,000; and
- Homeless households, 1,712,000–2,272,000.

THE POINT PREVALENCE OF DOUBLED-UP HOMELESSNESS. I would select 31.5 doubled-up individuals and 9.0 doubled-up households per 1,000 population, as this is the mean of the Boston (10) and the two New York figures (51,52). Since the data of at least one study (10) refer only to families with children, I assume that all households consist of families and that family size is 3.5, and that the U.S. population is approximately 240 million.

- National point prevalence of doubled-up individuals: 7.56 million; and
- National point prevalence of doubled-up households: 2.16 million

This estimate of the number of doubled-up households would be too low if there is a higher-than-expected number of one-person doubled-up households.

Suggestions for Future Research

The analysis presented in this chapter has highlighted causes of uncertainty in estimating the homeless population. Addressing these causes may lead to a more accurate estimate of the size of the homeless population.

The development of an appropriate scheme of stratified sampling across cities in studies designed to project the size of the national homeless population is, as discussed in this chapter, one of the most important problems. More research of the kind done by Tucker (25) with towns and cities as units of analysis is needed to find better predictors of their homelessness rates based on town or city size, RMA size, and various characteristics of the towns or cities such as poverty rate, housing characteristics, welfare policies, demographic composition, industrial base, and geographical location. Such data are readily available, as are estimates of the homeless populations in a large number of cities, so that a preliminary study could be done with secondary analysis of existing data.

Empirical studies of the yearly demand for shelter should be performed to obtain data on the frequency of recurrence of homelessness within the same year, multiple demand by the same individual during the same episode of homelessness, and variables accounting for the relative frequency of use of shelter versus street, doubling up, or other options. Season, geographic location, capacity and quality of shelters in the area, and availability of alternatives to shelter in the area are some of variables. With such data, one could identify the portion of the change in demand which is due to change in the point prevalence of homelessness and thereby estimate the latter more accurately.

Research is needed on methods of enumerating people who are homeless "on the street." Comparative studies of figures obtained by inspection and those obtained by questioning in certain selected sites might be a first step, along with intensive studies of the same sites to estimate the numbers of homeless people missed, as in Robinson's study (43). Qualitative, ethnographic studies of differing sites might help to better adapt enumeration methodology to the site under investigation. More intensive attention to intracity or intracounty sampling design may be desirable.

More investigations of service-using populations with the capture-recapture method would be helpful, particularly with more investigation of deviations from the assumptions used in the calculations (3) and more use of corrections to account for deviations from these assumptions.

Finally, research is also needed on methods of estimating the number of homeless people who are doubled up with other households. Comparative studies in a given geographic area with the two methods now available (social service agencies in the area and excess over expected water consumption) might be a first step. Replication in a large number of cities or counties is needed in order to study the distribution of doubled-up homeless households in U.S. cities or counties and to identify features of cities or counties which may be associated with differing prevalence of doubling up. Information is needed on the length and recurrence of doubling-up episodes of homelessness.

Appendix: Multipliers Used in Table 22.4

MULTIPLIER FOR GROWTH OVER TIME. In each series, the number of literally homeless people is extrapolated to spring 1990, assuming no increase since the data were collected (first value), an average yearly increase of 10 percent (second value), or on average yearly increase of 20 percent (third value). The multipliers differ in the three studies because of the different time interval between data collection and spring 1990.

MULTIPLIER FOR REMAINDER OF METROPOLITAN AREA. In each study, the data were collected in large cities, and the number of literally homeless people in the rest of the cities' metropolitan area, smaller cities, and nonmetropolitan areas was extrapolated using certain assumptions.

1. In the Alliance's study (8), the average homelessness rate in the principal cities of the Ranally Metropolitan Areas (RMAs) was estimated at 2.8 per 1,000, i.e., 210,000 homeless people among 75 million inhabitants of these cities. The average homelessness rate in all other areas was assumed to be one-third of that in the RMAs' principal cities, or 0.9 per 1,000, i.e., 145,000 homeless people among 161 million people, resulting in a national literally homeless population of 355,000 at the time of the study (first row, under "Low").

I reanalyzed the same data by breaking down further the cities and RMAs in categories according to size. The analysis presented in Table 22.3 shows that the size of the RMA rather than that of the city determines the homelessness rate. Therefore the data on individual cities and RMAs shown in the Alliance's report (8:53–54) were used to compute average homelessness rates in cities from RMAs of different sizes. The rates per 1,000 population were 4.8, 2.3, 1.2, and 0.9, respectively, in RMAs with more than 1 million inhabitants (total population, 147,239,664), RMAs with 250,000–1 million inhabitants (total population, 59,226,211), RMAs with less than 250,000 inhabitants (total population, 25,483,788), and nonmetropolitan areas (total population, 3,775,376). Multiplying the rates by the corresponding total populations yielded homeless populations of 706,750; 136,220; 30,581; and 3,398, respectively, adding up to a national homeless population of 876,949, or approximately 0.877 million at the time of the study (first row, under "High").

An intermediate set of assumptions was used to yield a middle estimate. The homelessness rates were assumed to be 3.2 per 1,000 in RMAs with more than 1 million inhabitants (i.e., two-thirds of the multiplier used above); 1.53 per 1,000 in RMAs with 250,000–1 million inhabitants (also two-thirds of the multiplier used above); 1.2 per 1,000 in RMAs with less than 250,000 inhabitants; and 0.9 per 1,000 in nonmetropolitan areas (same multiplier as above), yielding homeless populations of 471,167; 90,616; 30,581; and 3,398, respectively, in these area categories and adding up to a national literally homeless population of 595,762, or approximately 0.596 million, at the time of the study (first row, under "Middle").

2. Burt and Cohen (5,50) divided the U.S. population into: A, cities of 100,000 population or more (61.2 million inhabitants in 1986); B, the remainder of the metropolitan areas of these cities, and other metropolitan areas (123.5 million in 1986); and C, nonmetropolitan areas (53.6 million in 1986). Their sample of cities with 100,000 or greater population yielded, after adjustment for homeless children and non-service-using homeless people, a homelessness rate of 5.6 per 1,000, i.e., 343,005 homeless individuals in A. They assumed that the rate in areas B and C was one-third that in area A, i.e., 1.867 per 1,000, yielding estimated homeless populations of 230,945 in B and 105,281 in C, and therefore a national homeless population of 679,231 in March 1987 (fourth row, under "Low").

In analyzing the same data, I assumed that the homelessness rate in B was the same as that in A (based on the data of Table 22.3), yielding 691,600 homeless people in B, and I used the same A and C estimates as Burt and Cohen, thus yielding a national homeless population of 1,139,886 in March 1987 (fourth row, under "High").

For the intermediate set of assumptions, the homelessness rate in B was taken as two-thirds of that in A, i.e., 3.733 per 1,000, yielding 461,026 homeless people in B, and a national homeless population estimate of 909,312 in March 1987 (fourth row, under "Middle").

3. To extrapolate a national estimate from the seven-city data (10,40–45), I grouped the cities into those in RMAs with more than 1 million inhabitants (Phoenix, Pittsburgh, Washington, D.C., and Boston) and those in RMAs with 250,000—1 million inhabitants (Nashville, Omaha, and Birmingham). Two sets of estimates are available for each city: unadjusted count, and count adjusted for presumably missed homeless persons. Since there is no general agreement on the validity of this adjustment, I used the average of the adjusted and unadjusted mean in these computations. Thus I used 5.065 per 1,000 as the homelessness rate for cities in RMAs with more than 1 million inhabitants and 2.948 per 1,000 as that of RMAs with 250,000–1 million inhabitants. Since there were no data on the number of homeless people in RMAs with less than 250,000 inhabitants or in nonmetropolitan areas, the rates derived in the Alliance's report (8:54) were used, i.e., 1.2 per 1,000 and 0.9 per 1,000, respectively. I assumed that one-third of the large and medium RMAs' inhabitants were in the principal cities and two-thirds were in the remainder of the RMAs.

To estimate the national populations, I used the same estimates of the number of inhabitants of the three types of RMAs and the nonmetropolitan areas as in the Alliance's report (8). The national homeless population estimates were derived with three alternative assumptions—that the homelessness rate in the remainder of the RMA was one-third that of its principal city, two-thirds of it, or the same, yielding national homeless population estimates of 544,868 (seventh row, under "Low"), 749,291 (seventh row, under "Middle"), and 953,637 (seventh row, under "High"), respectively, for 1985.

References

1. Appelbaum RP. Counting the homeless. In Momeni J (ed.), *Homelessness in the United States: Data and Issues.* New York: Praeger, 1990, pp. 1–16.

2. General Accounting Office. *Homeless Mentally Ill: Problems and Options in Estimating Numbers and Trends.* GAO/PEMD-88-24. Washington, D.C.: Government Printing Office, 1988.

3. Cowan CD, Breakey WR, Fischer PJ. The methodology of counting the homeless. In Institute of Medicine, *Homelessness, Health, and Human Needs.* Washington, D.C.: National Academy Press, 1988, pp. 169–182.

THE SIZE OF THE HOMELESS POPULATION

4. Rossi PH, et al. The urban homeless: Estimating composition and size. *Science* *235*:1336–1341, 1987.

5. Burt MR, Cohen BE. *America's Homeless: Numbers, Characteristics, and Programs That Serve Them.* Washington, D.C.: Urban Institute, 1989.

6. Roth D, et al. *Homelessness in Ohio: A Study of People in Need.* Columbus: Ohio State Department of Mental Health, February 1985.

7. Farr RK, Koegel P, Burnam A. *A Study of Homelessness in the Skid Row Area of Los Angeles.* Los Angeles: Los Angeles County Department of Mental Health, 1986.

8. National Alliance to End Homelessness. *Housing and Homelessness.* Washington, D.C.: The Alliance, 1988.

9. Vernez G, et al. *Review of California's Program for the Homeless Mentally Disabled.* Santa Monica, Calif.: Rand Corporation, 1988.

10. City of Boston Emergency Shelter Commission. *The October Project: Seeing the Obvious Problem.* Boston: City of Boston, October 1983.

11. City of Boston. *Making Room: Comprehensive Policy for the Homeless.* Boston: City of Boston, 1986.

12. Lee BA. Homelessness in Tennessee. In Momeni J (ed.), *Homelessness in the United States: State Surveys.* New York: Praeger, 1989, pp. 181–203.

13. United States Conference of Mayors. *Status Report: Emergency Food, Shelter, and Energy Programs in 20 Cities.* Washington, D.C.: The Conference, January 1984.

14. Waxman LD, Reyes LM. *The Growth of Hunger, Homelessness, and Poverty in America's Cities, 1985.* Washington, D.C.: United States Conference of Mayors, 1986.

15. Reyes LM, Waxman LD. *The Continued Growth of Hunger, Homelessness, and Poverty in America's Cities, 1986.* Washington, D.C.: United States Conference of Mayors, December 1986.

16. Partnership for the Homeless. *National Growth of Homelessness, Winter 1987.* New York: The Partnership, March 1987.

17. Waxman LD, Reyes LM. *A Status Report on Hunger and Homelessness in America's Cities, 1988.* Washington, D.C.: United States Conference of Mayors, January 1989.

18. Reyes LM, Waxman LD. *A Status Report on Hunger and Homelessness in America's Cities, 1989.* Washington, D.C.: United States Conference of Mayors, December 1989.

19. Waxman LD, Reyes LM. *A Status Report on Hunger and Homelessness in America's Cities, 1990.* Washington, D.C.: United States Conference of Mayors, December 1990.

20. Hombs ME, Snyder M. *Homelessness in America: A Forced March to Nowhere.* Washington, D.C.: Community for Creative Non-Violence, 1982.

21. U.S. Department of Housing and Urban Development. *A Report to the Secretary on the Homeless and Emergency Shelters.* Washington, D.C.: HUD, May 1984.

22. House Committee on Banking, Finance, and Urban Affairs, and Committee on Government Operations. *HUD Report on Homelessness.* Joint Hearing before the Subcommittees on Housing and Community Development and on Manpower and Housing, 98th Cong., 2d sess., May 24, 1984. Washington, D.C.: Government Printing Office, 1984.

23. House Committee on Banking, Finance, and Urban Affairs. *HUD Report on Homelessness—II.* Hearing before the Subcommittee on Housing and Community Development, 98th Cong., 1st sess., December 4, 1985. Washington, D.C.: Government Printing Office, 1986.

24. Peroff K. Who are the homeless? And how many are there? In Bingham RD, Green RE, White SB (eds.), *The Homeless in Contemporary Society.* Newbury Park, Calif.: Sage Publications, 1987.

25. Tucker W. Where do the homeless come from? *National Review* (*September 25*): 32–43, 1987.

26. Walker L. *Homelessness in the States*. Lexington, Ky.: Council of State Governments, 1989.

27. Schwartz DC, Ferlauto RC, Hoffman DN. *A New Housing Policy for America*. Philadelphia: Temple University Press, 1988, p. 26.

28. New York State Department of Social Services. *Homeless in New York State*. Report to the Governor and the Legislature. Albany, N.Y.: The Department, October 1984.

29. Health and Welfare Council of Central Maryland. *Where Do You Go from Nowhere? Homelessness in Maryland*. Baltimore: The Council, 1986.

30. Morrow-Jones HA, van Vliet W. Homelessness in Colorado. In Momeni (ed.), *Homelessness: State Surveys*, pp. 21–37. See ref. 12.

31. Timmer DA, Knottnerus JD. Homelessness in Florida. In Momeni (ed.), *Homelessness: State Surveys*, pp. 39–56. See ref. 12.

32. Kivisto P. Homelessness in the frostbelt: The case of Illinois. In Momeni (ed.), *Homelessness: State Surveys*, pp. 57–71. See ref. 12.

33. Kunz JS. Homelessness in Missouri: Population, problems, and policy. In Momeni (ed.), *Homelessness: State Surveys*, pp. 92–112. See ref. 12.

34. Gioglio GR. Homelessness in New Jersey: The social service network and the people served. In Momeni (ed.), *Homelessness: State Surveys*, pp. 113–129. See ref. 12.

35. Hirschl T, Momeni JA. Homelessness in New York: A demographic and socioeconomic analysis. In Momeni (ed.), *Homelessness: State Surveys*, pp. 131–144. See ref. 12.

36. Blake GF, Abbott ML. Homelessness in the Pacific Northwest. In Momeni (ed.), *Homelessness: State Surveys*, pp. 166–180. See ref. 12.

37. Baker SG, Snow DA. Homelessness in Texas: Examination of population size and demographic configuration. In Momeni (ed.), *Homelessness: State Surveys*, pp. 206–217. See ref. 12.

38. Maurin JT, Russell L. Homelessness in Utah. In Momeni (ed.), *Homelessness: State Surveys*, pp. 219–231. See ref. 12.

39. Bromley DJ, et al. Homelessness in Virginia: Dimensions of the problem and the public reaction. In Momeni (ed.), *Homelessness: State Surveys*, pp. 234–250. See ref. 12.

40. Brown C, et al. *The Homeless of Phoenix: Who Are They? And What Should Be Done?* Phoenix, Ariz.: South Phoenix Community Mental Health Center, June 1983.

41. Winograd K. *Street People and Other Homeless: A Pittsburgh Study*. Pittsburgh, Pa.: Alleghany County MH-MR-DA Program, August 1983.

42. Wiegand RB. Counting the homeless. *American Demographics* 7(12):34–37, 1985.

43. Robinson FG. *Homeless People in the Nation's Capital*. Washington, D.C.: University of the District of Columbia, Center for Applied Research and Urban Policy, 1985.

44. Luke JS. *A Preliminary Study of the Homeless in Omaha-Douglas County*. Omaha, Neb.: University of Nebraska, Center for Applied Urban Research, August 1986.

45. La Gory M, et al. Homelessness in Alabama: A variety of people and experiences. In Momeni (ed.), *Homelessness: State Surveys*, pp. 1–20. See ref. 12.

46. Rossi PH, Fisher GA, Willis G. *The Condition of the Homeless in Chicago*. Amherst, Mass.: University of Massachusetts at Amherst, Social and Demographic Research Institute, 1986.

47. Tobier E. The homeless. In Brecher C, Horton RD (eds.), *Setting Municipal Priorities, 1990*. New York: New York University Press, 1989, pp. 307–336.

48. Momeni JA. No place to go: A national picture of homelessness in America. In Momeni (ed.), *Homelessness: Data and Issues*, pp. 165–183. See ref. 1.

49. Freeman R, Hall B. Permanent homelessness in America? *Population Research and Policy Review* 6:3–27, 1987.

50. Burt MR, Cohen BE. *Feeding the Homeless: Does the Prepared Meal Provision Help?*

Vol. 2, pt. 2, sect. B. Washington, D.C.: Urban Institute, 1988.

51. Stegman MA. Housing. In Brecher, Horton (eds.), *Setting Municipal Priorities,* pp. 197–219. See ref. 47.

52. Tobier E. The homeless. In Brecher, Horton (eds.), *Setting Municipal Priorities, 1990,* p. 336, n. 35. See ref. 47.

CHAPTER 23

The Design and Use of
Case-Control Studies to Guide
Public Policy for the Prevention
of Homelessness

James R. Knickman, Ph.D., and Beth C. Weitzman, Ph.D.

A n underlying goal of much research about homelessness is to provide information to help policy makers design public programs to reduce or eliminate
the incidence of homelessness. From a prevention viewpoint, perhaps, the key
social science information that must be learned relates to the dynamics of
homelessness: What factors predict homelessness in different populations?

Descriptive analysis of a homeless population in and of itself cannot provide
the answer to that question. In contrast, a comparison group analysis allows the
researcher to compare the prevalence of potentially causal factors in a homeless
population and a comparison population and to make inferences about the
importance of distinct factors in predicting homelessness.

If comparison groups are not present, it is easy for the researcher to slip into
spurious inferences. For example, if one looks only at the first major work
published by Bassuk and colleagues, it would be easy to infer that having been
raised in a female-headed household places women at risk of homelessness, as
one-third of the study's homeless mothers had never known their fathers (1).
However, this first study focused only on characteristics of a homeless population and did not include information on a comparison group. After reviewing
Bassuk and Rosenberg's subsequent study, which includes a comparison sample, it becomes apparent that female heads of the comparison families who have
permanent housing are even more likely to have been raised without a father: 48
percent of the housed mothers were born into female-headed households, as
compared to 29 percent of the homeless mothers (2). Clearly this is not a
contributing factor.

Studies involving explicit comparisons based on information from one sample of homeless individuals or families and one sample of housed individuals or families are often called case-control studies. The purpose of this chapter is to consider methodological issues and inherent difficulties related to the case-control approach as applied to research on homelessness.

To help in explaining these research issues, we review three examples of case-control studies of factors related to homelessness. We address research design issues such as how to identify comparison groups and groups of homeless individuals. We review issues related to appropriate statistical analysis of case-control data. Finally, we explain the public policy significance of case-control studies.

Although some of the conceptual and data-analytic issues addressed appear straightforward at first, our experience in conducting case-control studies suggests that potential pitfalls in design and implementation are numerous. An understanding of these potential problems is important for researchers who consider using this research approach or wish to critically interpret findings from case-control studies.

Examples of Case-Control Studies

Three major empirical studies of causes of homelessness have used case-control research (2–6). They vary substantially in research questions addressed, samples studied, and significance for public policy.

The study conducted by Bassuk and Rosenberg (2) is based on in-person interviews with 49 homeless and 81 housed female-headed families in Boston. It explores potential explanations or predictors of homelessness including demographic characteristics, social ties, relationships with men, social service utilization, and presence of health and mental health problems. In this study, the criterion for homelessness was residence at a family shelter at the time of interviewing, which was done at the shelter. The comparison sample was much more difficult to interview. To identify a comparison sample matched on two characteristics, low income and female head of household, the researchers identified blocks in Boston which according to the 1980 census had a high prevalence of poor families headed by women. Interviewers then went door-to-door on these blocks during daylight hours and managed to complete 81 surveys among 118 eligible families. This excluded 356 families who were not at home when the interviewers were on the block.

The study by Sosin et al. (3) involved interviews conducted at three types of sites in Chicago: shelters, meal programs, and inpatient treatment programs that serve indigent people. The last-named programs included some special mental health programs and some detoxification centers, but the vast majority of the treatment programs were for alcohol rehabilitation. At each site, meals were served both to homeless people and to housed individuals in financial crisis. Thus, the homeless sample and the comparison sample were obtained from the same basic sampling frame. Homelessness was defined as one of four residential states: temporary shelter (less than 14 days) with family or friends; public shelter; temporary residence in treatment center; or staying overnight in public places.

The sampling approach used by Sosin et al. (3) differs substantially from that of the other two studies in that the percentage of homeless families identified among the sample of meal program users provides a direct estimate of the incidence of homelessness in that population. For typical case-control studies that use distinct sampling frames for the homeless and housed samples, the percentage of homeless individuals studied reflects the sampling design rather than the true incidence of homelessness in the population studied. As discussed later, this fact greatly affects the analysis and interpretation of case-control data.

Data for the Sosin et al. sample were collected through in-person interviews conducted by professional interviewers and graduate students (3). The types of questions asked were similar to those asked by Bassuk and Rosenberg (2). The two studies differ in that Sosin et al. included both single individuals and families, while Bassuk and Rosenberg focused exclusively on families.

The third example of case-control studies, conducted by Knickman and colleagues (4–6), also focused exclusively on families. It involved interviews with 704 homeless families and 524 housed families, all of them residents of New York City. Its principal purpose was to help the city's Human Resources Administration to identify public assistance families at high risk of using the emergency housing shelter in the near future. Interviews with homeless families were conducted at the city's Emergency Assistance Units, where families go to request emergency housing. Thus, as in the Bassuk and Rosenberg study (2), the definition of homelessness focused on shelter use.

The interviews were done as the families awaited placement. Thus, they occurred at the start of an episode of homelessness rather than at random points during an episode, as in the other two studies. The comparison group was a representative sample of the 230,000 families on public assistance in New York City at a given point in time. Interviews with the comparison group were conducted at Income Maintenance Centers during the periodic recertification interviews required of all public assistance families. All interviews were conducted by Louis Harris and Associates.

These three studies represent useful examples for discussion, since each one used case-control methodology; yet they differ in some important sampling details and data-analytic approaches.

General Principles for a Case-Control Study

Epidemiology research texts provide a discussion of essential elements of case-control methodology. However, there are special problems and issues when these methodological standards are applied to studies of homelessness.

All case-control studies must begin with the identification of a representative sample. This task is difficult because it subsumes the complex and controversial issue of determining who is homeless. Are families who are doubled up to be included among the homeless, or only those who seek shelter? Do we limit our definition to those on the street, or do we include those living for months in welfare hotels? The purpose of the particular study should guide its definition of homelessness. However, the chosen definition will help shape the study's findings.

Once homelessness has been defined, researchers are still faced with the difficult task of locating and gaining access to a representative sample. At the risk of stating the obvious, there are no formal registries of homeless people. Unlike voters, taxpayers, car owners, and other groups that we can sample from existing lists, homeless people must be "found." Under such conditions, it is impossible for researchers to control completely the composition of their samples, and the definition of homelessness is often based on practical considerations. This leads to problems of external validity, in that findings cannot be generalized to all homeless people but apply just to those represented in the study.

In none of the three case-control studies under review was the sample selected to represent the entire homeless population. Each focused only on a subset of homeless people. Furthermore, each study took place in only one city, raising additional questions about its application to other sites. Sosin et al. (3) looked only at people using meal programs, excluding those who did not use such services and underrepresenting those who made sporadic use of them. Bassuk and colleagues' sample (1,2) was limited to families in selected shelters. The study by Knickman and colleagues (4–6) is, in fact, a study of shelter requesters rather than shelter users, and it is limited to public assistance families. The variability of homeless subpopulations under study makes it extremely difficult to compare and contrast the findings across studies. Are differences in findings due to differences between the three study cities, differences in sampling strategies, or differences in the way homelessness has been defined?

The selection of a representative comparison group is fraught with many of the same problems as that of the homeless group. Again, the definition of an appropriate comparison group is complex and controversial. Are we interested in comparing the homeless people to the average American, or are we interested in comparing them to poor people? The three studies under discussion used a sample of poor people, since this allows one to disentangle the effects of poverty from those of homelessness. However, finding a representative sample of low-income people is not simple. The complexity of this task is highlighted by the fact that the three studies' comparison samples differ dramatically from each other. Bassuk and Rosenberg used the broadest definition by focusing on housing site: if one lived in a poor neighborhood, one was poor (2). Knickman and colleagues' sample was limited to public assistance families (4–6). Sosin et al. only looked at those who used meal programs (3). How different homeless people look from people who are housed is a function of who is included in the comparison group.

Once the decision about whom to survey has been made, the timing of the survey must be determined. When to survey is a crucial but subtle research design decision that affects the representativeness of the chosen sample of the homeless and the ability to interpret study findings. Surveyors who interview a random sample of people who are homeless on a given day or during a given week include a disproportionately large number of "long-term" homeless people, who may well be different from short-term homeless people. Furthermore, when respondents are interviewed in the midst of an episode of homelessness, it is not possible to discern whether many characteristics preceded homelessness or resulted from it. For instance, did the high rates of depression found in Bassuk and colleagues' work (1,2) contribute to or result from the experience of being homeless?

The problem of interviewing homeless people in the midst of an episode, although not unique (a similar problem has long been noted in the study of populations of patients) has been ignored in much of the research on homelessness to date. A sample selected during an episode of homelessness is far easier to obtain than a sample of those first entering an episode of homelessness. In particular, it is extremely time-consuming to obtain a sample of newly homeless people because at any given time, the vast majority of those in shelters are in the midst of an episode of homelessness. In Knickman and associates' study (4–6), it took six months to get the sample. However, this strategy avoids the pitfall of overrepresenting those whose homeless period is unusually long, and it provides a better understanding of the population's characteristics before the experience of being in a shelter.

The findings from Knickman and associates' study (4–6) highlight the importance of distinguishing people who are undergoing their first episode of homelessness from those with previous episodes. In that study, important differences were found between first-episode families and those for whom this was a new, but not first, entry into the shelter system. For example, substance abuse problems were more prevalent among repeat shelter users than among first-time users. Given the study design, it is not possible to determine whether substance abuse elevated a family's risk of recurrent homelessness or whether the previous shelter stay(s) had resulted in higher rates of substance abuse.

From a policy perspective, it is critical that we obtain a clear picture of which problems may be tackled before a family or individual becomes homeless or enters a shelter, and which problems arise during the shelter experience and should be addressed before or while a family is being resettled. This requires a firm understanding that the point at which homeless families or individuals are interviewed determines what one will know about them.

Data-Analytic Issues

In case-control studies, the data analysis must consider the fact that the choice of the samples is based on the value of the dependent variable—in this instance, whether or not an individual or family is homeless. This is in contrast to the typical survey research study, in which a sample is drawn from some population, and then data analysis determines the distribution of a dependent variable across individuals who have varying values of some characteristics of interest.

A second complicating feature of case-control data is that the dependent variable of interest is dichotomous (e.g., a person is homeless or housed). The special distribution of a dichotomous variable must be considered in choosing data-analytic techniques.

CROSS-TABULATIONS

In presenting information about the characteristics of homeless and comparison samples, it is most useful to start with simple, descriptive statistics. For example, Table 23.1 presents cross-tabulations of variables measuring medical and psychiatric problems in the Bassuk and Rosenberg paper (2). The cross-tabulations make it clear that the homeless sample is somewhat more likely to have had medical problems and much more likely to have had substance abuse problems and psychiatric hospitalization than is the sample used for comparison. In this statement, the denominators are the numbers of homeless and housed families. Since each sample is expected to represent its underlying population, the statement is clear and accurate. However, it is not accurate to use these cross-tabulations to make statements where the denominator is the number of people with a given medical or psychiatric problem. For example, one cannot infer from Table 23.1 that 43 percent (13/30) of families with medical problems are homeless. This statement is not true because homeless families represent a larger share of the study sample than they do of the general population.

A valid approach to such questions compares the odds of homelessness for subgroups defined by the presence or absence of a problem. For example, Table 23.2 presents data from Knickman and Weitzman's report (6) concerning the parenting history of the homeless and housed samples. The odds of being homeless are 3.27 (183/56) for a family that has added a new child in the past year, but 1.13 (521/468) for a family without a new child. While these odds are

TABLE 23.1   CROSS-TABULATION OF DATA FROM THE BASSUK AND ROSENBERG STUDY

	Homeless		Housed	
Problem	N	%	N	%
Medical problems				
Present	13	27	17	21
Absent	36	73	64	79
Substance abuse problems				
Present	8	16	5	6
Absent	41	84	76	94
Psychiatric hospitalization or diagnosis				
Present	13	27	8	10
Absent	36	73	73	90

Source: Data from Bassuk EL, Rosenberg L, Why does family homelessness occur? A case-control study. *American Journal of Public Health* 78: 783–788, 1988.

TABLE 23.2   CROSS-TABULATIONS AND ODDS OF HOMELESSNESS FOR VARIABLES
FROM THE KNICKMAN AND WEITZMAN STUDY

	Shelter Requesters		Comparison Group		Odds of Homelessness[a]	Relative Odds
Characteristic	N	%	N	%		
Pregnant						
Yes	243	36	29	6	8.4	9.0
No	461	64	495	94	0.9	
Had baby in past year						
Yes	183	26	56	11	3.3	2.9
No	521	74	468	89	1.1	
Had child before age 18						
Yes	259	37	124	24	2.1	1.9
No	445	63	400	76	1.1	

Source: Data from Knickman JR, Weitzman BC, *Forecasting Models to Target Families at High Risk of Homelessness*. Final Report, vol. 3. New York: New York University Health Research Program, 1989.

[a]Sample calculations: Odds for pregnant subsample, 8.379 = 243/29; odds for nonpregnant subsample, 0.931 = 461/495; relative odds—pregnant v. nonpregnant, 9.0 = 8.379/0.931.

not meaningful in an absolute sense because of the oversampling of homeless families, they are meaningful in a relative sense, as explained by Schlesselman (7). Thus, the fact that the relative odds are 2.89 (3.27/1.13) suggests that families with new babies are much more likely to become homeless than are other families.

The presentation of relative odds is useful, but this statistic still does not present an easy-to-read risk of homelessness for different subgroups. The simple risk of homelessness can be calculated only if it is known what proportion of homeless families has been sampled, and what proportion of housed families. For example, in Knickman and colleagues' study (4–6), New York City was able to supply administrative information showing that about 300,000 families spend some time on public assistance during a given year (as compared with 230,000 who are on public assistance at any point in time). Also, 10,000 public assistance families apply for city-sponsored emergency housing at some point during a given year. Since the public assistance comparison sample included 524 families in the New York study, the probability of being in the sample for each of these families was 0.17 percent (524/300,000). For the homeless sample of 794 families, the sampling probability was 7.04 percent (704/10,000). Table 23.3 takes the sample distribution of Table 23.2, applies the population weights, and displays the estimated distributions for the New York City public assistance population. These weighted and estimated distributions can be used to compute the simple risks of homelessness. For instance, for families with new babies, the risk is 7.7 percent, while for those without new babies it is 2.8 percent. Note that the relative risks are similar to, but not identical with, the relative odds computed in Table 23.2.

Multivariate Analysis

When it is important to know the distinct effects of each characteristic on the risk of homelessness, one has to use multivariate statistical analysis. Multivariate analysis is particularly important if the homeless and housed samples are not perfectly matched on important demographic or background characteristics.

Ordinary least-squares regression analysis and logistic regression analysis offer convenient multivariate approaches to assessing the effects of a series of risk factors and demographic factors at one time. Table 23.4 shows the multivariate analysis presented in Knickman and Weitzman's paper (6), based on both weighted ordinary least-squares regression and weighted logistic regression.

Ordinary least-squares parameters are statistically consistent, but the variances of the parameters are estimated inefficiently (i.e., they generally are larger than they would be with more appropriate estimation techniques). This inefficiency is due to the fact that the linear model implied by ordinary least

TABLE 23.3   CROSS-TABULATIONS, ODDS, AND RISKS OF HOMELESSNESS, USING POPULATION ESTIMATES FROM THE KNICKMAN AND WEITZMAN REPORT

Characteristic	Shelter Requesters		Comparison Group		Odds of Homelessness[a]	Relative Odds	Simple Risk of Homelessness
	N	%	N	%			
Pregnant							
Yes	3,445	36	16,050	6	0.22	9.0	17.7
No	6,548	64	273,950	94	0.02		2.3
Had baby in past year							
Yes	2,599	26	30,992	11	0.08	2.9	7.7
No	7,401	74	259,008	89	0.03		2.8
Had child before age 18							
Yes	3,679	37	68,626	24	0.05	1.9	5.1
No	6,321	63	221,374	76	0.03		2.8

Source: Data from Knickman JR, Weitzman BC, *Forecasting Models to Target Families at High Risk of Homelessness.* Final Report, vol. 3. New York: New York University Health Research Program, 1989.

Note: Population estimates are calculated as number in sample subgroup times inverse of sampling probability.

[a]Sample calculations: odds for pregnant subsample, $0.2153 = 3,455/16,050$; odds for nonpregnant subsample, $0.0239 = 6,548/273,950$; relative odds, $9.0 = 0.2153/0.0239$; simple risk for pregnant subsample, $17.7 = [3,455/(3,455 + 16,050)] \times 100$; simple risk for nonpregnant subsample, $2.3 = [6,548/(6,548 + 273,950)] \times 100$.

squares generally will not fit the data well for individuals with unusually low or high predicted probabilities of homelessness.

The advantage of least-squares parameters is that they provide very intuitive and easily understandable information. The estimated regression parameters indicate the actual increment to the risk of homelessness for sample members having the risk factor associated with the parameter.

The distributional model underlying the logistic regression approach is generally more likely to fit data when the dependent variable is dichotomous (as in case-control studies). The parameters and their variances are estimated efficiently with maximum likelihood techniques, and the parameter estimates are statistically consistent.

However, one problem with the logistic regression approach is that the estimators appear to be more sensitive to intercorrelations among independent variables of the model than is the case in ordinary least-squares analysis. We find that a number of estimated parameters are statistically insignificant when estimated with logistic regression, even though the same parameters were quite significant when least squares were used. Those parameters that are insignificant with logistic regression (though not with least squares) become consistent-

TABLE 23.4 PREDICTORS OF HOMELESSNESS:
WEIGHTED LEAST-SQUARES AND WEIGHTED LOGISTIC MODELS

Variable	Least Squares Model		Logistic Model	
	Coefficients	T-Ratio	Coefficients	T-Ratio
Constant	0.012	0.562	−3.849	−4.391[a]
Prior shelter use	0.036	1.947	0.392	0.974
Age	0.000	−0.689	−0.035	−1.466
Disruptions	0.077	3.023[a]	1.082	1.763
Ever evicted	0.037	1.988[a]	0.807	1.848
Current pregnancy	0.120	6.019[a]	1.782	4.052[a]
Baby past year	0.026	1.639	0.676	1.524
Ever detoxified	0.080	2.395[a]	1.832	1.374
Ever had casework by Special Services for Children	0.058	1.667	0.907	0.969
Ever doubled	0.024	2.252[a]	1.033	2.164[a]
Two moves	0.066	2.941	0.582	1.383
Previously primary tenant	0.115	3.967[a]	1.707	2.743[a]
Stay with parents	0.013	0.625	0.326	0.561
Stay with others	0.007	3.645[a]	1.375	2.954[a]
Hispanic	−0.017	−1.564	−0.620	−1.642
White/other	−0.022	−1.187	−0.868	−1.228

Source: Data from Knickman JR, Weitzman BC, *Forecasting Models to Target Families at High Risk of Homelessness*. Final Report, vol. 3. New York: New York University, Health Research Program, 1989.
[a]Indicates significance at the 0.05 level.

ly significant when the specified models have two or three fewer independent variables.

A second problem with the logistic approach is more presentational. The estimated parameters do not reflect increments to risk, as with the least-squares parameters. Since the estimated relationships are inherently nonlinear, the increments to risk vary across subgroups of individuals depending on the presence or absence of other risk factors. However, Shlesselman explains how the estimated logistic parameters can be used to estimate the relative odds of homelessness depending on the presence or absence of a specific risk factor for a representative person in the sample (e.g., the person with the mean value of all other risk factors) (7). Knickman and Weitzman explain how increments to risk, analogous to the least-squares parameters, can be calculated for each risk factor for different subgroups of people (6). However, estimation of actual increments to risk, adjusting for other factors, requires knowledge of the sampling probabilities, as discussed in the section on cross-tabulations.

JAMES R. KNICKMAN AND BETH C. WEITZMAN

Policy Implications

No single research methodology can answer all questions. Case-control studies are especially effective for gaining comparative information on large samples of people. They should not be thought of as substitutes for ethnographic research or for studies of the magnitude of the population. Case-control methods cannot provide the depth of information on the lives of homeless people which typifies many qualitative studies. Nor can case-control studies, which are often based on narrowly defined samples of homeless people, be easily used to take a census of the homeless. However, for the purpose of understanding the distribution of various characteristics and conditions that influence the onset of homelessness, the case-control method is effective and appropriate.

The use of case-control studies allows us to test and explore some common assumptions about the nature of homelessness in our society. These studies allow us to disentangle the characteristics of homeless people from those of merely poor people, and to challenge many misconceptions regarding the factors that lead individuals to seek refuge in shelters or the streets. Case-control studies are particularly useful for generating information relevant to public policy that attempts to reduce the incidence of homelessness because these studies can point to factors that potentially explain the roots, dynamics, or causes of homelessness.

From a public policy perspective, a case-control study can make an important contribution by identifying target groups of families or individuals at high risk of becoming homeless. Multivariate models of risk factors which predict homelessness can be used to identify the estimated risk of homelessness for individuals or families with varying risk characteristics. These estimated risks can be used to target prevention initiatives to individuals or families who have the highest estimated risk of becoming homeless.

The study done by Knickman and colleagues for New York City focused on such targeting (4–6). The city's Human Resources Administration hoped to develop preventive services that could be targeted to high-risk families. These services would not have been cost-effective if all 230,000 families on public assistance at a given point in time were eligible for enhanced preventive services. The case-control data collected in the New York study was used to identify the 5 percent of the public assistance family population at highest risk of becoming homeless in the following 12 months. The analysis showed that this high-risk group of 15,000 families includes 5,000 of the 10,000 families who are expected to become homeless over the course of 12 months.

The first phase of case-control studies represented by the research reviewed in this chapter (2–6) is promising. At the very least, these disparate studies make it clear that in many ways, the homeless population looks less different from the housed population than one might have surmised. For example, when comparative data are considered, common misconceptions about the role of mental illness in homelessness are challenged (3). In order to develop more effective policies to prevent homelessness and assist homeless people, it is essential that additional case-control studies be undertaken to provide more insight into the roots of homelessness and the lives of homeless Americans.

References

1. Bassuk EL, Rubin L, Lauriat AS. Characteristics of sheltered homeless families. *American Journal of Public Health 76:*1097–1101, 1986.

2. Bassuk EL, Rosenberg L. Why does family homelessness occur? A case-control study. *American Journal of Public Health 78:*783–788, 1988.

3. Sosin MR, Colson P, Grossman S. *Homelessness in Chicago: Poverty and Pathology, Social Institutions and Social Change.* Chicago: Chicago Community Trust, 1988.

4. Knickman JR, Weitzman BC. *A Study of Homeless Families in New York City: Risk Assessment Models and Strategies for Prevention.* Final Report, vol. 1. New York: New York University, Health Research Program, 1989.

5. Knickman JR, et al. *A Study of Homeless Families in New York City: Characteristics and Comparisons with Other Public Assistance Families.* Final Report, vol. 2. New York: New York University, Health Research Program, 1989.

6. Knickman JR, Weitzman BC. *Forecasting Models to Target Families at High Risk of Homelessness.* Final Report, vol. 3. New York: New York University, Health Research Program, 1989.

7. Schlesselman JJ. *Case-Control Studies: Design, Conduct, and Analysis.* New York: Oxford University Press, 1982.

CHAPTER 24

Between Relevance and Rigor: Methodological Issues in Studying Mental Health and Homelessness

Anne M. Lovell, M.S.W., M. Phil., Ph.D. cand.,
Susan Makiesky Barrow, Ph.D., and Elmer L. Struening, Ph.D.

Definitions of mental health and psychiatric status are always affected by a multitude of factors, including cultural, historical, and environmental ones. Standardized methods of improving the reliability and validity of judgments about mental health and psychiatric status can help control some of these factors; yet in an area such as homelessness, the urgency of meeting basic human needs has often affected the methods by which and the care with which data could be collected. Unfortunately, careless or erroneous assessments of relevant dimensions of homelessness can affect general perceptions of and responses to the problem, as well as the relevance of the theoretical framework within which it is placed. Attention to issues of reliability and validity is important to assure both that serious psychiatric problems do not go ignored and that mental disorders are not attributed where they are nonexistent.

While progress has been made in assuring the reliability of measures in the fields of psychiatry and psychiatric epidemiology in the last few years, the validity of the definitions used is still being questioned. A similar problem is apparent in homelessness research, although the effort to define the mental and psychological status of people without homes is not new.

For example, although theories of homelessness, vagabondage, and vagrancy have shifted focus since at least the sixteenth century, sometimes emphasizing personal and moral characteristics and sometimes giving way to social and economic explanations, psychological and psychiatric theories have abounded since the beginnings of psychological medicine. Yet the particulars of such theories have more to do with the vagaries of the disciplines than with the reality of the homelessness that confronts them. Thus in late nineteenth-century France, under the sway of Charcot's elaborations on neurasthenia and hysteria, wide support was given to the definition of vagabondage as a "physical, moral and intellectual neurasthenia" and, in a different light, as a "psychic overexcitement . . . which prevents those so affected from dedicating themselves to regular work" (1). One hundred years later, when psychoanalysis dominated much of French psychiatry, the vagabond could be defined by his "search for an idealized and inaccessible object . . . [which] could well be the fantasized image of the mother" (2).

Conceptions about the psychiatric status of homeless people change radically within shorter time spans as well. Only 20 years ago, American psychiatrists put forth numerous theories of the "Skid Row personality," which they attributed to "deficient or arrested development"; to "deprivation of normal, social, familial relations early in life leading to insecurity, apathy, indifference, passivity and intellectual insufficiency"; or to a deficiency in relationships and in the ability to share, known as "undersocialization" (3:274). In contrast, today's studies of homelessness and mental health generally reflect less a concern with etiology than a concern with identifying psychiatric disorders that are discrete entities—surely a reflection of the centrality of a classification system such as DSM III-R (4) to the field.

This paper will discuss the reliability and validity of measures of mental health in homelessness research in the United States from 1980 on. The year 1980 has been chosen as the baseline because it marks a turning point in American public and professional awareness that the homeless population encompassed growing numbers of mentally disordered people (5) and was no longer confined to those geographically delimited areas known as Skid Rows (6). Thus we will leave aside the abundant literature on Skid Row alcoholism in the sixties and seventies.

The methods used to measure dimensions of mental illness in the studies and surveys examined here (7–32) differ in the degree to which they assure reliability and validity. The major instruments used since 1980 are summarized in Table 24.1. We begin with a discussion of reliability.

Reliability

Measurement in psychiatry must be concerned with two types of reliability, which concern the extent to which the observations are repeatable and errors of measurement have been excluded. The first, inter-rater reliability, involves the degree to which raters or interviewers agree on their measures, ratings, or diagnoses. The second, internal consistency reliability, is the extent to which the items or questions *within* a scale are correlated.

TABLE 24.1 PSYCHIATRIC AND PSYCHOLOGICAL INSTRUMENTS USED IN RESEARCH ON HOMELESSNESS AND MENTAL DISABILITY

Type of Evaluation	Instrument[a]	Used by[a]	Source(s) of Information	Areas Covered	Reliability and/or Validity with Homeless Population	Comments
Level of functioning	GAS[b] (7)	Baumann et al. (8)	Rating by interviewer	Overall level of functioning and symptomatology	Interrater reliability of interviewers was 80; shown to have postdictive validity (hospital records), convergent and discriminant validity	Level of functioning not separated from symptomatology
	GAS	Mulkern et al. (9)	Rating by interviewer	Overall level of functioning and symptomatology	—	—
	Level of Functioning Scale from the FACTS (10)	Baumann et al. (8)	Observation	Level of functioning in six areas: family relations; interpersonal relations; work, academic, economic; legal; thinking and feeling; substance abuse	—	Possible confounding of symptoms (e.g., thinking and feeling) with functioning
	Not specified	Mulkern et al. (9)	Interviewer judgment	Grooming, quality of speech, physical behavior, appropriateness of affect, effects of alcohol	—	Possible confounding of functioning abilities with consequences of homelessness
Diagnosis	Clinical evaluation	Arce et al. (11)	Interview	Not specified	—	DSM-III criteria used
	Clinical evaluation	Bassuk et al. (12)	Interview	Not specified	—	DSM-III criteria used

DIS (13)	Fischer et al. (14)	Interview by lay interviewers	Six categories of mental disorder for past month, past six months, and lifetime: substance abuse and/or dependence; schizophrenic disorders: affective disorders; anxiety and/or somatoform disorders; antisocial personality; cognitive impairment	—	Generates DSM-III diagnoses
DIS (13)	Koegel and Burnam (15)	Interview by lay interviewers	Six categories of mental disorder for past month, past six months, and lifetime: listed above.	—	Generates DSM-III diagnoses
SADS-L (16)	Barrow et al. (17)	Interview of subject by clinically trained interviewers	Major diagnostic categories: schizophrenia; schizoaffective disorders; affective disorders; anxiety disorders; personality disorders; alcoholism and/or drug abuse	Inter-rater reliability kappa for all diagnostic categories was .73	Generates RDC diagnoses
SCID (18)	Struening and Susser (19)	Interview by clinically trained interviewers	Major diagnostic categories: schizophrenia; schizophreniform; schizoaffective-depressed; schizoaffective-bipolar; depression with psychotic features; other psychiatric disorder	—	Generates DSM-III diagnoses

(continued)

TABLE 24.1 (*Continued*)

Type of Evaluation	Instrument[a]	Used by[a]	Source(s) of Information	Areas Covered	Reliability and/or Validity with Homeless Population	Comments
Symptomatology	PEF (20)	Chafetz and Goldfinger (21)	Clinical records and brief interview of clinician who did the evaluation	Nineteen symptoms, six summary scales: Disorganization; Grandiosity-Externalization; Withdrawal; Antisocial; Depression; Anxiety	—	Ceiling effect possible
	BSI (22)	Morse et al. (23); Morse and Calsyn (24)	Self-report to interviewer	Global Severity Index and nine subscales; Psychoticism; Somaticization; Obsessive-Compulsive; Interpersonal Sensitivity; Depression; Anxiety; Hostility; Phobic Anxiety; Paranoid Ideation	—	—
	Not specified	Solarz and Mowbray (25)	Self-report to interviewer	Global Severity Index and nine subscales, listed above	—	—
	Not specified	Mulkern et al. (9)	Self-report to interviewer	Presence or absence of seven symptoms, including auditory and visual hallucinations; suicidal ideation; suicide attempts	—	—

Scale	Source	Method	Description	Reliability	Modifications
Psychoticism Scale from PERI (26)	Struening (27)	Self-report rating scale	Ten items on psychotic beliefs, feelings, and perceptions	Internal consistency reliability was .88	Modified
SADS-C (16)	Barrow et al. (17)	Rating by clinically trained interviewers	Seven scales: Depressive Syndrome; Endogenous Features; Manic Syndrome; Anxiety; Delusions, Hallucinations, Disorganization; Extracted Hamilton; Miscellaneous Psychopathology	Inter-rater reliability based on interviews of homeless people and outpatients (intraclass correlation; .61–.74)	Modified; GAS eliminated; time frame is past two weeks
GHQ (28)	Fischer et al. (14)	Interview	Twenty items covering current distress	—	Modified
CES-D (29)	Struening (27)	Self-report rating scale	Sixteen depressive symptoms items and five "feeling good" items	Internal consistency reliability; .88 for depressive symptoms scales; .70 for "feeling good" scales	Seven items modified, one item added
CES-D (29)	Robertson et al. (30)	Self-report rating scale	Twenty items covering current distress	—	—
CES-D (29)	Koegel and Burnam (15)	Self-report rating scale	Twenty items covering current distress	—	—

(*continued*)

TABLE 24.1 (*Continued*)

Type of Evaluation	Instrument[a]	Used by[a]	Source(s) of Information	Areas Covered	Reliability and/or Validity with Homeless Population	Comments
	PSS (31)	Roth et al. (32)	Interview	Ten symptom areas: depression and/or anxiety; suicide and/or self-mutilation; speech disorganization; inappropriate affect, appearance, or behavior; interview belligerence and/or negativism; disorientation and/or memory impairment; retardation and/or lack of emotion; agitation and/or excitement; grandiosity; suspicion and/or ideas of persecution and/or hallucinations	No inter-rater reliability; postdictive validity indicated by modest correlation of subjective distress (depression and/or anxiety, and suicide and/or self-mutilation) and reality testing disturbance (grandiosity, and suspicion or persecution and/or hallucinations) with psychiatric hospitalization (.28, .24, .19, and .30); low correlation of behavioral disturbance (remaining six symptom areas) with psychiatric hospitalization (range, .03–.14).	Ten scales selected out of 23 first-level scales and used to provide indices of psychiatric severity, behavioral disturbance, and reality testing disturbance; no clinical diagnoses generated.

[a]Numbers in parentheses are reference citations.

[b]GAS, Global Assessment Scale; FACTS, Form for Assessment of Client Treatment Services; DIS, Diagnostic Interview Schedule; SADS-L, Schedule for Affective Disorders and Schizophrenia—Lifetime Version; RDC, Research Diagnostic Criteria; SCID: Structured Clinical Interview for DSM-III; PEF, Psychiatric Evaluation Form; PERI, Psychiatric Epidemiology Research Interview; SADS-C, Schedule for Affective Disorders and Schizophrenia—Change Version; GHQ, General Health Questionnaire; CES-D, Center for Epidemiological Studies Depression Scale; PSS, Psychiatric Status Schedule.

INTER-RATER RELIABILITY

Spitzer and Williams (33) have described three sources of error variance that affect inter-rater reliability: (a) *information variance,* or the different kinds and amounts of information available about the person of interest; (b) *observation* and *interpretation variance,* or differences in what observers notice and how they interpret this information; and (c) *criterion variance,* or disagreements as to what constitutes the presence of a disorder or symptom. While their discussion applies to situations in which two or more clinicians examine a series of individuals and make independent judgments about the individuals' psychiatric diagnoses, their scheme is useful for thinking about the reliability of other measures of psychiatric status as well, such as symptoms.

Reliability is potentially increased as we move from the least structured method (unsystematic observation) to the most structured method (diagnostic instrument), and from a single item or measure to several questions or even combined measures.

The nature of homelessness research, however, does not always allow for elaborate questioning. Because of limited time, the physical context in which they take place, and lack of resources, surveys (e.g., that done by Chaiklin [34]) and assessments made on the basis of limited contacts, such as the data provided by a mobile team or an outreach staff (e.g., the studies done by Barrow and Lovell [35,36] Cohen et al. [37]; and Putnam et al. [38]) may depend on unstructured and somewhat unsystematic observation. Staff training, manuals and guidelines, even the "culture" of a service may shape similar ways of seeing and interpreting behavior among staff members. This is somewhat analogous to the use of rigorously trained interviewers or observers as "instruments," a method that has precedents in more qualitative research (39). Nevertheless, reliability is affected because while many symptoms and behavioral patterns are readily observable, others take time to discern. For example, florid psychotic symptoms such as hallucinations are more easily perceived by the outsider than are so-called negative symptoms, such as blunted affect or illogical thinking. Similarly, sorting out whether a homeless woman's fear of being murdered is real or a paranoid delusion may require that the rater take the time to learn about the constraints of her habitat. Reliability in these cases will be affected by variations not only in the information available (e.g., whether the violent context of the street is taken into account, rather than only what a woman reports) but also in the interpretations different observers make of the same behavior. In the above example of a homeless woman's behavior, one observer may be quick to label as a delusion that which another with more street experience would interpret as a high level of justified fear.

The use of different observers at different sites also cuts down on repeatability. Information variance may have contributed to the higher rates of behavioral symptoms reported for certain sites in a multi-site study (17). Assessments were based on workers' first contact with a client; yet even a single contact in the shelter-based programs gave workers a better chance to get to know the client than did the street-based outreach programs or drop-in centers. Gender differences in rates of disorder in a multishelter study (40) may be explained similarly. Women were interviewed by workers from the shelter where they stayed; men were interviewed by outside interviewers who, for the most part, did not know them (M. Goldstein, personal communication). It is possible that higher rates of mental illness among the women were partly due to the greater amount of information that interviewers had about them.

Self-report has been used in several studies as a complement to observations or as the principal measure of mental disorders. The reliability of self-report for eliciting psychiatric status is questionable, as an underreporting bias might be assumed, given the stigma attached to mental illness and the fears many formerly institutionalized homeless people have of treatment (17,41). Particular types of biases may also be associated with particular subgroups of homeless people. For example, the higher rates of symptomatology many of the studies show for women (30,42), while possibly reflecting real gender differences, may also be due to a higher likelihood that women will report symptoms.

Some studies of mental illness among homeless people have used clinical interviews. While the psychiatric interview is sometimes upheld as the "expert standard" against which to compare other evaluations of psychiatric status, it poses its own problem of reliability. Three studies (11,12,43) based on clinical interviews of people in emergency shelters used the currently accepted diagnostic criteria found in DSM III. This reduces criterion variance, since all interviewers apply the same inclusion and exclusion criteria and technical definitions of signs and symptoms. However, in the absence of a structured set of questions, there is no guarantee that interviews will obtain the same types and amounts of information. Even clinicians' judgments may be unreliable, simply because differences in training and clinical experiences lead clinicians to have their own ways of seeing and interpreting human behavior. The results of a reliability study carried out as part of the Epidemiological Catchment Area nationwide survey (44) showed agreement between psychiatrists to be lower than that between lay interviewers (45). Tests of inter-rater reliability would thus seem to be useful mechanisms for pinpointing divergences between clinically trained interviewers before an actual study is undertaken.

When diagnoses are reported without specifying criteria, reliability is almost certainly lower because of criterion variance. This is the case for studies that base psychiatric diagnoses on hospital or clinic records (46,47), on interviews (12,43), and on observations (37,38). According to Spitzer and Williams:

> Generally, the reliability of diagnoses obtained by using case records is lower than the reliability of diagnoses based on live interviews. . . . The explanation may be that live interviews provide important diagnostic information that is left out of case

records or, conversely, that case records frequently provide ambiguous information that interferes with making a differential diagnosis. (33:597)

THE TESTING OF RELIABILITY: MENTAL HEALTH MEASURES USED WITH HOMELESS PEOPLE

Structured or semistructured questionnaires or interviews reduce information variance. Most of the instruments listed in Table 24.1 are standardized and were used reliably in a number of studies before being applied to the area of homelessness. Yet the populations on which reliability has been established—for instance, adolescents, college students, inpatients, and general communities—differ in several ways from people living in shelters, on the streets, or in makeshift arrangements. Only one instrument, the Form for Assessment of Client Treatment Services (FACTS), was developed specifically for a study of homeless people (8). For all other instruments, factors such as the conditions under which previous studies were carried out and the characteristics of their subjects may affect inter-rater reliability very differently than the factors at hand in studies of homeless people. For example, reliability studies of the Schedule for Affective Disorders and Schizophrenia (SADS), which have been carried out primarily on patients, excluded actively delusional, unmedicated, and/or somewhat uncooperative patients (48)—the very ones who might be found among mentally ill persons who are also homeless. The inter-rater reliability of the Diagnostic Interview Schedule (DIS) was good in studies limited mostly to patients and ex-patients (49,50) and poorer when administered in general population studies, where more subjects are on the threshold of "caseness" (51,52).

For these reasons, when interviewers are trained to use a scale or instrument on a "new" sample, such as homeless people, reliability studies are both instructive for training and methodologically important. Inter-rater reliability coefficients were reported for only two of the interview studies reviewed here. The first used a brief interval scale, the Global Assessment Scale (GAS), which measures overall symptomatology and level of functioning, in a survey of unsheltered people in Austin, Texas (8). The interviewers were students with some clinical interviewing knowledge, as well as experience with people of low socioeconomic background and minorities. After nine hours of training, interviewers rated cases. The overall inter-rater reliability correlation, a very acceptable .80, was based on vignettes (Baumann, personal communication, 1986), the least conservative test of agreement; videotapes, "live" people, or test-retest, in that order, are more conservative tests.

In the second study (17), inter-rater reliability was tested for three instruments to be used with mentally ill people staying in shelters or on the streets. One 60-hour training period covered both SADS-C (symptom scale for the past two weeks) and SADS-L (lifetime diagnosis). Interviewers had backgrounds in the social sciences or in social services with populations similar to that being studied. A reliability study was carried out on a sample of "street people" who had been assessed by service providers as being psychiatrically disabled and had been chosen for their similarities to the potential sample subjects. For all diagnostic categories generated by the SADS-L, the overall kappa (which corrects for chance agreement between ratings of nominal data) was .73, well within the range reported in published reliability studies with this instrument.

With SADS-C, the results of intraclass correlation ranged from acceptable (.61 for delusions, hallucinations, and disorganization) to excellent (.93 for manic symptoms). Those dimensions of behavior that could not be measured reliably are particularly informative with respect to assessing mental disorders among homeless people. For example, "bizarre behavior" was the item with the lowest intraclass correlation: .34. This is a difficult item to rate because it is so open to interpretation variance. Signs of bizarre behavior, such as eccentric dress or gestures, may seem adaptive on the streets or may be the only alternative given material constraints, whereas in other contexts (and even on the streets) they may be interpreted as manifestations of mental disorder. There was poor agreement between raters on delusions and hallucinations, possibly because the SADS instruments, initially developed for a study of depression in inpatient and clinic settings, might not provide detailed enough descriptions for the range of behaviors and symptoms seen in people with nonaffective, psychotic disorders.

A third instrument Scales for Level of Functioning (SLOF), was tested after four days of training with the same interviews. It consists of a series of interval rating scales based primarily on observation. Like most other level-of-functioning instruments, it was developed for use with inpatient and outpatient clinic populations. The SLOF was used to rate vignettes of persons who were homeless and manifested psychiatric problems. The intraclass correlation coefficient ranged from acceptable (.54 for "social acceptability") to excellent (.98 for "personal care skills"). However, the original scales had to be modified to drop items, such as "household responsibility" and "care of living space," which were inapplicable to severely mentally ill homeless people, and to add items, such as "intimidating behavior" and "eats nutritiously," considered to be relevant dimensions of functioning in the difficult circumstances of homelessness.

Although the scales and instruments used in studies of homeless people, such as the General Health Questionnaire (GHQ), the Center for Epidemiological Studies of Depression Scale (CES-D), SADS-C, SLOF, and the Psychiatric Status Schedule (PSS), have often been modified to assure the relevancy of items to what was being measured, most reports and articles do not specify what modifications were made, to the detriment of other researchers who may wish to consider the instruments for new studies.

THE INTERNAL CONSISTENCY RELIABILITY OF SCALES

Internal consistency, the correlation among items within a scale, is applicable to symptom scales and level of functioning. It is a standard applicable to measures that are additive or linear. Good internal consistency signifies that the individual items or questions reflect to some degree the construct or idea they were meant to measure. If internal consistency is low, either there are too few items or the items do not have much in common.

When scales are modified, they should be reexamined for the internal consistency of their items. Although instruments were modified for studies, internal consistency was tested in only two instances. In a random sample study of 1,400 people in 15 New York City municipal shelters (27), two instruments often used as screening scales were used to assess mental health, after slight revisions to take into account the unique living environment of shelter residents and to clarify or simplify the questions.

To screen for psychotic beliefs, feelings, and perceptions, 10 items were selected from the 13-item psychoticism scale of the Psychiatric Epidemiology Research Interview (PERI) (26). Based on a sample of 1,120 shelter residents, the internal consistency reliability of the 10-item scale was .88; the average correlation among the 10 items was .43. With multiple correlations squared as communality estimates, loadings on the first unrotated principal factor varied from .54 to .78.

The 20-item CES-D scale (29) was also revised by substituting 7 items and adding 1 item measuring positive feelings. Factor analysis of a 21×21 correlation matrix, computed from the responses of 1,130 shelter residents, revealed an orthogonal, two-factor solution measuring depressive symptoms and "feeling good." Factor loadings varied from .43 to .66 over the 16 depressive symptom items and from .39 to .72 over the 5 items defining "feeling good." The internal consistency reliability coefficients were .88 and .70 for the "depressive symptom" and "feeling good" scales, respectively. Reliability coefficients were higher than expected for the number of items involved in defining each factor scale. In other words, these psychometric characteristics indicate that items were meaningful to shelter residents and that responses were organized along two modestly correlated dimensions at the item level.

Internal reliability was also estimated for the SADS-C (53) and the SLOF (54) on a sample of the first 50 subjects in the study of clients of programs for psychiatrically disabled homeless people (55). Standardized alpha (used when variances among the items are great) for the seven subscales on the SADS-C ranged from .80 for the Extracted Hamilton Depression Scale to .56 for the Anxiety Scale (which comprises only three items).

Internal consistency correlations for the SLOF, which ranged from .57 to .83, were generally poorer than those reported when the SLOF was used on populations of inpatients and outpatients (56). The lowest alphas, for the Physical Functioning and Social Acceptability Scales, were nevertheless higher than those for the populations of patients. The physical functioning correlations may be explained by the lack of variance within the scale. These correlations are expected given that we would not expect most items of physical functioning (e.g., "use of arms and legs," "vision," "teeth") to be correlated. The items on the other scale, Social Acceptability, do not appear to be particularly related. In fact, the scale should be factor-analyzed with a larger sample to determine whether or not it is tapping more than one domain of functioning.

Validity

The validity of indicators of mental status has only rarely been addressed in the studies reviewed here. This is not surprising, because many of the instruments used had already been validated in earlier research on various populations. Furthermore, validation, which is a process of exploring the extent to which an instrument measures what it is supposed to be measuring, can never be complete. However, important and essential steps in that process can be taken. For example, the CES-D, used in two of the studies (27,30), has been shown to discriminate depressive symptoms from other psychiatric symptoms in several populations (29,57–59) when other instruments, medical records, or clinical assessments are used to measure symptomatology and/or generate diagnoses.

Only one study reviewed here attempted to analyze the validity of a symptom scale, at least in psychometric terms. Baumann et al. (8) estimated the degree to which scores on the GAS correlated with level-of-functioning scores on a second instruments, the FACTS. The GAS scores showed much higher correlation with those areas of the FACTS that the authors assume are more "psychological" in nature—interpersonal relations, .66; thinking and feeling, .62; and family relations, .47—than with substance abuse and trouble with the law (.19 each). However, the analysis does not clarify which construct—symptomatology or level of functioning—is being tapped.

The GAS also demonstrated predictive validity (or more accurately, postdictive validity): low GAS scores, indicative of lower functioning and more severe symptomatology, were found to be more closely associated with a history of mental problems than were scores at the other end of the scale, which indicate functioning a lay person would consider more "normal" and not indicating a need for help. However, evidence for concurrent validity was weakened by the fact that only 64 percent of the people who reported that they were currently experiencing mental problems had low GAS scores. This rather surprising divergence between an observer's rating on the GAS and an individual's self-report of psychological status may have to do with the fact that each is describing a different aspect of psychological status. The GAS, which was developed on patients, attempts to tap the level of symptomatology and functioning typical of people with severe mental disorders.

For example, the GAS rates at the severe end behavior such as "is unable to function in almost all areas (e.g., stays in bed all day) OR behavior is considerably influenced by either delusions or hallucinations." In contrast, the self-report questions that elicited mental problems tap a wide range of severity. Subjects were asked, for example, if they had ever felt as though they "wanted to see a counselor for mental problems" and whether they were "currently experiencing any mental problems other than from alcohol and drugs." Thus the limited overlap with GAS scores was not surprising.

If we have concentrated on a seemingly trivial example of a validity issue in a study of homeless people, it is to point out that the varied mental health indicators used in the studies reviewed here are probably measuring quite different types of psychiatric status. While researchers may have their own assumptions about the validity of their measures, in the absence of tests or even discussions of validity, the reader can only speculate as to what is being measured. In fact, the very framework used for examining the validity of our measures may be different from that traditionally used in psychiatry. It can be suggested that the theory inherent in constructs useful for research among homeless people concerns two dimensions in particular: temporality and the person-environment fit.

Reconceptualization of Constructs

When data produced by surveys of homeless people have been interpreted, attention is rarely paid to duration. All of the symptom scales and at least one of the level-of-functioning scales (the SLOF) used in the studies reviewed here measure behavior over a brief period, from one week to one month. In this sense, it is totally incorrect (invalid) to interpret their findings as indicators of mental disorders, unless other measures are used to validate such results. Duration of the symptom may also be directly related to environment. Feelings of sadness, having been "down" or "blue" during the past week or two, may be related to particular stressors at a particular time.[1] They do not tell us whether or not an individual has suffered from severe depression on and off throughout a lifetime. For example, first-time shelter users in a New York City survey showed higher scores on a depressive symptom scale (the CES-D) than did long-time residents (19). A similar argument can be made for psychotic symptoms, although this is less likely. Symptoms and signs may flare up and go away over a person's lifetime, or they may have been produced at one point in time by interrupted sleep patterns, malnutrition, and general disorientation due to geographical mobility.

The constructs that may contribute to a better understanding of the prevention of homelessness and mental distress and disorders concern the relationship between symptom and sign, on the one hand, and environment, on the other. Some constructs that could be used to explain what some of the instruments in the studies reviewed above are measuring are demoralization, reactive disorders, and shelterism.

DEMORALIZATION

One result of critiquing the validity of early psychiatric rating scales was the emergence of hypotheses that these scales, prevalent from World War II through the 1960s, might really be measuring some sort of nonspecific distress. Dohrenwend and Shrout (61) proposed that the construct "demoralization" might be the common denominator in all of these scales. Demoralization is "a condition that is likely to be experienced in association with a variety of problems . . . and perhaps conditions of social marginality as experienced by minority groups and persons such as housewives and the poor whose social positions block them from mainstream strivings" (62:115). The major facets of demoralization were operationalized in a 27-item scale derived from eight PERI scales, including those for self-esteem, helplessness-hopelessness, sadness, and anxiety.

Of the scales used thus far in research with homeless people, only one had previously been examined in relation to the screening scales that, according to findings by Dohrenwend and Shrout (61) measure demoralization. The CES-D was found to be highly related to a general symptom checklist (62). One might expect that especially among a group of people who were without homes and *not* selected (for a program or research) because of a known mental disorder, demoralization would be especially likely to be present, even if called something else, such as depression. Because some scales have been modified in other studies reviewed here, it is well worth considering whether the construct reflected in their scores might be measures of the dimension of demoralization.

The name we give a manifestation of behavior is not without importance. In the early years of the Depression, an "inability to earn a satisfactory living" was considered a sign of psychopathic defect; by 1936, when most people recognized the extent of unemployment and the effect of the Depression, "familiarity with unemployment had made it less a mark of defective character," and the diagnosis of "psychopathic personality" was resorted to less (Lewis, quoted by Hopper [63:3]). Because demoralization seems to be characteristic of people in certain situations—for instance, of poor people—it focuses our attention on the situations themselves rather than on individuals' reactions to them. While demoralization may call for treatment (e.g., crisis intervention or counseling) it also points to a preventive strategy to change a pathogenic situation. For the same reason, we may want to differentiate depressive symptoms, especially if they are likely to be situational or reactive, from depression.

REACTIVE SYNDROMES

There appears to have been an increase in reporting of personality disorders in recent studies of homeless people. In 1983, a Philadelphia emergency shelter study (11) found that almost 7 percent of the clients could be diagnosed as having personality disorders; a year later, a study in a Boston emergency shelter (43) found 21 percent of the clients to have personality disorders. Although both studies used DSM-III categories, their rates are not directly comparable, as neither used random samples or similar populations. However, when re-searchers report personality disorders for such a large proportion of clients in various types of settings, attention should be paid to the validity of the category itself. Recent critiques in the psychiatric literature are not irrelevant to studies of the homeless. Stangl et al. (64) have pointed to the poor inter-rater reliability of personality disorders in the DSM-III field trials and the low coefficients of correlation reported in the published literature for these disorders (median kappa = .23, highest kappa = .49). Without good reliability, it is not possible to assess validity.

Three relevant points have been made about personality disorders. First, the boundaries between what is normal and what is abnormal are not yet clearly established, even in DSM III. It is difficult for an observer to determine a threshold for severity of a disorder. Second, in practice, a time-limited reaction to stress (i.e., reactive syndrome) can be distinguished from a lifelong behavior pattern only with difficulty. For example, in an individual case, are the sus-piciousness, mistrust, hypersensitivity, and lack of feeling that are considered to be diagnostic criteria for "paranoid personality" actually situational de-fenses, or are they parts of a lifelong personality pattern? The same question may be asked about the criteria for dependent personality, passive-aggressive personality, and other diagnostic categories. A personality disorder, by defini-tion, must be characteristic of both current and long-term functioning. Yet even when interviewing is done by experienced clinicians, it is difficult to separate traits from states, and "normal" traits or personality style from maladaptive personality disorders (65,66).

One category of particular concern to researchers in the area of homelessness is "antisocial personality disorder." While in published research it tends to have good inter-rater reliability compared to other disorders, this does not per se establish its validity. Its criteria, as defined by DSM III, could easily describe a life-style that represents structured arrangements in a context of economic and other constraints, rather than reflecting a conscious violation of others' rights. The criteria that must have been met in adulthood (e.g., significant unemploy-ment, repeated thefts, irritability or aggressiveness [anger], failure to plan ahead "as indicated by travelling from place to place without a prearranged job or clear goal for the period of travel or clear idea about when the travel could terminate or lack of a fixed address for a month or more") also seem class-bound, or at least partly environmentally determined (4:321). In fact, they describe the lives of many homeless people. More work needs to be done on deciphering exactly what this category means.

There may be a similar confusion between symptoms associated with "post-traumatic stress disorder" (PTSD) and those associated with other constructs. The former label is used to describe a pattern of symptoms that follows exposure to a psychologically traumatic event that "would evoke significant symptoms of distress in almost everyone" (4:238). The trauma is reexperienced and is accompanied by a numbing of responses or reduced involvement with the external world, as well as other symptoms such as sleep disturbance, memory impairment, or difficulty in concentrating. Despite the attention given to PTSD because of the frequency of psychological problems experienced by Vietnam veterans, mental health practitioners reportedly confuse it with other disorders. For example, persons suffering PTSD may share the following characteristics with those diagnosed as having antisocial personality disorders: hostility, aggressiveness, projection of blame, suspicion of authority, and problems with interpersonal relationships (67). It is quite possible that symptoms of PTSD found among people who have lost their homes are also confounded with symptoms of other disorders.

"Shelterism"

Some of the characteristics and behavior (whether passive, apathetic, and despondent; or aggressive, suspicious, and "uncooperative") rated by interviewers, or even self-rated and self-reported, may be a reaction to the context in which the person is staying. A positive response to the question "Do you have mental problems?" may also reflect such a reaction. The construct we are suggesting may be what service providers working in shelters have called "shelter shock," or what we might call "shelterism," either of which may be produced by conditions in large, crowded, unsafe spaces where people sleep for want of more permanent quarters. Two authors surveying residents of the Chicago shelters during the Depression used the term *shelterization* to describe the despondency, apathy, and dependency provoked by such institutions (cited by Segal and Baumohl [68:115]).

A similar construct was examined empirically during the 1950s and 1960s, with reference to psychiatric institutions. The effects of institutionalization were often confused with chronicity as an inevitable course of psychiatric illness (69–71). Segal and Moyles (72) found a similar cluster of symptoms among residents of certain community-based shelter facilities that mimicked the management style of psychiatric institutions. Shelters differ in some ways from psychiatric institutions or even adult homes; for example, although they may develop cultures and delimited worlds of their own, shelters are also comparatively open, and current patterns of use range from long-term stays to alternation between shelters and streets or even the homes of friends and relatives (27). Institutionalization, as explicated in the studies of the 1950s and 1960s, could be explained by the nature of the total institution and its day-to-day functioning. For today's shelters, there may be specific clusters of symptoms found among clients which might be affected by the characteristics of shelters and in fact could disappear if the context were to change.

The validity of these three proposed constructs—demoralization, reactive syndromes, and shelterism, all of which may overlap—could be tested in several ways. However, the best test might involve some sort of diachronic reliability (73), determining whether the phenomena (behaviors) persist over time. Either follow-up studies or ongoing contact with homeless people would show whether or not the symptoms disappeared after the individuals left the pathogenic context. For example, once housing was provided, it can be hypothesized, many such symptoms could disappear.

Validity and the Environmental Contamination of Measures

Several researchers have pointed to a different order of problems with validity. We might call this, as have Frankfather et al., "the contaminating effects of environmental contingencies" (74:12). Baxter and Hopper (5), Barrow and Lovell (36), Chafetz and Goldfinger (21), and Baumann et al. (8) have noted a bias in ratings of functioning and/or symptomatology: a tendency to overestimate because the dishevelled, bizarre appearance of individuals in the street is confused with signs of mental disorder. What is being measured may be either a direct effect of the environment or a strategy of adaptation to the environment. Similarly, when instruments require a positive manifestation of behavior as an indication of good functioning, constraints of the environment may not allow for such manifestations. Aspects of the environment which have *direct* effects might include dangerous or noisome conditions, which affect sleep and concentration; food retrieved from garbage, donated food, or routinized meals, which affect appetite; a lack of recreational and other resources, which affects interest and pleasure; and overcrowded conditions and the characteristics of one's "fellow" shelter residents or other imposed persons in one's habitat, which affect an individual's interpersonal behavior (e.g., showing fear of others, or thinking people dislike him or her).

The validity of a diagnosis of psychiatric impairment must be questioned when signs of the impairment cannot be separated from signs of the effects of life on the street. For example, one survey included the following as "selective elements of mental status": "appearance—physically unkempt, dishevelled and dirty, clothing atypical bizarre"; posture ("slumped/rigid, tense/atypical, inappropriate"); facial expression ("suggesting anxiety, fear, apprehension/. . . bizarreness, inappropriateness"), and other aspects of behavior that could be reactions to both the environment and the interview situation (34:85). In the Ohio survey, 54 percent of the sample had characteristics or behavior related to psychiatric impairment but also to life on the streets, including dirty or dishevelled appearance, inappropriate behavior, and flattened affect (32). Chafetz and Goldfinger (21), looking at the relationship between residential stability and symptoms in a psychiatric emergency room population, found that on summary scales for the Psychiatric Evaluation Form (PEF) only "inappropriateness" was significantly related to homelessness.

A symptom that is maladaptive in one context may also be a source of strength or a sole means of survival in another. For example, paranoia may be a healthy response to having to share space with 1,000 other men. Uncooperativeness, such as refusal to take psychotropic medication, may ensure alertness when one has to live on the street in the face of potential robbery, physical and sexual assault, and arrest. Aggressive, even psychoticlike behavior, may keep people away or, if need be, attract them.

Level-of-functioning instruments present even more problems of environmental contamination than do screening scales and symptom scales. First, most criteria for what investigators consider to be good functioning are not easily met in the circumstances of street life, shelter existence, or having to stay on the move. On the SLOF, for example, almost every item is contingent on circumstance: the ability to manage money requires the availability of money; measures of interpersonal relationships assume relatively "normal" opportunities for interacting; and so forth.

The validity of the very concept of functioning, as borrowed from the field of social psychiatry, may be questioned in many instances. Long-term research or first-hand knowledge of the way homeless people live (e.g., knowledge gained through personal experience, advocacy, or direct services) invests "functioning" with a different meaning.

For example, poor hygiene, eccentric dress, soiled and tattered garments, and inability to keep track of possessions may be due to lack of access to shower and toilet facilities, lockers, and clothes. They may also reflect functional behavior in difficult circumstances. Just as in the thirties women "passed" as men in the male world of transiency (75), contemporary homeless women construct appearances to protect themselves from rejection and attack (76,77).

To understand the degree to which symptoms and levels of functioning are related to environmental contingencies, one can systematically collect qualitative data from observations of environmental indicators. While pathology cannot be teased out definitively from external circumstances, the data can suggest which behaviors may have environmental correlates.

Discussion

The first wave of studies from the current (post-1980) period of research on homelessness was often realized in a climate of urgency and expediency. States, cities, private agencies, foundations, and advocacy organizations commissioned surveys and reports, or carried them out themselves, often trading methodological rigor for rapidly gathered data of immediate relevance to questions about the numbers, characteristics, and needs of homeless people. The consequences of a lack of attention to operational definitions of homelessness and to sampling and other related issues of generalizability of findings, or external validity, have been discussed elsewhere (78). In this paper, we have been concerned with some of the problems that arise when unreliable measures of mental status are used, as well as with the lack of clarity surrounding what they are actually measuring. Certainly, poor reliability, differing definitions of mental status, and confusion as to the constructs of mental health contribute to the inconsistency in rates of mental disorder reported in earlier reviews of research on homelessness (e.g., that by Fischer and Breakey [79]).

More recent studies have taken greater care with instrumentation, in most cases using standardized instruments. Although diagnostic interviews have cut down on some problems of validity that are inherent in scales measuring behavior that—in certain contexts—may not be a sign of individual pathology, problems still arise when instruments developed on clinical populations are applied to marginal and highly mobile populations, and even more so when functioning and symptoms alone are measured. Tests of reliability and, where feasible, thoughtful discussion of what is possibly being measured should ensue. Without taking into consideration reliability and, in a more anthropological or qualitative sense, validity, researchers face a twofold risk: (a) The lack of attention to measurement problems, especially the potential confounding of psychological disorders and environmental factors, will prevent policy and services from being based on empirical knowledge of homelessness. As a result, real problems of mental illness may not be addressed. (b) If researchers do not attempt to separate out environmentally produced characteristics from symptoms of psychopathology, they risk medicalizing personal problems and life circumstances that are clearly social and economic in nature. Clarification of issues of reliability and validity will, it is hoped, improve future research on homelessness and mental health, as well as interpretations of the current body of data.

Note

1. Of course, stressors have been shown to be risk factors for major psychiatric disorders. Dohrenwend and colleagues have found that the pathogenic triad—the temporal clustering of

a fateful loss (e.g., of a person or a home), physical vulnerability (e.g., severe illness or injury), and loss of social support—are risk factors for depression, though not for schizophrenia (60).

References

1. Benedikt M. Le vagabondage et son traitement. *Annales d'hygiène publique 24:*496, 1890.

2. Millet L, Collet J-C, Durou B, Kulik J, Micas M, Pan J. Vagabondage, espaces, et philobatisme. *Annales medico-psychologiques 139(2):*219, 1981.

3. Goldfarb C. Patients nobody wants: Skid Row alcoholics. *Diseases of the Nervous System 31:*274–281, 1970.

4. American Psychiatric Association. *Diagnostic and Statistical Manual of Mental Disorders,* 3d ed., rev. Washington, D.C.: American Psychiatric Association, 1987.

5. Baxter E, and Hopper K. *Private Lives and Public Spaces.* New York: Community Service Society, 1981.

6. Lee BA. The disappearance of Skid Row: Some ecological evidence. Paper presented at the annual meeting of the American Sociological Association, San Francisco, Calif., 1978.

7. Spitzer RL, et al. The Psychiatric Status Schedule: A technique for evaluating psychopathology and impairment of role functioning. *Archives of General Psychiatry 23:*41–51, 1970.

8. Baumann DJ, et al. *The Austin Homeless.* Austin: University of Texas at Austin, May 1985.

9. Mulkern V, et al. *Homelessness Needs Assessment Study: Findings and Recommendations for the Massachusetts Department of Mental Health.* Boston: Massachusetts Department of Mental Health, August 1985.

10. Kenrick DI, et al. Form for Assessment of Client Treatment Services (FACTS). Report prepared for Arizona Department of Behavioral Health Services, July 1981.

11. Arce AA, et al. A psychiatric profile of street people admitted to an emergency shelter. *Hospital and Community Psychiatry 34(9):*812–817, 1983.

12. Bassuk EL, Rubin L, Lauriat A. Characteristics of sheltered homeless families. *American Journal of Public Health 76(9):*1097–1100, 1986.

13. Robins LN, et al. *National Institute of Mental Health Diagnostic Interview Schedule.* Washington, D.C.: Government Printing Office, 1979.

14. Fisher PJ, et al. Mental health and social characteristics of the homeless: A survey of mission users. *American Journal of Public Health 76(5):*519–524, 1986.

15. Koegel P, and Burnam A. The prevalence of specific psychiatric disorders among homeless individuals in the inner city of Los Angeles. *Archives of General Psychiatry 45:*1085–1092, 1988.

16. Endicott J, Spitzer RL. A diagnostic interview: The Schedule for Affective Disorders and Schizophrenia. *Archives of General Psychiatry 35:*837–844, 1978.

17. Barrow S, Lovell AM, Struening EL. *Evaluation of Programs for the Mentally Ill Homeless: A Progress Report.* New York: New York State Psychiatric Institute, 1984.

18. Spitzer RL, Williams JBW. *The Structured Clinical Interview for DSM III (SCID).* New York: New York State Psychiatric Institute, Biometrics Research, 1985.

19. Struening EL, Susser E. *First Time Users of the New York City Shelter System.* New York: New York State Psychiatric Institute, Epidemiology of Mental Disorders Research Department, 1986.

20. Spitzer RL, et al. *Psychiatric Evaluation Form*. New York: New York State Department of Mental Hygiene, Biometrics Research, 1986.

21. Chafetz L, Goldfinger M. Residential instability in a psychiatric emergency setting. *Psychiatric Quarterly 56(1):*20–34, 1984.

22. Derogatis LR, Melisaratos N. The Brief Symptom Inventory: Introductory report. *Psychological Medicine 13:*595–605, 1983.

23. Morse G, et al. *Homeless People in St. Louis: A Mental Health Program Evaluation, Field Study, and Follow-up Investigation*. Jefferson City: Missouri Department of Mental Health, 1984.

24. Morse G, Calsyn RJ. Mentally disturbed homeless people in St. Louis: Needy, willing, but underserved. *International Journal of Mental Health 14(4):*74–94, 1986.

25. Solarz A, Mowbray C. An examination of mental health problems of the homeless. Paper presented at the annual meeting of the American Public Health Association, Washington, D.C., November 17–21, 1985.

26. Dohrenwend BP, et al. Nonspecific psychological distress and other dimensions of psychopathology. *Archives of General Psychiatry 37:*1229–1236, 1980.

27. Struening EL. Psychosocial characteristics of the New York City shelter population. Paper presented at the New York State Psychiatric Institute Annual Scientific Conference, Tarrytown, N.Y., 1985.

28. Goldberg DP. *The Detection of Psychiatric Illness by Questionnaire*. London: Oxford University Press, 1972.

29. Radloff LS. The CES-D scale: A self-report depression scale for research in the general population. *Applied Psychological Measurement 1(3):*385–401, 1977.

30. Robertson MJ, Ropers RH, Boyer R. *The Homeless of Los Angeles County: An Empirical Evaluation*. Los Angeles: University of California School of Public Health, Basic Shelter Research Project, January 1985.

31. Spitzer RL, Endicott J, Nee J. The Psychiatric Status Schedule for epidemiological research. *Archives of General Psychiatry 37:*1193–1197, 1980.

32. Roth D, et al. *Homelessness in Ohio: A Study of People in Need*. Columbus, Ohio: Ohio Department of Mental Health, February 1985.

33. Spitzer RL, Williams JB. Classification of mental disorders. In Kaplan HI, Sadloff BJ, (eds.), *Comprehensive Textbook of Psychiatry IV*, vol. 1, 4th ed. Baltimore: Williams and Wilkins, 1985.

34. Chaiklin H. *Report on the Homeless: The Service Needs of Shelter Care Residents*. Baltimore: University of Maryland, School of Social Work and Community Planning, January 1985.

35. Barrow S, Lovell AM. *Evaluation of Project Reach Out, 1981–82*. New York: New York State Psychiatric Institute, 1982.

36. Barrow S, Lovell AM. *Referral of Outreach Clients to Mental Health Services*. New York: New York State Psychiatric Institute, 1983.

37. Cohen NL, Putnam JF, Sullivan AM. The mentally ill homeless: Isolation and adaptation. *Hospital and Community Psychiatry 35(9):*922–924, 1984.

38. Putnam JF, Cohen NL, Sullivan AM. Innovative outreach services for the homeless mentally ill. *International Journal of Mental Health 14(4):*112–124, 1986.

39. Brown GW, Harris T. *The Social Origins of Depression*. London: Tavistock Publications, 1978.

40. Crystal S, Goldstein M. *Correlates of Shelter Utilization One-Day Study*. New York: City of New York, Human Resources Administration, August 1984.

41. Bachrach LL. The homeless mentally ill and health services: An analytical review of the literature. In Lamb HR (ed.), *The Homeless Mentally Ill*. Washington, D.C.: American Psychiatric Press, 1985.

42. Crystal S, Ladner S, Towber R. Multiple impairment patterns in the mentally ill homeless. *International Journal of Mental Health 14(4):*41–77, 1981.

43. Bassuk EL, Rubin L, Lauriat A. Is homelessness a mental health problem? *American Journal of Psychiatry 141(12):*1546–1550, 1984.

44. Eaton WW, Kessler LG (eds). *Epidemiological Field Methods in Psychiatry: The NIMH Catchment Area Program.* Orlando, Fla.: Academic Press, 1985.

45. Robins LN. Epidemiology: Reflections on testing the validity of psychiatric interviews. *Archives of General Psychiatry 42:*918–924, 1985.

46. Lipton FR, Sabatini A, Katz SA. Down and out in the city: Homeless mentally ill. *Hospital and Community Psychiatry 34(9):*817–821, 1983.

47. Morrissey J, et al. *The Development and Utilization of the Queens Men's Shelter.* Albany: New York State Office of Mental Health, 1985.

48. Spitzer RL, Endicott J, Robins E. Research diagnostic criteria: Rationale and reliability. *Archives of General Psychiatry 35:*773–778, 1978.

49. Robins LN, et al. National Institute of Mental Health Diagnostic Interview Schedule: Its history, characteristics, and validity. *Archives of General Psychiatry 38:*381–389, 1981.

50. Robins LN, et al. Validity of the Diagnostic Interview Schedule, Version II: DSM-III diagnoses. *Psychological Medicine 12:*855–870, 1982.

51. Anthony JC, et al. Comparison of the lay Diagnostic Interview Schedule and a standardized psychiatric diagnosis. *Archives of General Psychiatry 42:*667–675, 1985.

52. Helzer JE, et al. A comparison of clinical and lay Diagnostic Interview Schedule diagnoses. *Archives of General Psychiatry 42:*657–666, 1985.

53. Endicott J, Spitzer RL. What, another rating scale? The Psychiatric Evaluation Form. *Journal of Nervous and Mental Diseases 154:*88–104, 1982.

54. Schneider LC, Struening EL. SLOF: A behavioral rating scale. *Social Work Research and Abstracts 19:*9–21, 1983.

55. Barrow S, Lovell AM, Struening EL. *Serving the Mentally Ill Homeless: Client and Program Characteristics.* New York: New York State Psychiatric Institute, 1985.

56. Schneider LC. The development and examination of the psychometric properties of a behavioral rating scale to assess the levels of functioning of the psychiatrically impaired. D.S.W. diss., Columbia University, School of Social Work, 1980.

57. Weissman MM, et al. Assessing depressive symptoms in five psychiatric populations: A validity study. *American Journal of Epidemiology 106(3):*203–214, 1977.

58. Roberts RE. Reliability of the CES-D scale in different ethnic contexts. *Psychiatry Research 2:*125–134, 1980.

59. Roberts RE, Vernon SW. The Center for Epidemiologic Studies Depression Scale: Its use in a community sample. *American Journal of Psychiatry 140(1):*41–46, 1983.

60. Dohrenwend BP, et al. Overview and initial results from a risk factor study of depression and schizophrenia. In Barrett JE (ed.), *Mental Disorders in the Community: Progress and Challenge.* New York: Guilford Press, 1986.

61. Dohrenwend BP, Shrout PE. Toward the development of a two-stage procedure for case identification and classification in psychiatric epidemiology. In Simmons RG (ed.), *Research in Community and Mental Health.* Greenwich, Conn.: JAI Press, 1982.

62. Link B, Dohrenwend BP. Formulation of hypotheses about the true prevalence of demoralization in the United States. In Dohrenwend BP, et al. (eds.), *Mental Illness in the United States.* New York: Praeger, 1980.

63. Hopper K. Rethinking the link between homelessness and psychiatric disorder: A limited goods perspective. Manuscript, 1985.

64. Stangl D, et al. A structured interview for the DSM III personality disorders. *Archives of General Psychiatry 42:*594–596, 1985.

65. Vaillant GE. The disadvantages of DSM-III outweigh its advantages. *American Journal of Psychiatry 141(4):*542–545, 1984.

66. Widiger TA, Frances A. Axis II personality disorders: Diagnostic and treatment issues. *Hospital and Community Psychiatry 36(6):*619–627, 1985.

67. Bailey JE. Differential diagnosis of posttraumatic stress and anti-social personality disorders. *Hospital and Community Psychiatry 36(8):*881–883, 1985.

68. Segal SP, Baumohl J. The community living room. *Social Casework 66(2):*111–116, 1985.

69. Martin DV. Institutionalism. *Lancet 2:*1188–1190, 1955.

70. Basaglia F. *Psychiatry Inside Out: Selected Writings of Franco Basaglia.* Ed. Scheper-Hughes N, Lovell A. New York: Columbia University Press, 1987.

71. Wing JK, Brown GW. *Institutionalism and Schizophrenia.* New York: Cambridge University Press, 1970.

72. Segal SP, Moyles EW. Management style and institutional dependency in sheltered care. *Social Psychiatry 14:*159–165, 1979.

73. Kirk J, Miller ML. *Reliability and Validity in Qualitative Research.* Sage University Paper Series on Qualitative Research Methods, vol. 1. Beverly Hills, Calif.: Sage Publications, 1986.

74. Frankfather D, Rick S, Caro F. Residential and service configurations for the chronically mentally impaired. Manuscript, n.d.

75. Minehan T. *Boy and Girl Tramps of America.* New York: Farrar and Rinehard, 1938.

76. Hand J. Shopping bag women of Manhattan. Ph.D. diss., New School for Social Research, 1982.

77. Stark L. Strangers in a strange land: The chronically mentally ill homeless. *International Journal of Mental Health 14(4):*95–111, 1986.

78. Lovell A, Barrow S, Struening EL. Measurement issues in services research on the homeless mentally ill. In Franks J, Levine MS (eds.), *Proceedings of the Eighth Annual MSIS National Users Group Conference.* Orangeburg, N.Y.: Nathan S. Kline Institute, 1984.

79. Fischer PJ, Breakey WR. Homelessness and mental health: An overview. *International Journal of Mental Health 14(4):*6–41, 1986.

INDEX

Abandonment of housing: definition, 275; initial step in, 278; neighborhood abandonment, 280

Abuse: in childhood, as antecedent of homelessness, 53, 98–99, 105, 290, 311; of homeless infants and children, 119; of homeless mentally ill persons, 98–99; by medical and mental health system, 123; of runaway youths, 99, 289; by shelter staff, 97; of welfare, 285

Access of homeless people: to advocacy, 288; to entitlements, 160; to health services, 114, 156, 174; to housing, 123; to legal aid, 304–305; to mental health treatment, 177; to special education, 185. *See also* Barriers

Adaptation to homelessness: by homeless people, 7, 104, 134–135, 148, 161, 390; by mental health system, 177; by psychiatrists, 209–210, 212–216

Adaptive skills: of homeless people, 134–135, 157–158; of SRO hotel residents, 148

Advocacy for homeless people, 18–19, 300–305; lack of, 288

Advocacy-empowerment, 208–209, 211–213

Advocacy literature, 33

Advocacy organizations, 329

Advocate-intensive work, 328

Affordable housing
—measures of: housing affordability gap, 273, 309–310; market-basket approach, 273–274
—shortage of, 273; role of federal government in, 281; role of upper/middle-class households in, 279

Aid to Families with Dependent Children (AFDC), 239, 246–249; fall in real value, 232, 234, 248–49; income of homeless people from, 45, 46–47; loss of eligibility after OBRA 1981, 248–249; and reimbursement of hotel costs for homeless families, 19. *See also* Federal benefit programs

Alcohol abuse in homeless people, 177–179;

alcohol dependence syndrome, 178; as crime, 34–35; decriminalization of, 34–35, 93; environmental, 178; as greatest risk factor for arrest, 93–94; overlap with mental illness, 69; prevalence among homeless adults, 34, 47

Alcohol abusers: definition of, 34; heterogeneity of, 177; homeless people stereotyped as, 34–35; at increased risk for arrest, 93; traditional and nontraditional, 178; visible lifestyle of homeless abusers, 36

Alcohol abuse services: alcohol-free living environments, 178; case comparison study, 179; nonmedical detoxification, 178; types, 178

Alcohol use, by hotel residents, 140–141, 146, 148

American Psychiatric Association, 57, 176

Annual prevalence of homelessness: definition, 340; extrapolated from point prevalence, 340; proposed estimates for planning, 353; recent estimates, 350

Antecedents of homelessness: abuse precipitating running away, 99; abuse of tenants to force eviction, 100; abuse of homeless adults in childhood, 98–99; adverse life events, 6; foster care, 12, 53–54; marginal living, 6; precarious housing, 6

Antisocial personality disorder, 387

Arrests of homeless people: categories of offenses, 91–92; criminal activity in homeless adolescents, 93; difference between homeless and domiciled adults, 92; distribution of criminal activity in homeless subgroups, 92–93; excess prevalence, 90; life patterns of, 90–91; rates, 90–91; ratio of jail to prison incarceration, 91

Arson, 92, 277

Assertive case management. *See* Case management

Attitudes of, toward homeless people: community residents, 180, 306; health care

—training programs for homeless people, 182

Council of Large Public Housing Authorities (CLPHA), 265

Counting homeless people: capture-recapture method, 345–346, 354; census, 343–344; doubled-up population, 337, 346, 354; duplication, 339, 342; literally homeless, 337–339; local sampling, 344–345; national sampling, 344–345, 353; service-using homeless people, 337, 344–346; in shelters, 337–338, 342–346; on the street, 337–339, 342–344, 354; timing of, 339; undercount, 339, 343–344

Criminal activity: among chronically mentally ill, 87; contribution to overall crime rate, 92; distribution across homeless subgroups, 92–93; drug trafficking, 89; drug use, 89–90; illegal income, 88–89; significance of, in homeless environment, 103–104; sources of information, 88; types of, 91–92

Definitions: case-control, 363; family, 114; gentrification, 275; homeless maker, 269; homeless-making process, 269; homelessness, 1–4; household, for food stamp eligibility, 171; mental health status, 372; poverty, revised definition, 241; poverty gap, 244; poverty rate, 239; pressure toward homelessness, 269; prevalence, annual, 340; prevalence, point, 340; prevention, primary, 11; prevention, secondary, 11; prevention, tertiary, 11; reliability, internal consistency, 373; reliability, inter-rater, 373; sheltering, 167; validity, 384

Deindustrialization, 232

Deinstitutionalization of mentally ill people: and homelessness, 232–233; lack of discharge planning, 35, 194; role of government, 289; social disaffiliation, 15

Democratic party, 7, 286, 331

Demoralization, 176, 386

Denial of health problems, 146, 158

Developers. See Financial institutions

Discharge planning, hospitals, 155

Discrimination against homeless people, 288–289

Disinvestment theory of homelessness, 15, 293

Disorders: of maternal bonding, 118; of place and service delivery settings, 130

Displacement from housing: benefits for displaced tenants, 261–262; Community Development Block Grants, 262; contractual, 270; direct, last tenant, 272; direct chain, 272; economic, 270; exclusionary, 272; intimidation, 270; physical, 270; population-based studies, 272–273; pressure, 272; rate of, in New York City, 272; retrospective studies, 273; and Urban Development Action Grants, 262; and vouchers, 259

Double vulnerability, 114

Doubled-up individuals, 2; estimated number for planning purposes, 353; estimated range, 12, 40, 316, 346, 351–352

Doubled-up homelessness, estimated cost of prevention, 319

Doubled-up households, 337; estimated number, 346, 351–352

Doubling up, 9; definition, 3; frequency, in homeless adult surveys, 50; frequency, in McK/HCH population, 41; initial response to loss of one's home, 6, 310, 311; as strategy to manage household income, 252

Drug abuse: by homeless adults, 47, 179; by homeless youths, 74; overlap with mental illness, 69

Drug addiction, in homeless pregnant women and newborn, 115

Drug use: among homeless people, 89–90; among hotel residents, 140–141, 146–148; and arrests of homeless people, 93–94, 105; by underclass, 285

Economic recession (1981–82), and social disaffiliation, 15

Economies of makeshift, 291

Education
—of homeless children, 183–184; bussing, 121, 222; cost of, 184; governmental intervention, 184; preschool programs, 222; school attendance, 121, 183; school program connected to shelter, 222; special education, 122, 183; state plan, 184; transfers among schools, 122, 183. See also Homeless children, school-age
—of homeless adults: adult education programs, 221; educational status, 43, 46; job training programs, 181

Emergency shelters. See Sheltering

14, 45; recurrent, 7, 12, 132–133; sociopolitical significance, 7–8; as strategy of poverty, 291–292

—causes, studies of 1890 to 1970: economic factors, 28–31; migration to find work, 28; role of technological change, 30

—causes, studies of 1980s: causal interactions, 53; classifications of causes, 52; perceived causes, 51

—predictors/risk factors: comparison studies, 53–54, 370; longitudinal studies, 54

—pressure toward, 270, 292: definition, 269; employment sector, 282–284; family sector, 290; health sector, 288; housing sector, 274–276; public assistance sector, 285–286

—theories of, 13–16; historical perspective, 372–373; homelessness by choice, by nature, or by personality, 13; housing and poverty, 15; implications of theories for prevention, 16; social disaffiliation, 14; societal disinvestment, 15

Homelessness prevention. *See* Prevention of homelessness

Homelessness prevention proposals: Hartman, 317–328; Lindblom, 325–326; Schwartz, 324–325; Sosin, 325; Wright, 325

—education sector: antidrug education, 329; education for homeless families, 124; preparation for job opportunities, 329; special education linked to supported work, 329

—employment sector: child care for working mothers, 328; emergency work relief, 325; employees as share-holders, 328; employer education, 325; increased low and minimum wages, 326; increased participation in and duration of unemployment compensation, 226, 325; reduction of unemployment, 226, 326; retraining of workers, 325, 328; work programs with adequate pay targeted to homeless people, 325

—family sector: early intervention in family conflicts, 329; economic freedom for all members of household, 329; improving foster care, 329; rehabilitation of homeless families, 124–125; strengthening families, 326; transition program on leaving foster family, 326, 329

—health sector: community-based support programs, 328–329; discharge to permanent housing after hospitalization, 124; im-

proved recognition of mental health and substance abuse as disability, 326; national health program, 37, 328; national insurance against income loss due to illness or disability, 328; special programs for people with special needs, 325; supported housing, 325; transition programs after discharge from institutions, 226, 326

—housing sector: adequate payments for relocation, 266; bridge loans, 325; deducting rent money from benefit payments, 325; eviction prevention, 325–326; federal homeownership program, 324; help for displaced households, 266, 325–326; governmental capital grants for nonprofit housing corporations, 328; housing rehabilitation for elderly, 324; more low-cost housing, 37, 324, 326; offsetting neighborhood resistance, 226, 326; organized resistance to displacement, 328; preserving public housing, 266, or SROs, 325–26; prohibiting destruction of federally assisted units, 266; public housing, 325–326; rent insurance, 325; rent subsidies, 266; revision of tax laws to assure equitable distribution of housing assistance, 266; Section 8 changes, 226, 326; shared housing, 326; simplified access to housing for families, 123–124; targeting rental subsidies to very-low-income families, 326; tenant-organized housing corporations, 328

—public assistance sector: advocacy and outreach in welfare, 325, 328; emergency financial aid for homeless, displaced, or others in crisis, 325; increase public benefit payments, 37, 226, 325–326, 328; protect against improper decertification, 326; raise income eligibility limits, 326; remove barriers to eligibility, 326

—taxation: raise earned income tax credit, 326; revise tax laws, 37, 266; tax hotel rooms for emergency housing, 226

Homeless parents: developmental hierarchy, 122; fear of losing their children, 123; people in crisis, 122; program for, 120; stress of testing, 120

Homeless persons: adaptation to homeless environment, 7, 134–135, 148, 161; extreme poverty of, 46, 238–239; identity concerns of, 147–150; resilience of, 7

Homeless population: heterogeneity of,

Middle-class perspective (*continued*)
of homeless people's behavior, 133; and
significance of homelessness, 14

National Alliance to End Homelessness's
analysis of HUD's 1984 national survey,
342
National Ambulatory Medical Care Survey
(NAMCS), 46
National Association for Community Health
Centers, 18
National Coalition for Jail Reform, 88
National Coalition for the Homeless, 323
National Council of State Housing Agencies
(NCHSA), 264
National Institute of Alcohol Abuse and Alco-
holism (NIAAA), 179
National Institute of Mental Health (NIMH):
Community Support System (CSS), 177,
211–212; homeless adults surveys, 20, 41–
51, 177; outreach programs, 204–205;
studies of service needs, 177
National Low Income Housing Information
Service, 255
Networking of services, 186; client-agency
linkage, 219; five-stage model of as-
sistance, 220; human service organization
networking, 219; interprofessional linkages, 219; natural support system, 218–
219; policies affecting, 226; with various
populations or problems, 218
New politics of inequality, 293
New York City, Department of Housing Preservation and Development, 19
New York City, homelessness policies, 18–
20, 312
New York City, Human Resources Administration, 19, 313
Nonaccelerating inflation rate of unemployment (NAIRU), 283
Nonorganic failure to thrive, 117–118

Omnibus Budget Reconciliation Acts
(OBRA). *See* Federal legislation, budget
Outreach: to alcohol abusers, 178–179; by
government administrators, 287–288; for
health services, 175; for legal services,
304–305; for mental health services, 197,
201–202, 204–205; programs for homeless
mentally ill people, 207–208, 216

PHA. *See* Public Housing Authorities
Planned shrinkage, 280
Point prevalence of homelessness
—local: by capture-recapture, 345–346; by
census, 342–344; changes over time, 340–
341, 348–349, 353–354; definition, 340;
of doubled-up households, 12, 316, 346;
from key informants, 341–342; of literally
homeless individuals, 12, 316, 342–344;
by sample, 340–345; of service-using
homeless individuals, 344–345; by site
within metropolitan area, 348; by size of
city, 342–343; by size of metropolitan
area, 348–349; street-to-shelter ratio, 340
—national: critique of assumptions related to
city size, site within metropolitan area, and
size of metropolitan area, and to change in
demand for shelter, 347–349; estimates for
planning, 352–353; estimates in recent
studies, 347; projections of doubled-up
population, 351–352; projections from key
informants' estimates, 346–347;
projections from national sampling of service users, 347; projections of service
using/literally homeless population, 346–
350; projections with standard and alternative assumptions, 346–350, 354–356; research needs, 353
Police: attitudes of homeless people toward,
102; harassment of homeless people by,
102; provider of health and social services
for homeless people, 105–106; relations
with homeless people, 102
Poor people: attitudes toward, 285; "deserving" and "nondeserving," 285; effects of
inflation, 286; government policies toward,
286; political isolation of, 284; as underclass, 285
Poverty, 4, 239–244; association with rate of
homelessness, 252; definition, 239; increased
severity in 1980s, 15, 252; number of people in, with standard definition, 240–241,
and with revised definition, 241; number of
people moved into, by federal tax changes,
242–244; number of people removed from,
by federal benefits programs, 241–243; revised definition of people in, 241
Poverty gap: definition, 244; effect of federal
benefit programs on, 244; magnitude of,
244
Poverty line, 239–241

Rent (*continued*)
275–277; Section 8 certificates, 256, 266;
Section 8 vouchers, 256
Rent control: moderate, 280; stringent, 280
Rent gap, 278
Residential hotels (SROs), 139–150; ethos,
140–141; norms, 140–141, 148
Resource people, 2, 3, 9, 40
Responsibility for homelessness: problem of,
294; role of government in, 294; role of
homeless people in, 291
Runaways, 289

San Francisco Tenderloin district, 139
Section 8 housing: construction, 256–257; existing certificates, 256–257, 265; housing
rehabilitation, 256–257; opting out, by
owners, 259; rent paid by tenants, 256;
small developers and, 223
Services for homeless families with children,
five-stage model: casework plan, 220–221;
casework support, 221; child care, 222;
community reintegration, 223–224; crisis
intervention, 220–221; employment program, 221–222; follow-up, 223–224; relocation, 222; school program, 222;
training sessions for parents, 221
Service-using homeless people, 337; estimated number, 344–345
Service utilization, by homeless people, 131
Sheltering: capacity in United States, 168;
cost of, 169–170; definition, 167; demand
for, 168–169; governmental intervention,
170; local surveys, 169; national surveys,
168–169; quality of shelters and hotels,
168; types of, 167–168
Shelters: decision to use, 6; evidence of crime
in, 96–97; incidence of victimization in,
97–98; mental health status of homeless
people in samples of, 69–72; utilization of,
by homeless people, 129. *See also* Hotel
residents
Single-room occupancy hotels (SROs): moratoria on SRO conversion, 20; programs to
open new SROs, 20
Snowballing, 338, 342
Social isolation: of homeless persons, 52; of
hotel residents, 142
Social praxis, 139
Social Security, 239; antipoverty effects of,
241–244

Social services for homeless people, 185; and
barriers to social benefits, 185; case management, 185–186; functions of, 185. *See
also* Networking of services
SROs. *See* Single-room occupancy hotels
Squatters, 2, 6
SSI. *See* Supplemental Security Income
State government, and housing sector, 281
State government, low-income housing programs: economic incentives, 324; eviction
prevention, 324; facilitation of new homeownership, 324; new financing methods,
324
Stereotyping: of homeless families and children, 121; of homeless people by professionals, 121, 123, 125; significance of, of
homeless people, 35–37
Stigmatization: as instrument of control
among hotel residents, 140–141, 144
Street: decision to use, 6; incidence of victimization of homeless people in, 97–98; mental health status of homeless people in
street samples, 72; sites used by homeless
people, 6, 339
Stressful life crises preceding homelessness,
49
Structural interests: challenging, 321, 323;
dominant, 321; repressed, 321
Stuart B. McKinney Homeless Assistance
Act. *See* Federal legislation, McKinney Act
Supplemental Security Income (SSI), 186,
246, 249–251; accelerated case review,
250–251; cuts in, 234; income of homeless
people from, 45; participation of homeless
people in, 45, 46–47; promotion of enrollment after 1983, 251; relation to poverty
line, 249; state supplement of, 250
Sweat equity, 317, 327
Symbolic interaction, 178

Tax: abatement on gentrifying property, 280;
breaks for investors, 264; credits for low-
income housing, 264; incentives for homeownership, 264; policies, 281; reduction in
1980s, 287; revenues not received by government, 264
Throwaways, 289–290
Treatment resistant: clients, 130–131, 289;
concept of, used to ignore concerns of
homeless people, 131; providers, 130–
131

Designed by Laury A. Egan

Composed by The Composing Room of Michigan, Inc.
in Times Roman text and Futura Bold display

Printed by The Maple Press Company, Inc.,
on 60-lb. Glatfelter Hi-Brite
and bound in Joanna Arrestox cloth